BRAIN INJURY – FUNCTIONAL ASPECTS, REHABILITATION AND PREVENTION

Edited by **Amit Agrawal**

Brain Injury – Functional Aspects, Rehabilitation and Prevention
Edited by Amit Agrawal

Published by InTech
Janeza Trdine 9, 51000 Rijeka, Croatia

Publishing Process Manager Bojan Rafaj

Technical Editor Teodora Smiljanic

Cover Designer InTech Design Team

Additional hard copies can be obtained from orders@intechopen.com

Brain Injury – Functional Aspects, Rehabilitation and Prevention, Edited by Amit Agrawal
p. cm.
ISBN 978-953-51-0121-5

Meet the editor

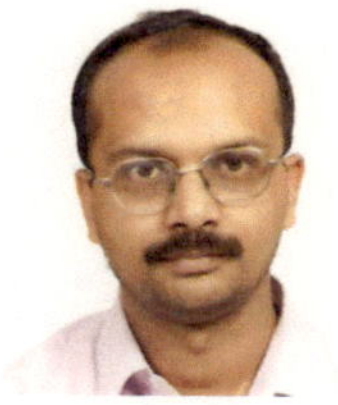

Dr Agrawal completed his neurosurgery training from National Institute of Mental Health and Neurosciences, Bangalore (India) in the year 2003. He is extremely enthusiastic, and result oriented professional with over 11 years of rich experience in Research & Development & Teaching & Mentoring in the field of neurosurgery. He has attended and participated in many international & national level symposiums & conferences and delivered lectures on vivid topics. He has published more than 300 articles in the medical field covering various topics in various national and international journals. He is the Editor-in-Chief of Journal of Neurosciences in Rural Practice. Presently he is Professor and head, Department of Neurosurgery, MM Institute of Medical Sciences and Research, Mullana (Ambala), India and promoting the concept of Neurosciences in Rural Practice through the Journal of Neurosciences in Rural Practice.

Contents

Preface

Brain injury remains one of the most difficult and challenging problems facing many researchers, clinicians and experts involved in care of these patients. The present two volume book "Brain Injury" is distinctive in its presentation and includes a wealth of updated information for professionals on the high quality research on many aspects in the field of brain injury as well as addresses the most difficult and challenging issues in the management and rehabilitation of brain injured patients. The Book One contains 5 sections and a total 26 chapters devoted to pathogenesis of brain injury, concepts in cerebral blood flow and metabolism, investigative approaches and monitoring of brain injured, different protective mechanisms and recovery and management approach to these individuals and Book Two contains (3 sections) 12 chapters devoted to functional and endocrine aspects of brain injuries, approaches to rehabilitation of brain injured and preventive aspects of traumatic brain injuries.

In Book Two chapters' discusses the issues of mental fatigue after brain injury, brain injury and cerebral lateralization, technology-based approaches to improve mental health outcomes in brain injured patients, endocrine sequel of traumatic brain injury. Many aspects of rehabilitation have been discussed and these include use of the international classification in brain injury rehabilitation, impact of community based rehabilitation, life Satisfaction following severe traumatic brain injury, cognitive recovery and rehabilitation, communicative impairment after traumatic brain injury, issues related to consequences and family needs, short, long, and very long-term vocational outcomes and safe driving.

I hope that collective contribution from experts in brain injury research area would be successfully conveyed to the readers and readers will find this book to be a valuable guide to further develop their understanding about brain injury. I am grateful to all of the authors who have contributed their tremendous expertise to the present book, my wife and daughter for their passionate support and last but not least I wish to acknowledge the outstanding support from Mr. Bojan Rafaj, Publishing Process manager, InTech Open Science, Croatia who collaborated tirelessly in crafting this book.

Dr Amit Agrawal
Professor of Neurosurgery Department of Neurosurgery
Narayna Medical College Hospital
Nellore, India

Part 1

Funtional and Endocrine Aspects

1

Mental Fatigue; A Common Long Term Consequence After a Brain Injury

Birgitta Johansson and Lars Rönnbäck
Institute of Neuroscience and Physiology, Sahlgrenska Academy, University of Gothenburg and Sahlgrenska University Hospital, Gothenburg
Sweden

1. Introduction

The aim of this chapter is to describe mental fatigue, and emphasize the need to consider its importance when discussing rehabilitation and return to work. It will include suggestions how mental fatigue can be assessed, both objectively and subjectively and how mental fatigue and cognitive functions may be related.

1.1 Why care about mental fatigue?

The less visible consequences such as cognitive, emotional and behavioural problems after a traumatic brain injury (TBI) are often not recognized immediately after an incident. In the beginning, the focus will be on the apparent problems as motor and language impairment, if the brain injury is more severe. After rehabilitation or when it is time to leave the hospital, which could occur pretty soon after a mild TBI, the person may feel rather well, although not recovered, but well enough to go home and rest, with the hope of returning to a productive everyday life after a while. This is the case for most people after a mild TBI. Patients will recover within days to weeks, but a significant minority develop persistent mental fatigue, and it will take a long time before they can accept the situation and find ways to lead their "new life". Until then, life can be very mentally tiring and for many it can be a great strain.

In the case of a slow recover, things might turn out not to work as smooth and easily as they used to. It is possible for patients to take walks in the forest, but reading, talking on the telephone or attending a meeting could be mentally very tiring and may require a prolonged rest afterwards. It is no longer a pleasure to go to parties, as they can't take part in conversations, and they soon become extremely tired and want to go home. It might also be shameful for the person to admit that the brain does not work properly. They also tend to experience difficulties concentrating, and it could be difficult to filter what they hear and see. Every unimportant detail is registered. Sensitivity to stress is also very common, even in minor situations which they are normally able to handle.

Many studies also report increased susceptibility to depression after brain injury (Ashman et al., 2004; Silver, Mc Allister, & Arciniegas, 2009; Whelan-Goodinson, Ponsfold, & Schönberger, 2008). Depression and mental fatigue can occur alone, but they sometimes occur simultaneously. Many symptoms overlap, but the core symptoms of the two states are different. For people with mental fatigue there is a clear picture of fatigue which is related to concentration and attention, and in particular the degree of mental load. The fatigue fluctuates over the day, and the recovery period can be long. Persons suffering from depression present low-spiritedness and a decreased interest in their surroundings. Many also find it difficult to feel pleasure, experiencing fatigue throughout the day. In most cases, the long-term post TBI problems relate to mental fatigue. It is also one of the most limiting, long-term consequences after TBI.

It can be very difficult for the person with mental fatigue, but also for relatives and fellow employees to understand the limitations caused by a brain injury. However, mental fatigue will become central to their lives and will have a significant impact on everyday life. They cannot continue with work or studies as they used to. There is a high risk that they will continue to work and pursue daily activities at an unsustainable level. Most people are eager to do what they are used to, but it takes a long time to change habits.

In case of mental fatigue there are often claims for incapacity benefit after a brain disorder, and the number of claims will increase significantly in our high-technology society, with the increasing demands on our mental capacity. Upon returning to work patients may need to seek renewed acceptance from fellow employees and colleagues who will need to be willing to change strategies and demands. In the beginning, this might be possible. After a while the injured brain is expected to become "normal" again. When this does not happen it can be a heavy burden involving stress and demands over and above tolerable levels. There is a risk to be totally exhausted or even of becoming losing one's job. However, people with mental fatigue is competent and can be well-educated and many have long-term experiences which are valuable in the work-place. With the high demands placed on efficiency and economical limitations of modern living, how can the skilled person's qualifications be used to maximum advantage when energy levels are not sufficient?

The long-term effects suffered by patients after a mild TBI can be illustrated by the example of a person who tried, for many years, to find explanations and treatments, but failed.

"After my summer holiday, I started to work again. I struggled for three weeks. I was sitting on the floor in my office crying, and I was extremely fatigued and I had a severe headache. My workload increased, as I could not do my work as efficiently as before. I was sent off for sick leave and I started to feel that I might never be able to continue with my work as before. This was a great disappointment and I became depressed. Life was not worth living and I didn't manage to take care of my children. My brain was not working properly.

After six long and difficult years, I finally met a doctor who understood my problems and who could explain to me why I was feeling this way. It helped a lot when I was given some useful information about my problems, and I started to understand things. I was no longer an awkward patient. This was a relief for me. From that moment on, I was able to lead my new life and I could do the things I found pleasurable and enjoyable, despite not being able to work".

2. What is mental fatigue?

2.1 Mental fatigue

Mental fatigue is common and it occurs after both a mild TBI as well as moderate to severe TBI. Mental fatigue is suggested to be a diffuse or a multifocal brain disorder (Chaudhuri & Behan, 2004; Hansson & L, 2004). The degree of the fatigue appears to have no relation to the severity of the trauma or time since injury and the extent of the fatigue seems to have no relation to the area of the brain that is primarily affected (Belmont, Agara, Hugeron, Gallais, & Azouvia, 2006).

Mental fatigue is characterized by pronounced mental fatigue after mental activity.
People suffering from this kind of mental fatigue may also experience rapid mental exhaustion which is disproportionate to the expected level following mental activity. Some people can continue to be productive in their jobs, but for others, problems connected to work and everyday activities are common. There are some people who are unable to work, who have obvious difficulties in everyday activities such as shopping, reading the newspaper as well as spending time with their family and friends. In today's society, we have to take in, process and handle a lot of information, which may be too taxing for those suffering from mental fatigue. This particular kind of fatigue can easily be mistaken for laziness or unwillingness. This is unfortunate as, in most cases people want to be able to accomplish more than they are actually capable of. Sometimes mental fatigue can also be mistaken for apathy, but a careful examination will show that most patients will be shown to have levels of high motivation, but the energy is missing.

Mental fatigue

- Mental exhaustion already after ordinary activities.
- Long mental recovery.
- Distinct 24h variation.

2.2 Mental recovery

A common symptom of mental fatigue is an extended time for recovering one's mental energy. If there is not enough time for rest, mental fatigue may increase over time and it is very common to experience/see an increase during the course of the day. Most people also have a clear 24-hour variation with the morning being the most productive time of the day and also the best time for taking on important tasks (figure 1).

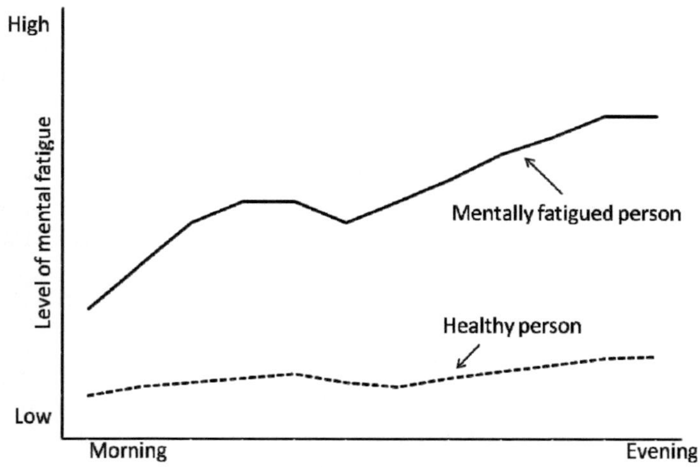

Fig. 1. The figure illustrates how fatigue can typically change over the day.

It is essential for the person to reserve extra time for rest, and most importantly, to avoid too many activities. It is crucial to consider the extended recovery time needed and this should be looked at in conjunction with working capacity. People suffering from mental fatigue are usually able to perform most tasks, but their patience is often limited. It is therefore sometimes difficult to understand that a person, who is normally able to perform tasks like any other person, is unable to accomplish tasks persistently long over a period of time.

2.3 Common associated symptoms

Other common associated symptoms often accompany mental fatigue. These symptoms include sensitivity to stress, even in situations where they previously had no problems. The symptoms can be very hard to handle. Memory problems are also common. However, in most cases the attention is decreased, with the result that the person is not being able to record activities being carried out by other people. Irritability and tearfulness are also common and could be embarrassing and difficult to manage. Sensitivity to light, and most frequently, noise is also common. Many also complain of decreased sleep, or disturbed sleep, while others sleep more than normal. Fatigue also impairs the ability to take initiative and make decisions. They also commonly report slowness of thinking. Many people suffer from headaches after activities involving deep concentration.

Common symptoms which often accompany mental fatigue

- Poor concentration
- Slowness of thinking and slow information processing speed
- Impaired memory
- Stress
- Emotional lability and irritability
- Sleeping problems
- Noise and light sensitivity
- Impaired ability to take initiative
- Headaches

3. Mental fatigue and cognitive functions

Mental fatigue also affects cognitive abilities. Increased subjective mental fatigue after TBI or mild TBI correlates to poor performance in attention tests and reduced processing speed (Belmont, Agar, & Azouvi, 2009). During a dual-task condition, reduced performance was also found with an increase in reaction time with a reported increase in subjective mental effort (Azouvi et al., 2004). TBI subjects also performed more slowly on a complex attention test, made more errors and reported a higher level of subjective fatigue (Ziino & Ponsfold, 2006a). Their performance was slower, but remained on the same level during a vigilance test, and a higher fatigue rating was associated with an increase in the number of errors made (Ziino & Ponsford, 2006b). Furthermore, practice increased the response speed for controls across time, while a lack of effect was found for subjects with mental fatigue after TBI (Ashman et al., 2008). Moreover, a simultaneous load on working memory that demands total control of the situation was more tiring than an automatic activity for TBI subjects (Park, Moscovich, & Robertson, 1999). Thumb pressing was used as an objective test of processing speed and the findings correlated with subjective fatigue (D. L. Lachapelle &

Finlayson, 1998). Mental fatigue has also been reported to correlate to decreases in processing speed and attention, both after mild and moderate TBI and processing speed was found to be the primary predictor for mental fatigue (Johansson, Berglund, & Rönnbäck, 2009).

An increased mental effort may be needed to compensate for a decreased cognitive capacity, or impaired neural network, resulting in an increase in mental fatigue. This has been explained by the "coping hypothesis", suggesting that the brain needs to work harder in order to compensate for impairments to cognitive functions such as attention and processing speed (Zomeren & van den Burg, 1985). This hypothesis has been supported by several authors (Belmont, et al., 2009; Ziino & Ponsfold, 2006a; Ziino & Ponsford, 2006b). This compensation after mild TBI or TBI has been measured during a memory and attention task and was suggested to be related to an increase in brain activity (Turner & Levine, 2008), and recruitment of brain areas outside the working memory network (Smits et al., 2009). This increased brain activity was measured using functional Magnetic Resonance Imaging (fMRI). Mental fatigue after TBI was also suggested to be related to an increased brain activity measured by fMRI for processing speed over time (Kohl, Wylie, Genova, Hillary, & Deluca, 2009). The neural network associated with diminished processing speed after a TBI was similar to the network used by healthy individuals and the network used was suggested to be partially related to reaction time. This indicates, according to the authors, that the neural network is the same as for healthy subjects, but the processing speed is slower. The prefrontal cortex plays a more important role in performing a cognitive task relating to the assessment of processing speed (Hillary et al., 2010). Reduced anisotropy in white matter after mild TBI was also detected by analysis using diffusion tensor imaging. At the same time abnormally slow functional connectivity patterns were detected in cortical grey matter using magnetoencephalography (Huang et al., 2009). Deficits in scores for complex visual information processing after mild TBI were found to be attributable to a reduced amplitude of event-related potential (J. Lachapelle, Bolduc-Teasdale, Ptito, & McKerral, 2008).

4. How common is mental fatigue after TBI?

It is difficult to have any clear figure as to how common mental fatigue is since it varies significantly in accordance with the methodological differences between studies and also how mental fatigue is defined. A majority of patients recover after a mild TBI within 1 to 3 months (Carroll, Cassidy, & Peloso, 2004; Lundin, de Boussard, Edman, & Borg, 2006), but for many individuals mental fatigue persists for a longer period. In follow-up studies, the frequency of prolonged fatigue varies from 30 to 73 %. One third of the patients who suffered from mild TBI complained of severe fatigue at 6 months as well as a decrease in physical and social activities (Naalt, Zomeren, Sluiter, & Minderhoud, 1999; Stulemeijer et al., 2006). After 5 years, 73 % reported still having a problem with fatigue, which affected their everyday life (Olver, 1996). Even after ten years, fatigue was still present, irrespective of injury severity (O´Connor, Colantonio, & Polatajko, 2005). Improvement was reported during the first year, after which time it was limited (Bushnik, Englander, & Wright, 2008).

Many participants were suffering from persistent mental fatigue, with mean time since injury of 6 years after mild TBI and 11 years after moderate TBI (Johansson, et al., 2009). The problem varied from those who could manage a position in full-time employment, to those who were extremely exhausted even after a short conversation or reading the newspaper. Mental fatigue is also dependent on the total activity as well as the demands of daily activities. We found a significantly increased subjectively reported mental fatigue among participants who had suffered a mild TBI but were working full-time compared to healthy controls. Their subjective report did not differ greatly from that given by the participants on sick leave. The differences reported between those on sick leave and those working full-time were found to be related to cognitive performance. Those subjects in full-time employment performed on similar level as the controls on cognitive tests, while those on sick-leave had primarily a decreased processing speed. Furthermore, no differences in relation to the prolonged cognitive effects as well as mental fatigue scores were found between mild TBI on sick leave and moderate TBI. According to a study carried out by Reitan and Wolfson some subjects with mild TBI may suffer a more severe injury, although this has not been diagnosed as such (Reitan & Wolfson, 1999). A study revealed that 30-year post-TBI follow-up, most patients presented a mild cognitive decline, but this was attributable to gender and age differences, with women and younger patients maintaining their cognitive level, and some younger subjects even improving their cognitive level, while older men showed a decline. It was suggested that there was a qualitative difference from the early sign of dementia of the Alzheimer type (Himanen et al., 2006).

The long-term effects after brain injury is today an area which is not covered in the research and one in which it has been difficult to produce concrete findings. Recent studies report long-term effects after recurring concussion among athletes actively engaged in their sport with a high incidence of head injuries. Whether or not this is similar to persistent post-concussion syndrome is unknown, but long-term or even deteriorating problems can occur after repeated head traumas (Gavett, Stern, & McKee, 2011). We also found a high frequency (44 %) among the mild TBI participants who had sustained more than one injury and had been on sick leave for several years, and were complaining of long-term mental fatigue and cognitive problems (Johansson, et al., 2009).

5. Assessment of mental fatigue

In clinical practice, fatigue is noticed, but not always as important and central as it could be. Mental fatigue has also been difficult to assess. Therefore, the problem has so far not generated any extensive research. It is treated by many professionals as an issue of secondary importance, one which has a specific diagnosis. The focus is on other problems, depending on the professional approach. Researchers report on incidences of depression, apathy, emotional problem, fatigue and impaired executive functions after mild TBI and TBI with a combination of these diagnosis/symptoms. A psychiatrist might focus on depression and anxiety, while a neuropsychologist will focus on executive functions and problems. It is possible to analyse all these symptoms with use of different scales or questionnaires, and all these symptoms could be significant.

As mental fatigue has such a great impact on many functions, it is important to consider the problem from a wide perspective and to look at the issue with an open mind, in order to develop an understanding of the cause of the problem. Mental fatigue is something specific, but it is easy to misunderstand symptoms if there is a limited amount of knowledge available. It could be mistaken for apathy if the person has difficulties with getting things done during the day, is not interested in learning new things and is not doing things that interest him or her. However, these problems could be the result if the energy levels are low. It might be too exhaustive to carry out activities that demand a high degree of concentration, as talking to friends, reading and learning new things. A good strategy is actually to be careful with the existing energy levels and to use it on fewer important activities.

5.1 Self-assessment of mental fatigue

Fatigue is usually assessed as a subjective problem with self-report questionnaires. It has been difficult to relate to objective assessment as a means of measuring it. There is, however, a dual problem as both the subjective scale and the objective test used must be sensitive and specific for mental fatigue.

A new self-assessment scale, the mental fatigue scale (MFS) was adapted from Rödholm et al. (Rödholm, Starmark, Svensson, & von Essen, 2001). The MFS contains 15 questions and these cover the most common symptoms occurring after brain injury (King, Crawford, Wenden, Moss, & Wade, 1995; Zomeren & van den Burg, 1985). The selection of items is based on many years of clinical experience and reports (Lindqvist & Malmgren, 1993). The questions include symptoms reported early on, as well as a long time after a brain injury or other neurological diseases. The questions relate to fatigue in general, lack of initiative, mental fatigue, mental recovery, concentration difficulties, memory problems, slowness of thinking, sensitivity to stress, increased tendency to become emotional, irritability, sensitivity to light and noise, decreased or increased sleep as well as 24-hour variations.

The items are based on common activities and the estimation relates to intensity, frequency and duration with exemplified alternatives. The intention was to make the scale more consistent between individuals and also between ratings for the same individual. Each item comprises examples of common activities to be related to four response alternatives. A higher score reflects more severe symptoms. A rating of 0 corresponds to normal function, 1 indicates a problem, 2 a pronounced symptom and 3 a maximal symptom. It is also possible to provide an answer which falls in between two scores (see example below).

The self-assessment scale for mental fatigue and related items was evaluated. Significant correlations were found between all the 14 questions (24-hour variation was not included as only 'yes' and 'no' responses were measured). The 14 questions had adequate internal consistency. The Cronbach's alpha scale was used, giving a reliability coefficient of 0.944 (Johansson, et al., 2009). This indicates that the core problem with mental fatigue comprises a broader spectrum of relevant items with either primary or secondary symptoms. The response alternatives are refined in such a way as to make the self reports more consistent. This might have resulted in a more definite deviation from the healthy controls (the scale can be downloaded at www.mf.gu.se).

The question relating to 24-hour variation was analysed separately as it was constructed differently. A majority of the participants with brain injury (about 70 %) stated that the morning time was best time and afternoon and evening was the worst. This shows the increase in fatigue due to mental load during the daytime, while this was not clearly noticed among healthy controls (10 % had a clear 24h variation, see also figure 1).

Individuals with mild TBI who were working full-time did not change their leisure and social activities, although they rated their mental fatigue and related items on the same level as the participants with mild TBI and TBI who were on sick leave and had decreased their

Example of a question from the self-assessment scale of mental fatigue.

Mental fatigue

Does your brain become fatigued quickly when you have to think hard? Do you become mentally fatigued from things such as reading, watching TV or taking part in a conversation with several people? Do you have to take breaks or change to another activity?

0 I can manage in the same way as usual. My ability for sustained mental effort is not reduced.

0.5

1 I become fatigued quickly but am still able to make the same mental effort as before.

1.5

2 I become fatigued quickly and have to take a break or do something else more often than before.

2.5

3 I become fatigued so quickly that I can do nothing or have to abandon everything after a short period (approx. five minutes).

leisure and social activities. Depending on their mental load during the day, subjects working full-time might need to devote more attention to mental load and use more energy than is normal. However, the scores for subjects in full-time employment did not reveal any significant differences compared to controls on cognitive tests, which indicates a difference in severity compared to mild TBI on sick leave.

Many participants gave spontaneous comments on the scale as it included important, key items which have been confusing for them. From a clinical viewpoint, the self-assessment scale can be a valuable therapeutic tool for the patient as it can clearly describe mental fatigue and common symptoms which co-occur. A better understanding of the problem is a very good starting point for further treatment.

5.2 Cognitive tests

With the intention of finding sensitive neuropsychological tests to assess mental fatigue, tests were chosen according to common problems after mild TBI. Tests included measured information processing speed (the time required to execute a cognitive task within a finite time period) (DeLuca & Kalmar, 2007), attention, working memory, verbal fluency and reading speed. The tests were digit symbol-coding from the WAIS-III NI (Wechsler, 2004), measuring information processing speed. Attention and working memory, both auditory and visual, were measured by means of the digit span and spatial span (Wechsler, 2004). Both tests included repetition of forward series of random numbers or blocks in order as well as in reverse. The verbal fluency test (FAS) measures the ability to generate as many words as possible beginning with a specific letter within one minute (Ellis, Kaplan, & Kramer, 2001). Parts A and B of the Trail Making Test (TMT), (Reitan & Wolfson, 1985) were used to measure visual scanning, divided attention and motor speed (Lezak, Howieson, & Loring, 2004). The test consists of a series of connect-the-circle tasks. The tasks in part A is to connect the circles in a sequence with a numerical order of 1 to 25. Part B comprise letters and digits in alternating numerical and alphabetical order, which have to be completed as quickly as possible. In order to evaluate higher demands such as dual tasks, a series of new tests was constructed with three and four factors, respectively. The same number of circles (25) was used in all parts. The alternation between factors was similar to part B but months was added in part C and both months and days of the week in chronological order in part D. In the latter, the order of letters and digits was changed. The reading speed was measured using the DLS reading speed test used for the screening of dyslexia (Madison, 2003).

Information processing speed and attention tasks were found to be most sensitive and were significantly decreased compared to healthy control, while no such effect was found for both visual and auditory working memory. The subjective rating of the mental fatigue scale was primarily linked to processing speed and attention and processing speed was found to be the primary predictor for mental fatigue. The total sum of scores also correlated significantly with percentages for sick leave (Johansson, et al., 2009). Information processing speed is also the cognitive function most likely to be affected after a brain injury (Frencham, Fox, & Maybery, 2005; Madigan, DeLuca, Diamond, Tramontano, & Averill, 2000; Martin, Donders, & Thompson, 2000).

The self-assessment scale in combination with tests that primarily measure information processing speed and a high cognitive load on attention might make it possible to evaluate problems described by patients with mental fatigue, as subjective mental fatigue after mild TBI and TBI are suggested to primarily correlate with objectively measured information processing speed. If cognitive decline within these neuropsychological regions are evident, the mental loading can be even higher. In addition, other cognitive impairments may also occur, which will also affect and interfere with a person's daily functioning.

6. Treatment

There is no known effective treatment for mental fatigue. When it persists, it can be very frustrating, leading to an increased risk of a depression. However, the situation can improve if the proper treatment and support are offered.

Rehabilitation should include information and advice on how to handle symptoms, offering counselling immediately after the trauma or illness. However, as the mental fatigue can be long-term, many years of support and rehabilitation may be needed.

A thorough examination will ensure that the patient has the necessary information about the problems concerning fatigue and the accompanying symptoms he or she is experiencing. With a better understanding of the situation, it is possible to find a balance between activities and rest, and this is essential. Time for rest during the day is necessary, as well as good strategies which conserve the energy levels. It is sensible to use the available energy for important tasks. It is also important to try to avoid stress as much as possible. For example, it is advisable to do one thing at a time, take more time for each activity, to avoid planning too many activities in a short period and to ensure that rest is included when planning the day's activities. Activities in everyday life and work can be managed more efficiently by keeping the total mental load under control.

It is recommended to avoid taking on more activities over longer periods in an attempt to improve mental endurance as this does not work. When the limits of mental activity are pushed, mental fatigue increases and there is a decrease in performance. Poor concentration and more mistakes can be the consequence if one's mental activities are not adapted to one's mental fatigue.

It is essential to stress that the individual's activity level in the majority of cases has to be profoundly reduced following the injury/disease. For some individuals affected by persistent mental fatigue, it can take a long time, sometimes several years, to find the right balance between rest and activity in daily life. It can also take time to find appropriate working strategies and to accept that the activity level must be greatly reduced compared to before the mental fatigue developed. However, once the person realizes the need for a more calm and stress-free way of living, he/she can start finding a new way of handling everyday activities, including a job.

Persons suffering from mental fatigue often feel better in an environment where it is possible to rest and keep the tempo low, although resting and sleeping do not resolve the problem. Going for walks in natural environments as well as doing calm and relaxing activities can provide mental rest.

Several substances have been tested, but no pharmacological therapy has been successful in treating mental fatigue in the acute phase nor for the alleviation of long-term cognitive and emotional problems (Arcinegas, Anderson, Topkoff, & McAllister, 2005; Beauchamp, Mutlak, Smith, Shohami, & Stahel, 2008). However, symptomatic treatments can be administered. Depression can be treated in various ways, for instance by administering selective serotonin reuptake inhibitors (SSRI) drugs and with psychotherapy. A low dose of an anti-depressant may also reduce the emotional lability and irritability in persons suffering from mental fatigue, but anti-depressants are not effective in treating the mental fatigue itself. If a pharmacological treatment is used, it is however, important to start on a low dose and increase gradually as people with TBI are particularly susceptible to adverse effects (Arcinegas, et al., 2005).

7. Future research

Mental fatigue is an extensive problem, and both mild TBI as well as TBI may have similar persistent problems with mental fatigue and long-term absence from work due to illness. About 2 % of the U.S. population is living with long-term consequences after TBI (Prevention, 2003). Accordingly, research on different aspects of mental fatigue is necessary. We need to increase our knowledge of the pathophysiological mechanisms underlying mental fatigue, and also our knowledge of the risk factors. It is also important to develop more specific and sensitive diagnostic tools. There is also an urgent need to find therapeutic methods for this group of people.

In our work we focus on different aspects of mental fatigue and we have recently started treatment studies. These include both non-pharmacological and pharmacological treatment. At present we are concentrating on exploring whether altered dopamine levels in the brain affect fatigue, as dopamine is to have an improved effect on attention. In addition, we have studied the effect of mindfulness-based stress reduction (MBSR) on persons who suffer from mental fatigue after traumatic brain injury and stroke. The intention is to assess whether the adaptation of a person's activity levels and improved stress management can lead to a reduction in mental fatigue. Promising results have been found in both studies and we will continue with further studies using these methods (unpublished data, in preparation).

8. References

Arcinegas, D. B., Anderson, C. A., Topkoff, J., & McAllister, T. W. (2005). Mild traumatic brain injury: a neuropsychiatric approach to diagnosis, evaluation, and treatment. *Neuripsychiatric Disease and Treatment, 1*(4), 311-327.

Ashman, T. A., Cantor, J. B., Gordon, W. A., Spielman, L., Egan, M., Ginsberg, A., et al. (2008). Objective measurement of fatigue following traumatic brain injury. *J Head Trauma Rehabil 23*(1), 33-40.

Ashman, T. A., Spielman, L. A., Hibbard, M. R., Silver, M. J., Chandna, T., & Gordon, W. A. (2004). Psychiatric challenges in the first 6 years after traumatic brain injury: Cross-sequential analyses of axis I disorder. *Arch Phys Med Rehabil, 85*(Suppl 2), S36-S42.

Azouvi, P., Couillet, J., Leclercq, M., Martin, Y., Asloun, S., & Rousseaux, M. (2004). Divided attention and mental effort after severe traumatic brain injury. *Neuropsychologia, 42*, 1260-1268.

Beauchamp, K., Mutlak, H., Smith, W. R., Shohami, E., & Stahel, P. F. (2008). Pharmacology of Traumatic Brain Injury: Where Is the "Golden Bullet"? *Mol Med, 14*(11-12), 731-740.

Belmont, A., Agar, N., & Azouvi, P. (2009). Subjective fatigue, mental effort, and attention dificits after severe traumatic brain injury. *Neurorehabil Neural Repair, 23*(9), 939-944.

Belmont, A., Agara, N., Hugeron, C., Gallais, B., & Azouvia, P. (2006). Fatigue and traumatic brain injury. *Ann Readapt Med Phys, 49*, 283-288.

Bushnik, T., Englander, J., & Wright, J. (2008). Patterns of fatigue and its correlates over the first 2 years after traumatic brain injury. *Head Trauma Rehabil, 23*(1), 25-32.

Carroll, L. J., Cassidy, J. D., & Peloso, P. M. (2004). Prognosis of mild traumatic brain injury: results of the WHO collaborating Centre Task Force on Mild Traumatic Brain Injury. *J Rehabil Med, 43*(suppl), 84-105.

Chaudhuri, A., & Behan, P. O. (2004). Fatigue in neurological disorders. *Lancet 363*, 978-988.

DeLuca, J. (2007). Information processing speed: How fast, how slow, and how come? In: *Information processing speed in clinical population,* DeLuca, J. and Kalmar, J.H., (Eds.), *265-273,* Taylor and Francis group, New York.

Ellis, D. C., Kaplan, E., & Kramer, J. H. (Eds.). (2001). *Delis-Kaplan Executive Function System – D-KEFS*. San Antonio, TX: The Psychological Corporation.

Frencham, K. A. R., Fox, A. M., & Maybery, M. T. (2005). Neuropsychological studies of mild traumatic brain injury: a meta-analytical review of research since 1995. *J Clin Exp Neuropsychol, 27*(3), 334-351.

Gavett, B. E., Stern, R. A., & McKee, A. C. (2011). Chronic traumatic encephalopathy: a potential late effect of sport-related concussive and subconcussive head trauma. *Clin Sports Med, 30,* 179-188.

Hansson, E., & L, R. (2004). Altered neuronal-glial signaling in glutamatergic transmission as a unifying mechanism in chronic pain and mental fatigue. *Neurochem Res, 29,* 989-996.

Hillary, F. G., Genova, H. M., Medaglia, J. D., Fitzpatrick, N. M., Chiou, K. S., Wardecker, B. M., et al. (2010). The Nature of Processing Speed Deficits in Traumatic Brain Injury: is Less Brain More? *Journal Brain Imaging and Behavior 4*(2), 141-154.

Himanen, L., Portin, R., Isoniemi, H., Helenius, H., Kurki, T., & Tenovuo, O. (2006). Longitudinal cognitive changes in traumatic brain injury A 30-year follow-up study. *Neurology, 66*(2187-192).

Huang, M. X., Theilmann, R. J., Robb, A., A, A., S, N., A, D., et al. (2009). Integrated imaging approach with MEG and DTI to detect mild traumatic brain injury in military and civilian patients. *J Neurotrauma, 26*(8), 1213-1226.

Johansson, B., Berglund, P., & Rönnbäck, L. (2009). Mental fatigue and impaired information processing after mild and moderate traumatic brain injury. *Brain Injury, 23*(13-14), 1027-1040.

King, N. S., Crawford, S., Wenden, F. J., Moss, N. E. G., & Wade, D. T. (1995). The Rivermead post concussion symptoms questionnaire: a measure of symptoms commonly experienced after head injury and its reliability. *J Neurol Neurosur Ps, 24,* 587-592.

Kohl, A. D., Wylie, G. R., Genova, H. M., Hillary, F., & Deluca, J. (2009). The neural correlates of cognitive fatigue in traumatic brain injury using functional MRI. *Brain Injury, 23*(5), 420-432.

Lachapelle, D. L., & Finlayson, M. A. J. (1998). An evaluation of subjective and objective measures of fatigue in patients with brain injury and healthy controls. *Brain Injury, 12*(8), 649-659.

Lachapelle, J., Bolduc-Teasdale, J., Ptito, A., & McKerral, M. (2008). Deficits in complex visual information processing after mild TBI: electrophysiological markers and vocational outcome prognosis. *Brain Injury, 22*(3), 265-274.

Lezak, M. D., Howieson, D. B., & Loring, D. W. (Eds.). (2004). *Neuropsychological assessment* (4th ed.). New York: Oxford University Press.

Lindqvist, G., & Malmgren, H. (1993). Organic mental disorders as hypothetical pathogenetic processes. *Acta Psychiatr Scand, 88*(suppl 373), 5-17.

Lundin, A., de Boussard, C., Edman, G., & Borg, J. (2006). Symptoms and disability until 3 months after mild TBI. *Brain Injury 20*(8), 799-806.

Madigan, N. K., DeLuca, J., Diamond, B. J., Tramontano, G., & Averill, A. (2000). Speed of information processing in traumatic brain injury: modality-specific factors. *J Head Trauma Rehabil 15*(3), 943-956.

Madison, S. (2003). *Läsdiagnos*. Lund: Läs och skrivcentrum.

Martin, T. A., Donders, J., & Thompson, E. (2000). Potential of and problems with new measures of psychometric intelligence after traumatic brain injury. *Rehabil Psychol, 45*(4), 402-408.

Naalt, J. v. d., Zomeren, v., A H, Sluiter, W. J., & Minderhoud, J. M. (1999). One year outcome in mild to moderate head injury: the predictive value of acute injury characteristics related to complaints and return to work. *J Neurol Neurosur Ps, 66*, 207-213.

O´Connor, C., Colantonio, A., & Polatajko, H. (2005). Long term symptoms and limitations of activity of people with traumatic brain injury: a ten-year follow-up. *Psychological reports, 97*, 169-179.

Olver, J. H. (1996). Outcome following traumatic brain injury: a. comparison between 2 and 5 years after injury. *Brain Injury, 10*, 841-848.

Park, N. W., Moscovich, M., & Robertson, I. H. (1999). Divided attention impairments after traumatic brain injury. *Neuropsychologia 37*(10), 1119-1133.

Prevention, C. f. D. C. a. (2003). Report to congress on mild traumatic brain injury in the United States: Steps to prevent a serious public health problem. *Atalnta: Centres for disease control and prevention.*

Reitan, R. M., & Wolfson, D. (1999). The two faces of mild head injury. *Arch Clin Neuropsych, 14*(2), 191-202.

Reitan, R. M., & Wolfson, D. (Eds.). (1985). *The Halstead-Reitan neuropsychological Test Battery. Theory and clinical interpretation*. Tucson. AZ: Neuropsychology Press.

Rödholm, M., Starmark, J.-E., Svensson, E., & von Essen, C. (2001). Asteno-emotional disorder after aneurysmal SAH: reliability, symptomatology and relation to outcome. *Acta Neurol Scand, 103*, 379-385.

Silver, J. M., Mc Allister, J. W., & Arciniegas, D. B. (2009). Depression and cognitive complaints following mild traumatic brain injury. *Am J Psychiatry, 166*(6), 653-661.

Smits, M., Dippel, D. W. J., Houston , G. C., Wielopolski, P. A., Koudstaal, P. J., Hunink, M. G. M., et al. (2009). Postconsussion syndrome after minor head injury: brain activation of working memory and attention. *Hum Brain Mapp, 30*(9), 2789-2803.

Stulemeijer, M., van der Werf, S., Bleijenberg, G., Biert, J., Brauer, J., & Vos, P. E. (2006). Recovery from mild traumatic brain injury: a focus on fatigue. *J Neurol Neurosur Ps, 253*(8), 1041-1047.

Turner, G. R., & Levine, B. (2008). Augmented neural activity during executive control processing following diffuse axonal injury. *Neurology 71*(11), 812-808.

Wechsler, D. (Ed.). (2004). *Wechsler Adult Intelligence Scale – third edition, WAIS-III NI, Swedish version*. Stockholm: Pearson Assessment.

Whelan-Goodinson, R., Ponsfold, J., & Schönberger, M. (2009). Validity of hopsital anxiety and depression scale to assess depression and anxiety following traumatic brain injury as compared with the structured clinical inteview for DSM-IV. *J Affect Disorder*, 114, 94-102.

Ziino, C., & Ponsfold, J. (2006a). Selective attention deficits and subjective fatigue following traumatic brain injury. *Neuropsychology 20*, 383-390.

Ziino, C., & Ponsford, J. (2006b). Vigilance and fatigue following traumatic brain injury. *J Int Neuropshychol Soc, 12*(1), 100-110.

Zomeren, A. H. v., & van den Burg, W. (1985). Residual complaints of patients two years after severe head injury. *J Neurosurg Psychiatry, 48*(1), 21-28.

2

Brain Injury and Cerebral Lateralization

Şenol Dane
Fatih University, Medical Faculty, Ankara
Turkey

1. Introduction

The aim of my manuscript will be to explicate the associations among cerebral lateralization, especially left-handedness, decreased longevity, the age of menopause, asymmetries in the bone mineral densities, the asymmetries in common carotid artery intima-media thickness and the risk of sudden death of brain infarction.

2. Left-handedness and decreased longevity

Life span studies[1,2,3,4,5,6,7,8] have shown that the population percentage of left-handers diminishes steadily, so that they are drastically underrepresented in the oldest age groups. This population trend suggests the reduced longevity of left-handers[9]. Coren and Halpern (1991) suggest that some of the elevated risk for left-handers is apparently due to environmental factors that elevate their accident susceptibility. Also, left-handedness may be a marker for birth stress related neuropathy, developmental delays and irregularities, and deficiencies in the immune system due to the intrauterine hormonal environment. Halpern and Coren (1990) have argued that left-handedness is associated with a younger age at death[10].

Coren (1989) and Halpern and Coren (1991) reported that left-handers were more susceptible to accident-related injuries and more left-handers died in accidents than right-handers[11,12]. Zverev and Adeloye (2001) reported that left-handedness as a risk factor for head injuries obtained during confrontation activities[13]. Also, an increased prevalence of left hand preference was noted in a population of patients having traumatic brain injuries (MacNiven, 1994)[14]. Dane, Karsan and Can (1999) showed that left-handers may be more susceptible to sport-related injuries[15]. Graham and Cleveland (1995) and Wright, Williams, Currie and Beattie (1996) suggested that left-handedness appears to be a risk factor for injury among adolescent school athletes[16,17]. Also, left-handed locomotive drivers were more likely to be involved in accidents (Bhushan & Khan, 2006)[18].

Also, Canakci, Akgul, Akgul, and Canakci (2003) reported that left-handed participants had a significantly higher dental trauma risk than right-handedness[19]. Dagistan, Gursoy, Cakur, Miloglu, Harorli, and Dane (2009) also studied the relation of left-handedness and risk of dental trauma in professional boxers[20]. The left-handed boxers had the higher dental trauma risk than right handed ones. Also, the rate of left-handedness was elevated in men diagnosed with fractures than for all other male patients (Stellman, Wynder, DeRose & Muscat, 1997)[21] and it was demonstrated that the non right-handers were at greater risk for bone breaks and fractures (Coren & Previc, 1996)[22].

Coren (1989) suggested that environmental biases against left-handers were the most likely reason for the increased injury risk in left-handers[23]. Really, furniture, doors of homes, playground apparatus for children, and automobile designs are based on right-handed world. Also, it has been suggested that the biological differences between right- and left-handers might play a role in increased injury risk of left-handers. Graham, Dick, Rickert and Glenn (1993) reported that the proportion of hospitalized left-handed children for injury treatment was larger than the proportion of right-handers and suggested that left-handedness is a risk factor for unintentional injury in children and adolescents in a pediatric emergency department population[24].

It has been claimed that the biological differences in terms of ear advantage[25,26] (Dane & Bayirli, 1998; Aydin, Dane, Ozturk, Uslu, Gumustekin, & Kirpinar, 2001), eye preference[27,28,29] (Dane & Gumustekin, 2002; Dane, Gumustekin, Yazici, & Baykal, 2003; Dane, 2006), nasal cycle[30,31] (Dane & Balci, 2007; Searleman, Hornung, Stein, & Brzuszkiewicz, 2005), and reaction time[32] (Dane & Erzurumluoglu, 2003) between right- and left-handers may contribute to the higher rate of injury in left-handers than in right-handers. Because, contradistinctions in intrinsic biological factors such as ear advantage, eye preference, nasal cycle and reaction time in left-handers may be associated with reversal perception of environment in comparison with right-handers and therefore increased accident related injuries.

However, there are also studies which show no elevated injury risk[33,34] (Peters & Perry, 1991; Hicks, Pass, Freeman, Bautista, & Johnson, 1993). Also, it has been reported that the risk of hand injury was similar for right- and left-handers and individuals with consistent hand preference, regardless of side, were more likely to injure their preferred hand when compared to mixed preference types[35] (Porac, 1993).

3. The age of menopause and left-handedness

It was reported that the early menopause occurs more often in left-handed than right-handed women[36,37,38,39] (Leidy, 1990; Nikolova, Negrev, Stoyanov, & Nikolova 1996; Dane, Reis, & Pasinlioglu, 1999; Dane, Kumtepe, Pasinlioglu, & Aksoy, 2004). It has been suggested that the early menopause in left-handed women may result from the differences in the immune activity between the right- and left-handers[39]. The cell-mediated immune activity and cell-mediated immune hypersensitivity (tuberculin reaction) were stronger in left-handed than right-handed women[39]; the age of menopause negatively correlated with tuberculin reaction and percentages of CD4+ and CD8+ lymphocytes[39], indicating that autoimmune reactions against hormone receptor sites[40] (Escobar et al., 1982) or oocytes[41,42] (Maclaren & Blizzard, 1985; Rabinowe et al., 1989) may cause early menopause. In some studies, it has been also reported that immune activity was powered in left-handed persons than in right-handed ones[43,44,45,46] (Dane & Tan, 1994; Köylü et al., 1996; Battcock et al., 1990; Ertunç et al., 1997).

4. The bone fractures and left-handedness

The bone mineral density is a marker of the collagen content of bones. Therefore, the higher bone mineral densities in the right-handers compared to the left-handers may be associated with the higher collagen content of bones of the right-handers. Dane, Akar, Hacibeyoglu, and Varoglu (2001), Akar, Sivrikaya, Canikli, and Varoglu (2002) and Gumustekin, Akar,

Dane, Yildirim, Seven, and Varoglu (2004) reported that hand preference may be related to the right-left asymmetry in femoral bone mineral density[47,48,49].

In a resent study, the bone mineral densities of both right and left proximal femur regions except Ward's region were higher in right-handed subjects compared to left-handed ones[50]. It can be stated that right-handed subjects have decreased risk of bone fracture than left-handed subjects.

The decreased bone mineral densities in left-handed participants compared to right-handers may be associated with the increased risk of bone breaks and fractures in left-handers[21, 22] (Stellman, et al., 1997; Coren & Previc, 1996) because the decreased bone mineral density is a good marker of bone fractures. Also, it can be stated that left-handed wictims will have more severe consequences during accident.

The decreased bone mineral density in left-handers may also associated with higher injury risk of smaller traumas. The measured bone mineral densities were within normal ranges in all subjects. The effect sizes of sex and handedness are similar. Therefore, left-handedness and female sex can be considered possible risk factors for bone fractures.

In above mentioned study, the bone mineral densities of both right and left all proximal femur regions were higher in men than in women[50]. The rate of left-handedness was elevated for men diagnosed with bone fractures when compared with all other male patients in a case-control study of 8.801 hospitalized patients with cancer and those with other conditions, but this relation was absent in women patients[21] (Stellman, et al., 1997). Aggleton, Kentridge, and Neave (1993) and Aggleton, Bland, Kentridge, and Neave (1994) reported that the left-handed men, but not the left-handed women, were more likely to die prematurely in accidents or in warfare[5,6]. Also, Dagistan, et al. (2009) reported that left-handed boxer men had higher dental trauma risk than right-handed boxers[20].

Coren and Previc (1996) reported the results of two studies[22]. On study 1 retrospective responses were used from medical history checklists completed by 1064 males on active duty with the United States Air Force. The left-handers were at significantly higher risk for knee problems, elbow and shoulder problems, and also swollen and painful joints, although there was no difference in the incidence of broken bones. On study 2 an expanded handedness scale and retrospective reports of both bone breaks and fractures for a predominantly university sample of 1.716 (975 women, 741 men) whose median age was 20 years, indicated that non right-handers were at greater risk for bone breaks and fractures.

In another study[51], ambidextrous men had slightly elevated risk of traffic and home injury, whereas ambidextrous women had slightly elevated risk of work injury compared with right-handers (Pekkarinen, Salminen & Järvelin, 2003).

Boote, Hayes, Abahussin, and Meek (2006) reported that fibrillar collagen in the human cornea and limbus is arranged anisotropically, and left and right corneas are structurally distinct[52]. Also, Dane, Aslankurt, and Yazici (2007) reported the cataracts formed earlier in the dominant eye for both right- and left-eye dominant patients[53]. This difference by handedness may also be associated with asymmetry in collagen content or structure of the lens by handedness in patients.

As a consequence, the higher susceptibility of the left-handed subjects for accident-related injuries such as bone fractures may be associated with lower bone mineral density in the left-handed participants than in the right-handed. Also, sex related differences in accident-related injuries may be explained by differences in bone mineral density by handedness in women.

5. Asymmetry in carotid artery

Arterisclerosis is a chronic disease of the arterial system characterized by abnormal thickening and hardening of the wessel walls. In arterosclerosis, the tunica intima undergoes a series of changes that decrease the artery's ability to change lumen size. Smooth moscle cells and collagen fibers migrate into the tunica intima, causing it to stiffen and thicken. This process gradually narrows the arterial lume. Common carotid intima-media thickness (CCA-IMT) has been shown to be associated with atherosclerosis and stroke[54,55,56,57,58,59,60,61,62]. Increased CCA-IMT determined by B-mode ultrasonography has been shown to be directly associated with an increased risk of myocardial infarction and stroke in older adults without a previous history of cardiovascular disease[62,63].

It has been reported that left-handed, not right-sided, brain infarction was associated with increased risk of sudden death and left-handed or ambidextrous patients have a lower risk of sudden death than right-handed patients[64].

Rodriguez-Hernandez et al. (2003) compared left and right common carotid artery intima-media thickness as measured by B-mode ultrasonography and reported that the difference between both sides was significant (left, 0.75 ± 0.11 mm, right, 0.71 ± 0.11 mm)[65]. Also, they reported that the incidence of nonlacunar cerebrovascular stroke was significantly higher at the left side and suggested a predilection for cerebrovascular disease at the left side, which may be related to greater hemodynamic stres and intimal damage in the left carotid artery. Also, Denairo et al. (2000) have reported that CCA-IMT was lower on the right side than on the left side in both sexes[66].

Bogren et al. (1994) have reported that all right-handed subjects in their study had higher flow rates in the left internal carotid artery than in the right, and all left-handed subjects had higher flow rates in the right internal carotid artery than in the left[67].

In the study performed by Onbas et al. (2007), there was a difference between ıntima media thicknesses of the left and right common carotid artery, with higher values on the left side[68]. In some earlier studies, CCA-IMT was also higher on left side than on right side[65,66,69,70].

Rodriguez-Hernandez et al. (2003) reported that the incidence of nonlacunar cerebrovascular stroke was significantly higher at the left side[65]. Algra et al. (2003) reported that left-sided, not right-sided, brain infarction was associated with increased risk of sudden death[64]. In the light of these studies, it can be speculated that there is a predilection for cerebrovascular disease at the left side, which may be related to greater hemodynamic stress and intimal damage in the left carotid artery.

But, a common pathophysiological mechanism associated with the higher IMT in the left CCA and the more frequent occurrence of stroke in the left hemisphere is unclear. The higher IMT in the left CCA may result from the fact that the cell-mediated (T cell-dependent) hypersensitivity was higher in the left side of the body than the right side[71,72,73].

Because atherosclerosis is a chronic inflammatory disease[74,75], its pathogenesis involves disturbed lipoprotein metabolism, the formation of proinflammatory lipid peroxidation products, and the host's immune responses[76,77]. Oxidized LDL is present in atherosclerotic lesions and contains a wide variety of lipid peroxidation products, which in turn can form neo-self determinants recognized by specific innate and adaptive immune responses[78,79]. During atherogenesis, LDL is oxidized, generating various oxidation-specific neopeptides, such as malondialdehyde-modified LDL or the phosphorylcholine head group of oxidized phospholipids. These epitopes are recognized by both adaptive T cell-dependent and innate T cell-independent type 2 immune responses[80,81].

In the study performed by Onbas et al. (2007), the difference in CCA-IMT between right and left sides was statistically significant in the left handers, but not in the right-handers[82]. The greater difference in the left-handers may be due to a more active and effective immune system in the left-handers than in the right-handers[39, 43, 44, 45, 46].
Also, in the study performed by Onbas et al. (2007), handedness related differences in CCA-IMT demonstrated. Both right and left CCA-IMTs were lower in the left-handers than in the right-handers. They speculated that a lower risk of sudden death in the left-handed or ambidextrous patients than the right-handed patients in brain infarction[64], may be associated with the lower IMT in the left-handers. The lower CCA-IMT on both sides for the left-handers may result from the handedness related differences in carotid artery blood flow in healthy subjects measured with MR velocity mapping[67].

6. References

[1] Porac C, Coren S, Duncan P. Life-span age trends in laterality. Journal of Gerontology, 1980, 35, 715-721.

[2] Porac C, Coren S. Lateral preferences and human behavior. New York: Sprinter. 1981.

[3] Halpern DF, Coren S. Do right-handers live longer? Nature, 1988, 333, 213.

[4] Coren S. The left hander syndrome: the causes and consequences of left-handedness. New York: Free Press. 1992.

[5] Aggleton JP, Bland JM, Kentridge RW, Neave NJ. Handedness and longevity: an archival study of cricketers. British Medical Journal, 1994, 309, 1681-1684.

[6] Aggleton JP, Kentridge RW, Neave NJ. Evidence for longevity differences between left handed and right handed men: an archival study of cricketers. Journal of Epidemiology and Community Health, 1993, 47, 206-209.

[7] Coren S. The diminished number of older left-handers: differential mortality or social-historical trend? International Journal of Neuroscience, 1994, 75, 1-8.

[8] Davis A, Annett M. Handedness as a function of twinning, age and sex. Cortex, 1994, 30, 105-111.

[9] Coren S, Halpern DF.Left-handedness: a marker for decreased survival fitness. Psychol Bull. 1991 Jan;109(1):90-106.

[10] Halpern DF, Coren S. Laterality and longevity: is lef-handedness associated with a younger age at death? In S. Coren (Ed.), Left-handedness: behavioral implications and anomalies. Amsterdam: Elsevier Science. Pp. 1990, 509-545.

[11] Coren, S. (1989) Left-handedness and accident related injury risk. American Journal of Public Health, 79, 1040-1041.

[12] Halpern, D. F., & Coren, S. (1991) Handedness and life span. New England Journal of Medicine, 324, 998.

[13] Zverev, Y., & Adeloye. A. (2001) Left-handedness as a risk factor for head injuries. East African Medical Journal, 78, 22-24.

[14] MacNiven, E. (1994) Increased prevalence of left-handedness in victims of head trauma. Brain Injury, 8, 457-462.

[15] Dane, S., Karsan, O., & Can, S. (1999) Sports injuries in right and left handers. Perceptual and Motor Skills, 89, 846-848.

[16] Graham, C. J., & Cleveland, E. J. (1995) Left-handedness as an injury risk factor in adolescents. Journal of Adolescent Health, 16, 50-52.

[17] Wright, P., Williams, J., Currie, C., & Beattie, T. (1996) Left-handedness increases injury risk in adolescent girls. Perceptual and Motor Skills, 82: 855-858.

[18] Bhushan, B., & Khan, S. M. (2006) Laterality and accident proneness: a study of locomotive drivers. Laterality, 11, 395-404.

[19] Canakci, V., Akgul, H. M., Akgul, N., & Canakci, C. F. (2003) Prevalence and handedness correlates of traumatic injuries to the permanent incisors in 13-17-year-old adolescents in Erzurum, Turkey. Dental Traumatology, 19, 248-254.

[20] Dagistan, D., Gursoy, G., Cakur, B., Miloglu, O., Harorli, E., & Dane, S. (2009) Handedness differences in dental traumatic injuries of boxers. Turkish Journal of Medical Science, 39(5), 803-807.

[21] Stellman, S. D., Wynder, E. L., DeRose, D. J., & Muscat, J. E. (1997) The epidemiology of left-handedness in a hospital population. Annals of Epidemiology, 7, 167-171.

[22] Coren, S., & Previc, F. H. (1996) Handedness as a predictor of increased risk of knee, elbow, or shoulder injury, fractures and broken bones. Laterality, 1, 139-152.

[23] Coren, S. (1989) Left-handedness and accident related injury risk. American Journal of Public Health, 79, 1040-1041.

[24] Graham, C. J., Dick, R., Rickert, V. I., & Glenn, R. (1993) Left-handedness as a risk factor for unintentional injury in children. Pediatrics, 92(6), 823-826.

[25] Dane, S., & Bayirli, M. (1998) Correlations between hand preference and durations of hearing for right and left ears in young healthy subjects. Perceptual and Motor Skills, 86, 667-672.

[26] Aydin, N., Dane, S., Ozturk, I., Uslu, C., Gumustekin, K., & Kirpinar, I. (2001) Left ear (right temporal hemisphere) advantage and left temporal hemispheric dysfunction in schizophrenia. Perceptual and Motor Skills, 93, 230-238.

[27] Dane, S., & Gumustekin K. (2002) Correlation between hand preference and distance of focusing points of two eyes in the horizontal plane. International Journal of Neuroscience, 112, 1141-1147.

[28] Dane, S., Gumustekin, K., Yazici, A. T., & Baykal, O. (2003) Correlation between hand preference and intraocular pressure from right- and left-eyes in right- and left-handers. Vision Research, 43, 405-408.

[29] Dane, S. (2006) Sex and eyedness in a sample of Turkish high school students. Perceptual and Motor Skills, 103, 89-90.

[30] Dane, S., & Balci, N. (2007) Handedness, eyedness and nasal cycle in children with autism. International Journal of Developmental Neuroscience, 25, 223-226.

[31] Searleman, A., Hornung, D. E., Stein, E., & Brzuszkiewicz, L. (2005) Nostril dominance: differences in nasal airflow and preferred handedness. Laterality, 10, 111-120.

[32] Dane, S., & Erzurumluoglu, A. (2003) Sex and handedness differences in eye-hand visual reaction times in handball players. International Journal of Neuroscience, 113, 923-929.

[33] Peters, M., & Perry, R. (1991) No link between left-handedness and maternal age and no elevated accident rate in left-handers. Neuropsychologia, 29, 1257-1259.

[34] Hicks, R. A., Pass, K., Freeman, H., Bautista, J., & Johnson, C. (1993) Handedness and accidents with injury. Perceptual and Motor Skills, 77, 1119-1122.

[35] Porac, C. (1993) Hand preference and the incidence of accidental unilateral hand injury. Neuropsychologia, 31, 335-362.
[36] Leidy, L. E. (1990). Early age at menopause among left-handed women. Obstetrics and Gynecology, 76, 1111–1114.
[37] Nikolova, P., Negrev, N., Stoyanov, Z., & Nikolova, R. (1996). Functional brain asymme try, handedness and age characteristics of climacterium in women. International Journal of Neuroscience, 86, 143–149.
[38] Dane, S., Reis, N., & Pasinlioglu, T. (1999). Left-handed women have earlier age of menopause. Journal of Basic and Clinical Physiology and Pharmacology, 10, 147–150.
[39] Dane, S., Kumtepe, Y., Pasinlioglu, T., & Aksoy, A. (2004) Relationship between age of menopause and cell-mediated immune hypersensitivity in right- and left-handed women. International Journal of Neuroscience, 114, 651-657.
[40] Escobar, M. E., Cigorraga, S. E., Chiauzzi, V. A., Charreau, E. H., & Rivarola, M. A. (1982). Development of the gonadotrophic resistant ovary syndrome in myastenia gravis: Suggestion of similar autoimmune mechanisms. Acta Endocrinologica, 99, 431–436.
[41] Maclaren, N. K., & Blizzard, R. M. (1985). Adrenal autoimmunity and autoimmune polyglandular syndromes. In N. R. Rose & I. R. Mackay (Ed.), The autoimmune diseases (pp. 201–225). New York: Academic Press.
[42] Rabinowe, S. L., Ravnikar, V. A., Dib, S. A., George, K. L., & Dluhy, R. G. (1989). Premature menopause: Monoclonal antibody defined T lymphocyte abnormalities and antiovarian antibodies. Fertility and Sterility, 51, 450–454.
[43] Dane, S., & Tan, Ü. (1994). Tuberculin reaction is stronger in left-handed than right-handed children. Turkish Journal of Medical Science, 21, 23–25.
[44] Köylü, H., Sengül, A., Özlan, L., Dalçik, H., & Etlik, Ö. (1996). Lymphocyte subsets in cerebral lateralization. Turkish Journal of Medical Science, 26, 249–251.
[45] Battcock, T. M., Finn, R., Barnes, R. M. R. (1990). Observations on herpes zoster: 1. Residual scarring and post-herpetic neuragia; 2. Handedness and the risk of infection. British Journal of clinical Practice, 44, 596–598.
[46] Ertunç, V., Dane, S., Karakuzu, A., & Deniz, O. (1997). Higher herpes zoster infection frequency in right-handed patients and more appearance in left body side of females. Acta Dermato-Venerologica, 77, 245.
[47] Dane, S., Akar, S., Hacibeyoglu, I., & Varoglu, E. (2001) Differences between right- and left-femoral bone mineral densities in right- and left-handed men and women. International Journal of Neuroscience, 111, 187-192.
[48] Akar, S., Sivrikaya, H., Canikli, A., & Varoğlu, E. (2002) Lateralized mineral content and density in distal forearm bones in right-handed men and women: relation of structure to function. International Journal of Neuroscience, 112, 301-311.
[49] Gumustekin, K., Akar, S., Dane, S., Yildirim, M., Seven, B., & Varoglu, E. (2004) Handedness and bilateral femoral bone densities in men and women. International Journal of Neuroscience, 114, 1533-1547.
[50] Sahin A, Dane S, Seven B, Akar S, Yildirim S. Differences by sex and handedness in right and left femur bone mineral densities. Percept Mot Skills. 2009 Dec;109(3):824-30.

[51] Pekkarinen, A., Salminen, S., & Järvelin, M. R. (2003) Hand preference and risk of injury among the Northern Finland birth cohort at the age of 30. Laterality, 8, 339-346.

[52] Boote, C., Hayes, S., Abahussin, M., & Meek, K. M. (2006) Mapping collagen organization in the human cornea: left and right eyes are structurally distinct. Investigative Ophthalmology & Visual Science, 47, 901-908.

[53] Dane, S., Aslankurt, M., Yazici, A. T. (2007) The formation of cataract is earlier in the dominant eye. Laterality, 12(2), 167-171.

[54] Ebrahim S, Papacosta O, Whincup P, Wannamethee G, Walker M, Nicolaides AN, Dhanjil S, Griffin M, Belcaro G, Rumley A, Lowe GD.Carotid plaque, intima media thickness, cardiovascular risk factors, and prevalent cardiovascular disease in men and women: the British Regional Heart Study. Stroke. 1999 Apr;30(4): 841-50.

[55] Zannad F, Visvikis S, Gueguen R, Sass C, Chapet O, Herbeth B, Siest G. Genetics strongly determines the wall thickness of the left and right carotid arteries. Hum Genet. 1998 Aug;103(2):183-8.

[56] Iannuzzi A, Wilcosky T, Mercuri M, Rubba P, Bryan FA, Bond MG. Ultrasonographic correlates of carotid atherosclerosis in transient ischemic attack and stroke. Stroke. 1995 Apr;26(4):614-9.

[57] Cuspidi C, Lonati L, Sampieri L, Pelizzoli S, Pontiggia G, Leonetti G, Zanchetti A.Left ventricular concentric remodelling and carotid structural changes in essential hypertension. J Hypertens. 1996 Dec;14(12):1441-6.

[58] Allan PL, Mowbray PI, Lee AJ, Fowkes FG.Relationship between carotid intima-media thickness and symptomatic and asymptomatic peripheral arterial disease. The Edinburgh Artery Study. Stroke. 1997 Feb;28(2):348-53.

[59] Bots ML, Hoes AW, Koudstaal PJ, Hofman A, Grobbee DE.Common carotid intima-media thickness and risk of stroke and myocardial infarction: the Rotterdam Study. Circulation. 1997 Sep 2;96(5):1432-7.

[60] Veller MG, Fisher CM, Nicolaides AN, Renton S, Geroulakos G, Stafford NJ, Sarker A, Szendro G, Belcaro G.Measurement of the ultrasonic intima-media complex thickness in normal subjects. J Vasc Surg. 1993 Apr;17(4):719-25.

[61] Cupini LM, Pasqualetti P, Diomedi M, Vernieri F, Silvestrini M, Rizzato B, Ferrante F, Bernardi G.Carotid artery intima-media thickness and lacunar versus nonlacunar infarcts. Stroke. 2002 Mar;33(3):689-94.

[62] O'Leary DH, Polak JF, Kronmal RA, Manolio TA, Burke GL, Wolfson SK Jr. Carotid-artery intima and media thickness as a risk factor for myocardial infarction and stroke in older adults. Cardiovascular Health Study Collaborative Research Group. N Engl J Med. 1999 Jan 7;340(1):14-22.

[63] Baldassarre D, Amato M, Bondioli A, Sirtori CR, Tremoli E. Carotid artery intima-media thickness measured by ultrasonography in normal clinical practice correlates well with atherosclerosis risk factors. Stroke. 2000 Oct;31(10):2426-30.

[64] Algra A, Gates PC, Fox AJ, Hachinski V, Barnett HJ; North American Symptomatic Carotid Endarterectomy Trial Group. Side of brain infarction and long-term risk of sudden death in patients with symptomatic carotid disease. Stroke. 2003 Dec;34(12):2871-5. Epub 2003 Nov 20.

[65] Rodríguez Hernández SA, Kroon AA, van Boxtel MP, Mess WH, Lodder J, Jolles J, de Leeuw PW. Is there a side predilection for cerebrovascular disease? Hypertension. 2003 Jul;42(1):56-60. Epub 2003 Jun 16.

[66] Denarié N, Gariepy J, Chironi G, Massonneau M, Laskri F, Salomon J, Levenson J, Simon A. Distribution of ultrasonographically-assessed dimensions of common carotid arteries in healthy adults of both sexes. Atherosclerosis. 2000 Feb;148(2):297-302.

[67] Bogren HG, Buonocore MH, Gu WZ.Carotid and vertebral artery blood flow in left- and right-handed healthy subjects measured with MR velocity mapping. J Magn Reson Imaging. 1994 Jan-Feb;4(1):37-42.

[68] Onbaş O, Dane S, Kantarci M, Koplay M, Alper F, Okur A. Clinical importance of asymmetry and handedness differences in common carotid artery intima-media thickness. Int J Neurosci. 2007 Apr;117(4):433-41.

[69] Simon A, Gariepy J, Chironi G, Megnien JL, Levenson J. Intima-media thickness: a new tool for diagnosis and treatment of cardiovascular risk. J Hypertens. 2002 Feb;20(2):159-69.

[70] Lemne C, Jogestrand T, de Faire U. Carotid intima-media thickness and plaque in borderline hypertension. Stroke. 1995 Jan;26(1):34-9.

[71] Dane S, Erdem T, Gümüştekin K.Cell-mediated immune hypersensitivity is stronger in the left side of the body than the right in healthy young subjects. Percept Mot Skills. 2001 Oct;93(2):329-32.

[72] Gontova IA, Abramov VV, Kozlov VA.The role of asymmetry of nervous and immune systems in the formation of cellular immunity of (CBaxC57Bl/6) F1 mice. Neuroimmunomodulation. 2004;11(6):385-91.

[73] Gontova IA, Abramov VV, Kozlov VA.Asymmetry of delayed type hypersensitivity reaction in mice. Bull Exp Biol Med. 2003 Jan;135(1):67-9.

[74] Steinberg D. Atherogenesis in perspective: hypercholesterolemia and inflammation as partners in crime. Nat Med. 2002 Nov;8(11):1211-7. No abstract available.

[75] Glass CK, Witztum JL. Atherosclerosis. the road ahead. Cell. 2001 Feb 23;104(4):503-16.

[76] Binder CJ, Hartvigsen K, Chang MK, Miller M, Broide D, Palinski W, Curtiss LK, Corr M, Witztum JL.IL-5 links adaptive and natural immunity specific for epitopes of oxidized LDL and protects from atherosclerosis. J Clin Invest. 2004 Aug;114(3):427-37.

[77] Binder CJ, Chang MK, Shaw PX, Miller YI, Hartvigsen K, Dewan A, Witztum JL. Innate and acquired immunity in atherogenesis. Nat Med. 2002 Nov;8(11):1218-26.

[78] Hansson GK, Libby P, Schönbeck U, Yan ZQ.Innate and adaptive immunity in the pathogenesis of atherosclerosis. Circ Res. 2002 Aug 23;91(4):281-91.

[79] Binder CJ, Chang MK, Shaw PX, Miller YI, Hartvigsen K, Dewan A, Witztum JL. Innate and acquired immunity in atherogenesis. Nat Med. 2002 Nov;8(11):1218-26.

[80] Hansson GK, Libby P, Schönbeck U, Yan ZQ.Innate and adaptive immunity in the pathogenesis of atherosclerosis. Circ Res. 2002 Aug 23;91(4):281-91.

[81] Binder CJ, Hartvigsen K, Chang MK, Miller M, Broide D, Palinski W, Curtiss LK, Corr M, Witztum JL.IL-5 links adaptive and natural immunity specific for epitopes of oxidized LDL and protects from atherosclerosis. J Clin Invest. 2004 Aug;114(3):427-37.

[82] Onbaş O, Dane S, Kantarci M, Koplay M, Alper F, Okur A. Clinical importance of asymmetry and handedness differences in common carotid artery intima-media thickness. Int J Neurosci. 2007 Apr;117(4):433-41.

3

Technology-Based Approaches to Improve Mental Health Outcomes for Patients with Traumatic Brain Injury

Jane Topolovec-Vranic, Svetlena Taneva,
Justin Shamis and Donna Ouchterlony
Trauma and Neurosurgery Program, St. Michael's Hospital, Toronto, Ontario
Canada

1. Introduction

Every year approximately 1.4 million people sustain a traumatic brain injury (TBI) in the United States (Langlois J.A. et al., 2006). Mental health disorders such as depression, anxiety, and post-traumatic stress disorder are commonly observed in these individuals. The prevalence of depression following TBI has been reported to range from 14-77% (Ashman et al., 2004). The rate of major depressive disorder within the first year after TBI is 7.9 times greater than in the general population (Bombardier et al., 2010). Mental health conditions can affect the individual for years, even decades after the initial trauma (Dikmen et al., 2004; Holsinger et al., 2002). Further, depression after TBI can lead to worse global outcomes (Fedoroff et al., 1992), poorer social functioning (Bourdon et al., 1992; Jorge et al., 1993; Schoenhuber & Gentilini, 1988), lower health-related quality of life, including an inability to return to work (Christensen et al., 1994; Rutherford, 1977), and suicide (Hesdorffer et al., 2009).

Post-TBI mental health conditions must be treated promptly as they can impair individuals from engaging in the rehabilitation process: these individuals experience poorer recoveries compared to individuals with TBI without mental health conditions (McAllister & Arciniegas, 2002; Mooney et al., 2005; Mooney & Speed, 2001). Although mental health disorders are a major cause of disability, many individuals, particularly those with depression do not receive adequate treatment (Andrews & Henderson, 1999; Bebbington et al., 2000; Kessler et al., 2001). One strategy to address this problem has been the development of technology-based mental health treatment programs. The recent widespread adoption of various computers and handheld devices in everyday life activities presents an opportunity to examine how these technologies can best facilitate various types of mental health treatments for individuals with TBI. Such programs utilize established and emerging technologies such as the Internet, handheld devices, downloadable computer programs, telephones, virtual reality, and video teleconferencing. In addition to providing an adjunct to traditional psychotherapy, technology-based approaches have the potential to deliver self-help interventions to people who do not seek or receive help for their condition (Kaltenthaler et al., 2002; Proudfoot et al., 2003). Further, technology-based treatment programs may have several advantages compared to conventional psychotherapy (Christensen & Griffiths, 2002; Garcia et al., 2004; Gega et al., 2004):

- they can reach a mass audience;
- they are likely to be cost-effective;
- they are capable of supporting individually tailored programs: users can take assessments and complete interactive workshops at their own pace;
- they are capable of supporting automated applications that guarantee intervention fidelity;
- they provide a convenient platform for delivering booster sessions;
- unlike most if not all clinic settings with predetermined hours of operation, such resources are available around the clock;
- they can be conveniently accessed from home, eliminating transportation difficulties and addressing lack of access to face-to-face mental health services in rural areas;
- they are available immediately: the demand for treatment for anxiety and depressive disorders exceeds the supply of suitably trained therapists, so waiting lists are often long;
- they can be delivered privately and anonymously: many sufferers prefer to avoid the stigma commonly incurred by seeing a therapist.

For people with TBI, the potential to use technology-based approaches to self-treat has several additional advantages. Often, victims of TBI are young and may be more familiar with technology-based approaches and may prefer using them to traditional psychotherapy. Further, the fact that individuals can access the Internet and other technologies from their home renders this medium more accessible, cheaper and private. Accessibility is particularly important for these individuals as many of them may also have additional injuries affecting mobility and their depressed mood and anxiety may decrease their motivation to leave the home to seek therapy.

This first objective of this chapter is to describe the results of a scoping review of the literature related to the implementation of technology based approaches for mental health care of patients with TBI and their families/caregivers. The second objective is to present the results of an original survey of TBI patient attitudes towards technology based-approaches to mental health care.

2. Background

Technology-based approaches to mental health treatment are effective, accessible and available means of relaying information or therapeutic interventions to individuals in the population. At present, there is a multitude of *informational* Internet sites that provide a rich variety of resources related to depression, anxiety, post-traumatic stress disorder and other mental health conditions (Griffiths et al., 2009; Ipser et al., 2007; Szumilas & Kutcher, 2009). Such information portals typically target the general user population. Additionally, Internet-based *treatment programs* have emerged in the last decade. Examples of such programs include treatment for insomnia (Ritterband et al., 2009; Strom et al., 2004), excessive alcohol consumption (Linke et al., 2004), panic disorder (Carlbring et al., 2003), post-traumatic stress disorder (Knaevelsrud & Maercker, 2007), social phobia (Andersson et al., 2006), smoking cessation (Feil et al., 2003), headache (Andersson et al., 2003), assertion training and stress management (Yamagishi et al., 2007), and tinnitus (Andersson & Kaldo, 2004).

Although these have primarily been feasibility studies, some have reported successful treatment outcomes (e.g. (Knaevelsrud & Maercker, 2007; Knaevelsrud & Maercker, 2009). Griffiths and colleagues (Griffiths et al., 2010) recently published a review of all the available randomized control trials (RCTs) of internet-based interventions for depression: the first trial was published in 2002 (Clarke et al., 2002), with nine additional trials published in the subsequent years (Billings et al., 2008; Christensen et al., 2004; Clarke et al., 2005; Meyer et al., 2009; Patten, 2003; Perini et al., 2009; Spek et al., 2007; van Straten et al., 2008; Warmerdam et al., 2008). Seven of the trials were community based (Christensen et al., 2004; Meyer et al., 2009; Patten, 2003; Perini et al., 2009; Spek et al., 2007; van Straten et al., 2008; Warmerdam et al., 2008), two were undertaken in the context of a health care organization (Clarke et al., 2002; Clarke et al., 2005), and one in the workplace (Billings et al., 2008). The sample sizes ranged from 48-786 patients with an average age of the participants from 30-50 years. Seven of the trials demonstrated efficacy of the intervention with effect sizes ranging from 0.42 to 0.65 as compared to placebo or wait list controls (Griffiths et al., 2010). Only four of the depression-related websites reviewed were available in the English language: ODIN, MoodGYM, and Bluepages are publicly accessible on the web without charge to consumers and the fourth program, Sadness, is available under restricted license at a small cost. All of the programs employ at least some component of cognitive behavioural therapy (CBT).

While some of these evaluations of technology-based treatment programs have demonstrated positive results on mental health outcomes, the extent of work in this area is limited when the focus is set on the TBI population. As summarized in the following section, very few technology-based resources have been developed and evaluated specifically for the TBI patient.

3. Scoping literature review

This section will present the results of a scoping literature review that aimed to identify the current state of progress in the implementation of technology-based approaches for mental health treatment in patients with TBI. Given the limited amount of literature identified for the TBI patient alone, the scope of the review was expanded to include interventions targeted for the patient's family/caregiver as family conflict due to caregiver burden may impact a TBI patients' quality of life and rehabilitation success. In addition, studies of both adult and pediatric populations were included. We will first summarize the preliminary feasibility and pilot studies. Next, studies describing the evaluation of the intervention using validated mental health outcome measures will be presented.

3.1 Methods used for the scoping literature review

The literature review identified peer-reviewed studies using the phrases of "traumatic brain injury", "mental health", "depression", "anxiety", "post-traumatic stress disorder", "mood disorder", "technology", "Internet", "telephone", "telemedicine", and "ehealth". The exclusion criterion was publication prior to the year 2000. Searches were conducted using PubMed, CINAHL, ProQuest, PsychINFO, Web of Science, and Google Scholar. The reference lists from identified studies were also reviewed. Case studies, pilot/feasibility studies, and randomized controlled trials were all included in the review. Since only a few studies specifically focused on the TBI patient, studies with a focus on the caregiver or family of the TBI patient were included as well. The following elements were extracted from each article: patient descriptors, sample size, treatment descriptors, outcome measures collected, and results summary. Articles were grouped in two categories: 1. *preliminary feasibility studies* (i.e. those that evaluated the ease of use and/or acceptability of the

intervention); 2. *efficacy studies* (i.e. those that evaluated the effectiveness of the intervention using a validated mental-health outcome measure).
Two reviewers concurrently reviewed the title, abstract, and results of each study yielded by the search to determine eligibility of each study. A third reviewer conducted an independent evaluation of the eligibility of the articles. Attempts were made to contact the corresponding authors of the identified articles to ensure that all of their relevant work was captured, and to ascertain whether they had any relevant unpublished, or in-press articles.
Each of the second category of articles (efficacy studies) were classified according to the American Academy of Neurology (AAN) levels of scientific evidence: *level I* included prospective, randomized, controlled clinical trials that controlled for drop-outs, had clear inclusion and exclusion criteria, and presented clear baseline characterization of the patient population; *level II* included prospective, randomized, controlled clinical trials that did not meet the criteria for level I; *level III* included controlled trial studies of natural history where the outcome assessment was independent of the treatment; and *level IV* included all uncontrolled studies, case studies, and expert opinions (Ben-Menachem, 2005).

3.2 Results of the scoping literature review

3.2.1 Feasibility studies

The earliest feasibilty studies in this field focused on the utilization of technology for the mental health treatment of the *caregivers* of TBI patients. Depression occurs not only in individuals with TBI, but it also frequently occurs in their caregivers (Harris et al., 2001). Family dysfunction has also been associated with post-TBI depression (Groom et al., 1998). By using behaviour coping strategies and problem solving, family dysfunction after TBI can be ameliorated (Leach et al., 1994).
Five published articles were identified which described the feasibility of implementing technology-based treatment programs for patients with TBI. These studies utilized telephone, Internet, computer, and video conferencing technologies (see Table 1 for summary).
Rotondi and colleagues examined the feasibility of using an interactive web-based intervention as a resource for psycho-social information and support for female spouses of patients with TBI (Rotondi et al., 2005). Seventeen spouses used the website for six months. The website offered them seven modules: support group, ask an expert, questions and answers library, reference library, community resources library, calendar of community events, and technical support. The interactions of the participants with the website were logged and coded for analyses. The support group module was the most used (68.6%), followed by the community services library module (20.1%). The website was used frequently over the six months of the study (838 times on average, where the median was 454 times and the range was 26-3679 times), was highly valued at the end of the period (75% found that the website was extremely satisfying and extremely helpful) and was rated as relatively easy to use (84%). The results of this study suggested that supportive and psychosocial services can be offered effectively via a website to families who have a member with a TBI. One of the strengths of the study, as discussed by the authors, was that it was the first evaluation of an online psychosocial intervention for female significant others of persons with TBI. Future work in this area would help determine and evaluate the needs of other caregivers.
A more recent study by Glang et al. examined the efficacy of an interactive multimedia CD-ROM program called Brain Injury Partners: Advocacy Skills for Parents of children who

have sustained a TBI (Glang et al., 2007). The program provided parents with information and training in educational advocacy skills. The study found a very large overall effect of the program, especially in the areas of skill application, knowledge, and attitudes. In addition, parents felt that the information was concise and useful.

Authors	Participants	Design and Intervention	Results and Conclusions
Rotondi et al., 2005	17 female spouses of individuals who sustained a TBI	Website containing seven modules: support group, ask an expert questions, questions and answers library, reference library, community resources library, calendar of community events, and technical support	75% found the website to be extremely satisfying and helpful; 84% stated that the website was relatively easy to use.
Glang et al., 2007	31 parents of children from Kindergarden to Grade 8 who had a TBI	CD-ROM programme Brain Injury Partners (control group - alternate CD-ROM)	Parents in the treatment group felt the CD-ROM was concise and useful.; significant improvements in knowledge, attitudes and application measures but not intentions and self-efficacy compared to the control group.
Bergquist et al., 2008	10 individuals with TBI and memory impairment	Internet-based cognitive rehabilitation program	All patients were able to use the program providing evidence that individuals with TBI are capable of using online resources.
Wade et al., 2009	9 families with adolescents who had a TBI	TOPS program with 10 online modules as well as video conferencing with a therapist	Website and video conferencing were rated as moderately to highly helpful and easy to use by the parents and by adolescents.
Martin et al., 2010	Military service members with moderate to severe TBI	8 weeks of telephone support from a pyschiatric neuroscience nurse	93% had improvements in their symptoms compared to 84% in the control group.

Table 1. Overview of feasibility studies for family members and individuals with TBI.

Focusing on the patient with TBI, Bergquist and colleagues evaluated the potential for patients with a documented acquired brain injury and memory impairment to learn to use an Internet-based cognitive rehabilitation program (Bergquist et al., 2008). Ten individuals were trained to use an instant messaging system and were asked to participate in weekly online cognitive rehabilitation therapy sessions. The authors reported that all participants successfully learned to use the system despite their cognitive challenges.

Wade and colleagues tested the feasibility and satisfaction with an online family problem-solving intervention for adolescents who had experienced a TBI (Wade et al., 2009). Nine adolescents utilized the Teen Online Problem Solving program (TOPS), which consisted of ten web-based sessions providing information and interactive exercises on cognitive, social, and behavioral skills typically affected by TBI. Video conferences with a therapist were also made available. The participants reported that the website and videoconferences were moderately to highly helpful and easy to use for both parents and adolescents. Teen satisfaction with the program suggested engagement in the treatment program and process. In addition, the teens stated that the mode of delivery was acceptable and the program length and structure were feasible.

Martin and colleagues demonstrated the feasibility of monitoring military service members with moderate to severe TBI via the telephone (Martin et al., 2010). The home rehabilitation program provided eight weeks of telephone support facilitated by a psychiatric neuroscience nurse. The results indicated that 93% of the participants in the telephone support group had improvements in their symptoms by the end of the study, compared to 84% in the control group (statistical significance of this finding was not indicated). Although no specific information on the types of symptoms improved was reported (cognitive, behavioral, affective, etc.) the study supported the notion that patients could be monitored safely and effectively at home via telephone.

The studies described above, and summarized in Table 1, laid the groundwork for subsequent evaluations of the efficacy of these various approaches to treatment in patients and/or their caregivers following TBI. Collectively they have demonstrated that various technologies (Internet, downloadable computer program, videoconferencing, telephone) show promise in the delivery of treatment programs that are feasible, helpful, and satisfactory for patients with TBI, including those with cognitive impairments, and their families.

3.2.2 Efficacy studies

Seven original research articles were identified that evaluated the implementation of a technology-based intervention program, and incorporated at least one validated mental health outcome measure (see Table 2 for summary). Five of the studies were randomized controlled trials (note: two articles were based on data from one study) and two were case series. Four studies reported the use of an Internet- or computer-based intervention and three reported on telephone counseling and education. Of the seven studies, four evaluated interventions specifically for the TBI patient, and three examined outcome measures in both the patient and their family members/caregivers.

Scheduled telephone counseling and education. Bell and colleagues conducted one of the early studies exploring the effectiveness of a scheduled telephone intervention on behavioral outcomes (Bell et al., 2005). The intervention offered counseling and education to patients with moderate to severe TBI. A two-group randomized prospective clinical trial was conducted with 171 participants. The control group received contact with the researchers only during the initial assessment and at the one-year follow-up interview whereas the intervention group received seven regular, scheduled telephone calls over the nine month study period. The telephone calls included motivational interviewing techniques, counseling, and education. The results of the study demonstrated better scores on the behavioral index, quality of wellbeing, and emotional state measures in the intervention group as compared to the control group. A separate analysis of the data from the study specifically focused on symptoms of depression (Bombardier et al., 2009). At the one year follow up assessment individuals in the intervention group scored significantly lower on all depression symptom measures than those in the control group. Further, in the subgroup of individuals who scored high on depression severity at baseline, those who received the intervention improved their depression scores at study completion, while the scores of those in the control group worsened.

Authors	Participants	Sample size	Design and Intervention	Outcome measures	Results	AAN level
Bell et al., 2005	Patients with moderate to severe TBI, discharged from an acute rehabilitation unit; age 36 yrs (range 18–70 yrs)	171	2-group double-blind RCT; telephone follow-up versus usual care over 9 month intervention period.	primary outcome composite (FIM, DRS, CIQ, FSE, GOS-E, EuroQol, NFI, PQOL, SF-36, and BSI); funtional status composite (FIM, DRS, CIQ, FSE, GOS-E, and EuroQol.); quality of well being composite (PQOL and SF-36 mental subscore); BSI	▲primary outcome composite: p=0.002, ▲functional status composite: p=0.003, ▲quality of well being composite: p=0.006, ▲EuroQol: p=0.008, ▲GOS-E: p=0.04, ■ FSE: p=n.s. ■ DRS: p=n.s. ▲PQOL: p=0.04, ▲SF-36 mental: p=0.01, ▲BSI: p=0.005	I
Bombardier et al., 2009	See Bell et al., 2005	171	Secondary analysis of data from Bell et al., 2005.	BSI-D, NFI-D, MHI-5	▲BSI-D: p=0.017, ▲NFI-D: p=0.002, ▲MHI-5: p=0.009	I
Bell et al., 2008	Patients with mild TBI, enrolled in the emergency departmen; age 32.5 yrs (SD=13 yrs)	366	2-group double-blind RCT; telephone follow-up versus usual care over 3 month intervention period.	post-traumatic symptom composite (Head Injury Symptom Checklist and 12 functional areas), general health composite (SF-12 Physical, PQOL, PHQ-Depression, PHQ-Anxiety/Panic, PHQ-Anxiety/Other, SF-12 Mental, major role and community integration)	▲post-traumatic symptoms composite: p=0.016, ■ general health composite: p=0.417	I
Wade et al., 2005	Families with children who had moderate to severe TBI; age 9.4 yrs (range 6.7-15.8 yrs); sustained TBI 16 mo prior to enrollment (range 15-29 mo).	6 children, 8 parents, 5 siblings	Pilot case study; Family Problem Solving program (12 sessions - weekly videoconferences with a therapist and self-guided Web exercises)	PSI, FBII, SCL-GSI, CES-D, SCL-90, AI, CES-D, BRIEF GEC, CDI, HCSBS-AB	Parent outcomes: ▲PSI: p<0.05, ▲FBII: p<0.01, ▲SCL-90: p<0.05, ■ AI: p=n.s. ▲CES-D: p < 0.05 Child outcomes: ■ BRIEF-GEC: p=n.s. ■ CDI: p=n.s. ▲HCSBS-AB: p<0.05	IV
Wade et al., 2006	Families with children who had moderate to severe TBI; age 10.8 yrs (SD 3.1 yrs); sustained TBI 13.7 mo prior to enrollment (SD 7.1 mo).	46	2-group RCT; FPS intervention (14 sessions - weekly videoconferences with a therapist and self-guided Web exercises)	SPSI-short version, SCL-90-R, GSI, CES-D, AI	Parent outcomes: ■ SPSI-short: p=n.s. ▲CES-D: p<0.05, ▲AI: p < 0.05, ▲SCL-90-R: p<0.05	II
Wade et al., 2008	Families with adolescents who had moderate to severe TBI; age 15.0 yrs (range 11.7-18.2 yrs); sustained TBI 9.3 mo prior to enrollment (range 2-20 mo).	9 families	2- group single blind RCT (audio and non-audio groups); TOPS intervention (14 sessions - weekly videoconferences with a therapist and self-guided Web exercises)	CBCL, BRIEF GEC, CDI, SCL-90 GSI, CES-D, CBQ, Issues checklist	Teen outcomes: ■ CBCL: p=n.s. ▲CBCL internalizing behavior: p=0.03, ■ BRIEF GEC: p=n.s. ▲ CDI: p=0.02, Parent outcomes: ■ SCL-90 GSI: p=n.s. ▲CES-D: p=0.01 Parent-teen interactions: ▲CBQ: p=0.04, ▲Number of issues: p=0.01	IV

Authors	Participants	Sample size	Design and Intervention	Outcome measures	Results	AAN level
Topolovec-Vranic et al., 2010	Mild to moderate TBI; age 42.5 yrs (range 19.3-72.3 yrs); sustained TBI 2.1 yrs prior to enrollment (range 0.1-7.3 yrs).	21	Pilot case study; MoodGym training program (5 weekly sesssions - Web exercises)	CES-D, PHQ-9	▲CES-D: p<0.05, ▲PHQ-9: p<0.05	IV

Legend: ▲, significant improvement compared to control group/baseline; ■, no significant difference compared to control group/baseline.
Abbreviations: AI, 10-item Anxiety Inventory; BRIEF GEC, Behavior Rating Inventory of Executive Function Global Executive Composite; BRIEF, Behavior Rating Inventory of Executive Function; BSI, Brief Symptom Inventory; BSI-D, Brief Symptom Inventory-Depression subscale; CBCL, Child Behavior Checklist; CBQ, Conflict Behaviour Questionnaire; CDI, Children's Depression Inventory; CES-D, Center for Epidemiologic Studies Depression Scale; CIQ, Community Integration Questionnaire; DRS, Disability Rating Scale; EuroQol, Quality of Life Measure; FAD, Family Assessment Device; FBII, Family Burden of Injury Interview; FIM, Functional Independence Measure; FPS, Family Problem Solving; FSE, Functional Status Examination; GOS-E, Glasgow Outcome Scale–Extended; GSI, Global Severity Index; HCSBS-AB, Home and Community Social Behavior Scale-Antisocial Behavior; MHI-5, Mental Health Index-5; NFI, Neurobehavioral Functioning Inventory; NFI-D, Neurobehavioral Functioning Inventory-Depression subscale; PHQ, Patient Health Questionnaire; PHQ-9, Patient Health Questionnaire for depression; PQOL, Modified Perceived Quality of Life; PSI, Parenting Stress Inventory; SCL-90 GSI, Global Severity Index of the Symptom Checklist-90; SCL-90-R, Symptom Checklist-90-Revised; SCL-GSI, Global Severity Index - Global Psychological Symptoms; SES, The Hauser–Warren Socioeconomic Index; SF-12, Short Form Health Survey-12; SF-36, Medical Outcomes Study 36-Item Short-Form Health Survey; SPSI-short version, Social Problem-Solving Index;

Table 2. Overview of efficacy studies for technology-based approaches and mental health outcomes for the TBI patient population.

In a follow up study, Bell and colleagues examined the effectiveness of scheduled telephone counseling on clinical symptoms and general health, including mental health, in 336 patients with mild TBI (the preceding study population consisted of patients with moderate to severe TBI (Bell et al., 2008)). Participants were recruited within three months of their TBI and the assessments were performed at six months post-injury. As in the preceding study, the researchers implemented a two-group parallel randomized clinical trial, utilizing motivational interviewing techniques in the conduct of the telephone counseling and educational intervention, and contacted the participants at 2 days and 2, 4, 8 and 12 weeks post-discharge from the emergency department where they were recruited. The researchers reported improvements in clinical post-traumatic symptoms but not the composite variable reflecting mental health in the intervention group. The authors commented on this unexpected outcome by highlighting the fact that the intervention specifically targeted symptom management. The secondary mental health outcomes were unaffected by the utilization of the telephone medium.

Bell et al.'s work represents the first large randomized intervention studies that allowed for sound scientific and generalizable results for a TBI population. The initial studies revealed that telephone-based interventions are an effective tool in ameliorating depressive symptoms. These positive outcomes could be attributed to targeted training of the caregivers in the intervention group which enhanced implementation of the recommendations provided as part of the standard of outpatient care. It also provided the matching of the intervention to individual needs in timing and content. The follow-up post-TBI symptom-focused study did not find a positive mental health outcome, but reported improved symptomatology. The differing outcomes highlight the critical role that the focus of the intervention plays, regardless of the medium. The studies also demonstrate that telephone technology is effective in delivering various types of interventions for the TBI population. Further research is required to evaluate optimal timing and frequency of the contacts, as well as cost-efficacy analyses of telephone-based follow-ups of patients post-TBI.

Online Family Problem Solving program. Wade and colleagues developed the *Family Problem Solving* (FPS) online treatment program for families of children with TBI (Wade et al., 2005; Wade et al., 2006). The original program, which was designed to be used by members of the family together, was comprised of a homepage with links to announcements, contact information, resources and the session materials. The program offered twelve sessions including eight "core" sessions teaching skills related to problem-solving, communication, and TBI specific behaviour management, and four sessions addressing stressors and burdens including stress management, working with the school, sibling concerns, and marital communication. The interactive sessions were completed by the families in advance of a videoconference with a trained therapist who reviewed the completed exercises and implemented a problem-solving process to address a problem or goal identified by the family. Validated quantitative pre- and post-outcome measures were completed aimed at assessing parental stress and burden, distress, depression, anxiety, as well as child behaviours and depression.

In the pilot evaluation study, a convenience sample of six families was recruited to assess the efficacy of the intervention (Wade et al., 2005). All families successfully completed the program with 10.3 (range 7-12) and 10.1 (range 7-14) web sessions and videoconferences completed, respectively. Even with the small sample size significant improvements were observed from pre- to post-intervention on parental adjustment (injury related stress and burden, parenting stress, depression, global psychological symptoms) and child adjustment (antisocial behaviour). There were no significant differences in self-reported depressive symptoms of the injured child. The authors identified the small sample size, lack of a control group, and potential bias by social desirability factors (participants were given the computer to keep after study completion) as limitations in their study. Nevertheless, the findings suggested that a computer-based intervention might successfully be used to improve both parent and child outcomes following TBI in children. This study contributed to the early work in this area by expanding the spectrum of technological solutions explored for treating mental health in the TBI population to include online interventions.

To address some of the limitations of their pilot study Wade and colleagues conducted a larger randomized clinical trial to evaluate the efficacy of the FPS intervention on parental anxiety, depression, and psychological outcomes, following pediatric TBI (Wade et al., 2006). Eligible families (child 5-16 years of age who had sustained a moderate-to-severe TBI between 1 and 24 months previously) were randomly assigned to the FPS group (n=26) or an Internet resources comparison (IRC) group (n=20). In addition to usual psychosocial care, all participating families received a computer (which they were allowed to keep at the end of the study), printer, high-speed Internet access, and a home page with links to brain injury web sites. Families in the FPS group also received a web camera for the duration of the study. Two additional supplemental sessions were added to the FPS website from the pilot study: anger management and pain management.

Baseline demographic and injury characteristics did not differ between the two groups. Attrition was 12% in the FPS group versus 0% in the IRC group (not significant). After controlling for baseline symptom levels, parents in the FPS group reported significantly less depression, anxiety, and general psychiatric symptoms as compared to those in the IRC group. The study, the first randomized controlled trial to combine a web-based intervention and synchronous videoconferencing with a trained therapist, also demonstrated that neither demographic nor injury characteristics moderated the treatment response. This suggested that even parents of lower socioeconomic status, or families with children of any age, injury severity, or time since injury could benefit from an online skill-building intervention. The main limitations of the study were a relatively small sample size that was skewed towards less severe injuries, the reliance on self-report measures, and the lack of an extended follow-up period. Moreover, based on the study design it was not possible to disentangle whether the treatment effect was a result of the problem solving intervention, or having access to a trained therapist, or both. An additional study with an attention control would be required to address this limitation.

Teen Online Problem Solving intervention. Wade and colleagues subsequently expanded their program to create modules aimed at adolescents (Wade et al., 2008). The Teen Online Problem Solving Intervention (TOPS intervention) emphasized the development and/or remediation of primary executive function skills (e.g. self-awareness, self-regulation, planning, and problem solving) and training in language pragmatics and social information processing to improve social competencies. The TOPS intervention was comprised of ten core sessions and six supplemental sessions including the four sessions from the original program plus "planning for high school" and "talking with your adolescent". Participants were randomized to audio or no-audio versions of the online components.

Children 11 to 18 years of age who had sustained a moderate-to-severe TBI in the previous 24 months were eligible to participate. Nine out of 17 eligible families (53%) agreed to participate. All nine families completed the ten core sessions with six completing one or more supplemental session. Significant improvements were reported on child internalizing symptoms and self-reported depression as well as parental depression. Moreover, significant reductions in parent-adolescent conflicts, number of problem issues, and severity of the family's problems were observed. There were no differences in outcomes between the audio versus non-audio groups.

The authors proposed that the cognitive reframing and problem solving skills developed through the TOPS intervention enabled parents and adolescents to resolve issues that otherwise could have contributed to anxiety and depression. They also discussed several benefits of technology-based approaches to treatment: information can be provided in a variety of modalities and may be more cost-effective than traditional approaches. Similar limitations were cited to those of their previous work, including a small sample size, lack of control group, reliance on self-report measures, and inability to disentangle the most effective component of the intervention. In addition, the need for longer-term follow up to ascertain maintenance of gains, was noted.

Online cognitive behaviour training program - MoodGym. Topolovec-Vranic et al. recruited 21 patients with mild or moderate TBI to evaluate the acceptability and efficacy of the Internet-based MoodGym training program (http://moodgym.anu.edu.au; Topolovec-Vranic et al., 2010). The MoodGym program was developed at the Australian National University to treat and prevent depression in a community-based population, primarily youth. The program consists of five cognitive behaviour training modules, a personal workbook, an interactive game, and a feedback evaluation form. Of the 21 patients who consented to participate in the study, 16 completed at least one module and 13 completed all of the modules. Using an intention-to-treat analysis, scores on the Center for Epidemiological Studies-Depression Scale (CES-D) were shown to decrease by 1.03 points for each module of the workshop completed. Significant decreases from baseline on both the CES-D and the Patient Health Questionnaire-9 (PHQ-9) were found at the 12-month follow-up assessment.

Although preliminary efficacy of the MoodGym training program was demonstrated for patients with TBI and symptoms of depression, this study was limited by its small sample size, lack of control group, and low completion rates for the intervention. While many participants commented that the program was enjoyable and that they would recommend it to others, some participants identified challenges such as concentration and memory challenges, and understanding some of the content on the website. A customized program addressing the cognitive deficits experienced by some patients with TBI may be more appropriate for this population.

3.3 Concluding remarks on the literature review

The scoping literature review of technology-based treatment programs for patients with TBI and/or their caregivers revealed limited scientific data to date. Only four treatment programs were identified that were evaluated with a TBI population (see Table 3). These four programs were presented in five feasibility studies, and seven evaluation studies which utilized a mental health outcome measure. Six of the seven efficacy studies demonstrated significant improvements in at least one of these measures for the patient or their caregiver. Depression was the primary mental health related outcome assessed.

Technology	Description	Audience	Study Authors
Telephone intervention	Teletherapy through motivational interviewing, counselling and education.	Individuals with TBI	Bell et al. 2005, 2008; Bombardier et al. 2009
Family Problem Solving (FPS) online treatment program	Website designed for families of children who had TBI. Several different modules on the website aim at helping families cope with a child who is recovering from a TBI.	Families with a child who sustained a TBI	Wade et al. 2005, 2006
Teen Online Problem Solving (TOPS) Intervention	Website designed for familes with an adolescent who sustained a TBI. Similar to FPS but geared towards issues pertinent to teenagers.	Families with an adolescent who sustained a TBI	Wade et al. 2008, 2009
MoodGym training program	Website designed to help treat depression in the youth population, using cognitive behavioural training modules, interactive games and a feedback evaluation form.	Individuals with TBI	Topolovec-Vranic et al. 2010

Table 3. Overview of technologies evaluated for the treatment of mental health conditions for TBI patients and caregivers.

Given the limited work in this area there is a need for further studies to establish the types of technologies and treatments that are effective for this population. Much of the work reported is characterized by small sample sizes, feasibility studies, unclear differentiation of the effect of the treatment medium versus the actual therapeutic technique utilized, and lack of ethnic or geographic diversity. There is little information to identify which patients with TBI are most likely to adopt and adhere to various technology-based treatment approaches. No cost-efficacy data are available and few studies describe the practical limitations of using such approaches (e.g. stress placed on families as a result of technical difficulties or lost Internet connectivity; lack of personal contact; constant upgrading and maintenance of the technologies and equipment).

Even with these potential barriers, the recent widespread adoption of various computers and handheld devices in everyday life activities presents an opportunity to examine how these technologies can best facilitate various types of mental health treatments customized for the TBI population. While the studies reviewed in this section identified some promising programs delivered by telephone or internet, there are great opportunities for leveraging up and coming technologies such as handheld devices and virtual reality. In an effort to motivate a systematic approach to the study of different types of technologies, the next section of this chapter will present the results of a survey that investigated patients' attitudes towards and willingness to use various technologies as part of their mental health treatment post-TBI.

4. Survey: attitudes towards technology-based approaches to mental health care in a traumatic brain injury population

The literature review described in the preceding section of this chapter has identified several technology-based treatment programs which have been evaluated for patients with TBI. While the technological provision of mental health services may be well suited for these patients, no studies have specifically addressed this question. The purpose of the following study was to examine, using a survey-based approach, the knowledge and attitudes of patients with mild or moderate TBI towards using technology to access mental health care. A better understanding of patients' experience with the use of technologies and their attitudes towards using such technologies for treatment may aid in the development of more tailored and useful interventions in the future.

4.1 Methods used for the survey

A convenience sample of all patients attending an out-patient Head Injury Clinic in Toronto, Canada, specializing in mild to moderate TBI, were recruited to participate in the study. Patients were invited by a research assistant to complete the "Technology Access and Knowledge Survey", adapted from a previous survey (Wilson et al., 2008) while they waited to be seen by the Clinic physicians. The adapted survey captured:

- basic demographic information about the patient (age, gender, education level, marital status, current employment status);
- information related to the injury (time since injury, mechanism of injury, any intracranial computed tomography diagnoses);
- data regarding the respondent's use of computers and the Internet, their knowledge and comfort with various technologies (e.g. chat room, online banking, personal

electronic device, virtual reality, mp3 player), and their comfort with using a computer or computer program to receive personal mental health information/treatment.

Study participants also completed the PHQ-9, a nine-item depression module taken from the PHQ (a screening tool for mental health diagnoses used in the primary care setting). The PHQ-9 has been demonstrated in the primary care setting to be sensitive to both diagnosis of depression according to the DSM-IV criteria and to measurement in depressive symptom severity (Nease, Jr. & Maloin, 2003). It has also been demonstrated to be sensitive in screening for depression in TBI patients (Fann et al., 2005). Scores from the PHQ-9 range from 0-27 with a sum score of 12 or above being the best screening criterion for major depression in this population (Fann et al., 2005).

Some participants did not complete all of the questions on the survey. The number of participants completing each question is indicated in the tables. This study was reviewed by the Research Ethics Board of the participating institution and informed consent was obtained from all participants.

4.2 Results of the survey

4.2.1 Description of the study sample

Study participants. A total of 422 of 520 patients who were approached (81% response rate) consented to participate in the study between May 2010 and June 2011. The average age of participants was 42 years (range 17-86 years) and 59% were male. The majority of the participants had completed some college, were never married or married/common-law, and were employed full-time. Detailed demographic characteristics of the study participants are provided in Table 4.

Characteristic	Responses
Gender (N=378)	
Male	223 (59%)
Education Completed (N=390)	
Grade School	66 (17%)
High School	79 (20%)
Some College/Trade School	125 (32%)
Undergraduate Degree	83 (21%)
Postgraduate Degree	36 (9%)
Marital Status (N=384)	
Never Married	158 (41%)
Married/Common Law	158 (41%)
Separated/Divorced	58 (15%)
Widowed	12 (3%)
Employment Status (N=398)	
Student	40 (10%)
Unemployed	82 (21%)
Employed	131 (33%)
Retired	36 (9%)
Other	107 (27%)

Table 4. Demographic characteristics of study participants.

Injury characteristics. The average time since injury for the patient sample was 17 months (range 0-166 months). The main mechanism for the injury was a motor vehicle collision. Most participants reported a loss of consciousness following the injury and having had a computed tomography (CT) scan completed with one third reporting that abnormalities were observed on the scan. Detailed injury characteristics of the study participants are provided in Table 5.

Characteristic	Responses
Mechanism of Injury (N=406)	
Motor Vehicle Collision	204 (50%)
Bicycle	17 (4%)
Violence	23 (6%)
Fall or hit by object	101 (25%)
Pedestrian	26 (6%)
Suicide attempt	1 (0.2%)
Work-related	19 (5%)
Sports	15 (4%)
Loss of consciousness (N=375)	
None reported	53 (14%)
Less than 30 minutes	160 (43%)
More than 30 minutes	83 (22%)
Unknown	79 (21%)
CT Scan Results (N=371)	
Positive	130 (35%)
Negative	120 (32%)
Not done	32 (9%)
Unknown	89 (24%)

Table 5. Injury characteristics of study participants.

Mental health status. The average PHQ-9 depression score for all respondents was 11.4 (median = 12). A score of 12 or above is considered an indication for major depression in this population. In our sample, half of the respondents scored at 12 or above (51%) indicating major depression. Forty two percent of respondents indicated that they were receiving treatment for a mental health condition at the time of survey completion.

4.2.2 Experience with computers

Access to computers and the Internet. Only 8% of the survey respondents did not have a computer at home. Eighty one percent indicated that they accessed the Internet at least one time per day. While at home, most individuals reported spending significant time on the computer and Internet: more than 4 hours per day (13% on the computer and 11% on the Internet), 1-4hours per day (36% and 35%), or less than 1 hour per day (32% and 35%). In addition to using a computer at home, over half of the respondents also had access to a computer (62%) and/or the Internet (58%) at work.

Specific experiences with using the Internet. More than half of respondents had *extensive experience* (*i.e.* "have done it many times") using the Internet for email (77%), online banking (52%), and downloading files (60%). However, less than half of participants (42%) had similar experience using handheld devices for various purposes – *extensive experience* with handhelds for accessing the Internet was reported by 43% of respondents, for downloading files by 33%, and for watching videos by 33%. Based on their experience with using the Internet in general, the majority of respondents (61%) felt that even with precautions (*e.g.* encryption, password protection, etc.) their information online was not private.

4.2.3 Attitudes towards web-based approaches to mental health

Despite their belief that information online is not completely private even with precautions, most respondents (63%) reported that they would be willing to enter personal mental health information online (e.g. age, gender, medical history, completing questionnaires).

Attitudes towards using a computer for mental health programs. An overwhelming proportion of the respondents (82%) endorsed that they would use a *computer/computer program* as an aid to their mental health care if it were available. When broken down into various components, approximately half of the survey respondents felt very comfortable using the computer for various mental-health related purposes: to access specific mental health information (48%), to complete exercises as an aid to their regular mental health treatment (55%), to receive personal feedback on exercises (50%), and to receive personal feedback from a counselor (52%). A significant proportion of respondents also indicated that they felt comfortable using a computer to complete exercises as their *main* form of mental health treatment (39%).

Attitudes towards using a handheld device for mental health programs. Although not as high as for computer-based programs, a significant proportion of respondents (65%) reported that they would be willing to use their handheld device as an aide to mental health care if it were available. Specifically, 36% indicated they would use their handheld device to access specific mental health information, 35% to complete exercises as an aid to their regular mental health treatment, 37% to receive personal feedback on exercises, and 39% to receive personal feedback from a counselor. In addition, 27% of the respondents felt comfortable using a handheld to complete exercises as their *main* form of mental health treatment.

Types of online mental-health related activities of interest. Participants were asked to indicate their preferred mode of communication with a counselor. The largest proportion (85%) indicated *in person* as a preferred option, followed by *over the phone* (52%), via *email* (40%), via *teleconference* (31%), and via *chat* (30%). A considerable portion of the patients in this survey also indicated that they would be willing to access mental health information online (56%), they would install a treatment program on their home computer (51%), and they would log into a secure Internet treatment program (46%). A smaller segment of the sample reported that they would use a virtual reality treatment program (40%) or that they would be willing to respond to anonymous mental health questions on the Internet (39%).

4.3 Concluding remarks on the survey findings

This survey of 422 patients with mild to moderate TBI revealed that half of the individuals (51%) in this sample met the screening criteria for major depression (PHQ-9 greater than or equal to 12) and 42% were currently receiving treatment for a mental health condition. A large proportion of the respondents (82%) indicated that they were interested in receiving further mental health treatment with the help of technological solutions. This result implies that there is a need in this patient population for additional mental health care that could be made accessible through the use of various technologies.

The majority of the patients surveyed owned a computer and had Internet access at their home (92%), while some also used a computer and the Internet at their workplace (62% and 58% respectively). Most of the respondents reported significant experience with the use of a computer and the Internet for various purposes, such as email (77%), banking (52%), downloading files (60%). A relatively smaller proportion reported extensive experience with the use of handheld devices for accessing the Internet (43%), downloading files (33%) or watching videos (33%). Overall, approximately 80% reported having extensive experience using a computer, while only 42% reported such experience using handheld devices. However, given the rapid changes in the field and that more and more individuals are acquiring handheld devices such as smart-phones, we anticipate that this proportion will significantly increase over time.

Even if they indicated a willingness to use a computer or a handheld device, patients seemed reluctant to use technology-based treatments as their main or only treatment. They were, however, very interested in utilizing technology-based interventions as an aid to traditional mental health treatment. While patients indicated that their preferred way of speaking to a counselor was in person, many were also willing to utilize the telephone, email, chat, computer and the Internet to connect to a counselor. They were also open to installing treatment programs on their home computer or using secure website treatment programs.

The findings of this survey highlight the importance of patient preferences in selecting a treatment for post-TBI depression. While previous research has reported the significance of TBI patient preferences for treatment modalities such as physical exercise, counseling, antidepressants, and others (Fann et al., 2009), the present study clarifies the extent of patients' willingness to utilize a variety of different technological solutions in their mental health treatment, reveals patient preferences to that effect as well as barriers to adoption that need to be considered. The survey did not ask patients to indicate their relative acceptance of technology-based approaches to mental health treatment as compared to pharmacological or alternative treatment options. This would be an interesting and important question for the future. Moreover, the survey did not discern whether respondents were being treated for a pre- or post-injury mental health condition. Pre-injury psychiatric disorder has been shown as a predictor of post-injury disorders (Gould et al., 2011) and these individuals may have different needs and preferences from patients with new-onset mental illness post-injury.

The results of the present survey are aligned with previous reports from the broader acquired brain injury literature: patients expressed strong interest in using telerehabilitative services to assist with problems in memory, attention, problem-solving, and others (Ricker et al., 2002). These studies collectively demonstrate that there is a need and demand for future work in this area.

5. Discussion

This chapter reviewed the current state of science regarding technology-based approaches for mental health care for people who have experienced a TBI. The literature review revealed that work in this area is at initial stages. Many of the reports fall within the scope of feasibility and pilot studies and do not offer scientific validation of the effectiveness of using technology with respect to mental health outcomes (only three papers received an AAN level I rating and two of these papers were based on the same study) . The scoping review identified a total of seven studies that utilized a scientific approach towards the evaluation of efficacy. These studies, however, presented unclear differentiation of the effect of the treatment medium versus the actual therapeutic technique utilized. In addition, three of the studies were characterized by small sample sizes (N<25 participants). Thus, there is a need for future work to further corroborate the existing evidence on the utility of technology-based approaches for the treatment of mental health conditions in the TBI population. Future comparative studies are needed to address some of the gaps related to technology implementation: which technologies are most effective; what is the optimal coupling between a particular type of mental health treatment (*e.g.* cognitive behaviour therapy) and a particular type of technology (*e.g.* teletherapy); what are the costs associated with the development and delivery of such resources; and what are the potential barriers to adoption by this particular population (social, physical, economical, etc.).

The technology access and attitudes survey highlighted that patients with TBI are a receptive audience for the implementation of technological solutions to help their mental health care with 82% of the participants expressing a willingness to do so. It is important to note that the sample studied was predominantly patients with mild, and some moderate TBI. The results from this sample are not necessarily translatable to a population of patients with severe TBI who have greater cognitive deficits. Moreover, the patients sampled in the study were those presenting to an out-patient Head Injury Clinic with persisting post-concussive symptoms (on average 17 months post-injury). This could represent a group that is highly invested in alternative treatment options, and more willing to utilize such approaches than individuals in the acute and sub-acute stages post-injury. On the other hand, the participants in this study may be less interested in using technology-based approaches as they have persisting medical concerns to deal with, and may be skeptical of new treatment options after years of trying to manage their symptoms. Additionally, all participants were recruited from a single centre and may not accurately represent the general TBI population.

The survey identified several specific issues to be considered in the design of technology-based solutions for mental health care for the patient with TBI:

- Since only 63% of patients stated that they would enter personal health information online, having a guest/anonymous option on websites would allow for a wider reach within this population. Websites should clearly describe the safety and protection of the users' privacy and the limitations to such.
- Most respondents indicated a preference for access to a counselor and would primarily be willing to use technology-based approaches as an adjunct to traditional therapy. However, a solid proportion of patients also indicated that they would use such resources as their main form of mental health treatment (39% would use a computer and 27% would use a handheld). Understanding the patient's preferences and providing access to face-to-face resources if needed is critical especially given the preliminary and relatively scarce data available to support the efficacy of stand-alone technology-based programs. There is an inherent risk in relying upon technology-mediated interventions in that patients may feel that self-management alone is sufficient when they need specialized treatment.
- The safety considerations for those who are severely depressed or suicidal must be recognized as there is a lack of monitoring of the individual when they access online resources, while a healthcare provider would be able to identify risk factors and intervene if necessary.

- Patients' responses also indicated a preference towards using computers compared to handheld devices for their online mental health treatment. While the survey did not directly identify the underlying reason for this preference, it is likely that lack of exposure to or experience with handheld devices is a barrier to adoption potential - the survey found a considerable difference in experience with using computers (80%) versus handheld devices (42%). We anticipate with the rapid uptake of handheld devices in the consumer market, the latter number will steadily rise in the coming years. Thus researchers and developers should strongly consider designing treatment programs that will be accessible on such devices.
- The results from some of the studies reviewed suggest that programs should be tailored for this patient population to take into consideration the cognitive, somatic, and affective deficits they may be experiencing (e.g. poor memory, difficulty with concentration, vision disturbances, apathy). Modularizing exercises into smaller components is one way to address this problem. Further, in addition to video, audio components may allow for better assimilation and internalization of intervention materials by helping to alleviate problems with concentration (Wade et al., 2006).

6. Conclusion

The recent widespread adoption of various computers and handheld devices in everyday life activities presents an opportunity to examine how these technologies can best facilitate various types of mental health treatments for individual with TBI. The results of the survey presented in this chapter indicate that patients are willing and enthusiastic about using such approaches to aid in their mental health care. While there is limited research to date in this field, the innovative studies available suggest that technology-based approaches are feasible, acceptable, and effective in improving mental health outcomes of patients with TBI and their caregivers. In this chapter we have also aimed to identify some points of consideration during the development of technology-based treatment programs for patients with TBI. Overall, the potential benefits of technological approaches to mental health care in this patient population are numerous and deserve further research attention and efforts.

7. Acknowledgments

The authors would like to thank all of the survey respondents for their participation in the study. We also wish to acknowledge the support of the St. Michael's Hospital Head Injury Clinic Team (Cheryl Masanic, MD, Kiloran Distin, MD, Alicja Michalak, MSN) and particularly Patricia Johnson, PhD, Mary Ann Pollmann-Mudryj, PhD, Naomi Ennis, BA(c), Michael Taylor, BA for their assistance with data collection, entry and results interpretation. We would also like to express our gratitude to Patricia Johnson, PhD for her insightful comments in reviewing this chapter.

8. References

Andersson, G., Carlbring, P., Holmstrom, A., Sparthan, E., Furmark, T., Nilsson-Ihrfelt, E. et al. (2006). Internet-based self-help with therapist feedback and in vivo group exposure for social phobia: a randomized controlled trial. *J.Consult Clin.Psychol., 74,* 677-686.

Andersson, G. & Kaldo, V. (2004). Internet-based cognitive behavioral therapy for tinnitus. *J.Clin.Psychol., 60,* 171-178.

Andersson, G., Lundstrom, P., & Strom, L. (2003). Internet-based treatment of headache: does telephone contact add anything? *Headache, 43,* 353-361.

Andrews, G. A. & Henderson, A. S. (1999). *Unmet Need in Psychiatry : Problems, resources, responses.* Cambridge: Cambridge University Press.

Ashman, T. A., Spielman, L. A., Hibbard, M. R., Silver, J. M., Chandna, T., & Gordon, W. A. (2004). Psychiatric challenges in the first 6 years after traumatic brain injury: cross-sequential analyses of Axis I disorders. *Arch.Phys.Med.Rehabil, 85,* S36-S42.

Bebbington, P. E., Brugha, T. S., Meltzer, H., Jenkins, R., Ceresa, C., Farrell, M. et al. (2000). Neurotic disorders and the receipt of psychiatric treatment. *Psychol.Med., 30,* 1369-1376.

Bell, K. R., Hoffman, J. M., Temkin, N. R., Powell, J. M., Fraser, R. T., Esselman, P. C. et al. (2008). The Effect of Telephone Counseling on Reducing Post-Traumatic Symptoms after Mild Traumatic Brain Injury: A Randomized Trial. *Journal of Neurology, Neurosurgery, and Psychiatry, 79,* 1275-1281.

Bell, K. R., Temkin, N. R., Esselman, P. C., Doctor, J. N., Bombardier, C. H., Fraser, R. T. et al. (2005). The Effect of a Scheduled Telephone Intervention on Outcome After Moderate to Severe Traumatic Brain Injury: A Randomized Trial. *Archives of Physical Medicine and Rehabilitation, 86,* 851-856.

Ben-Menachem, E. (2005). AAN/AES Guidelines on Use of New AEDS. *Epilepsy Currents, 5,* 30-32.

Berger, M., Wagner, T. H., & Baker, L. C. (2005). Internet use and stigmatized illness. *Soc.Sci.Med., 61,* 1821-1827.

Bergquist, T., Gehl, C., Lepore, S., Holzworth, N., & Beaulieu, W. (2008). Internet-based cognitive rehabilitation in individuals with acquired brain injury: A pilot feasibility study. *Brain Injury, 22,* 891-897.

Billings, D. W., Cook, R. F., Hendrickson, A., & Dove, D. C. (2008). A web-based approach to managing stress and mood disorders in the workforce. *J.Occup.Environ.Med., 50,* 960-968.

Bombardier, C. H., Bell, K. R., Temkin, N. R., Fann, J. R., Hoffman, J., & Dikmen, S. (2009). The efficacy of a scheduled telephone intervention for ameliorating depressive symptoms during the first year after traumatic brain injury. *J.Head Trauma Rehabil., 24,* 230-238.

Bombardier, C. H., Fann, J. R., Temkin, N. R., Esselman, P. C., Barber, J., & Dikmen, S. S. (2010). Rates of major depressive disorder and clinical outcomes following traumatic brain injury. *JAMA., %19;303,* 1938-1945.

Bourdon, K. H., Rae, D. S., Locke, B. Z., Narrow, W. E., & Regier, D. A. (1992). Estimating the prevalence of mental disorders in U.S. adults from the Epidemiologic Catchment Area Survey. *Public Health Rep., 107,* 663-668.

Carlbring, P., Ekselius, L., & Andersson, G. (2003). Treatment of panic disorder via the Internet: a randomized trial of CBT vs. applied relaxation. *J.Behav.Ther.Exp.Psychiatry, 34,* 129-140.

Christensen, B., Ross, T., Kotasek, R., Rosenthal, M., & Henry, R. (1994). The role of depression in rehabilitation outcomes in the acute recovery of patients with TBI. *Adv.Med.Psychother., 7,* 23-38.

Christensen, H. & Griffiths, K. M. (2002). The prevention of depression using the Internet. *Med.J.Aust., 177 Suppl:S122-5.,* S122-S125.

Christensen, H., Griffiths, K. M., & Jorm, A. F. (2004). Delivering interventions for depression by using the internet: randomised controlled trial. *BMJ, 328,* 265.

Clarke, G., Eubanks, D., Reid, E., Kelleher, C., O'Connor, E., DeBar, L. L. et al. (2005). Overcoming Depression on the Internet (ODIN) (2): a randomized trial of a self-help depression skills program with reminders. *J.Med.Internet.Res., 7,* e16.

Clarke, G., Reid, E., Eubanks, D., O'Connor, E., DeBar, L. L., Kelleher, C. et al. (2002). Overcoming depression on the Internet (ODIN): a randomized controlled trial of an Internet depression skills intervention program. *J.Med.Internet.Res., 4,* E14.

Dikmen, S. S., Bombardier, C. H., Machamer, J. E., Fann, J. R., & Temkin, N. R. (2004). Natural history of depression in traumatic brain injury. *Arch.Phys.Med.Rehabil., 85,* 1457-1464.

Fann, J. R., Bombardier, C. H., Dikmen, S., Esselman, P., Warms, C. A., Pelzer, E. et al. (2005). Validity of the Patient Health Questionnaire-9 in assessing depression following traumatic brain injury. *J.Head Trauma Rehabil., 20,* 501-511.

Fann, J. R., Jones, A. L., Dikmen, S. S., Temkin, N. R., Esselman, P. C., & Bombardier, C. H. (2009). Depression treatment preferences after traumatic brain injury. *J.Head Trauma Rehabil., 24,* 272-278.

Fedoroff, J. P., Starkstein, S. E., Forrester, A. W., Geisler, F. H., Jorge, R. E., Arndt, S. V. et al. (1992). Depression in patients with acute traumatic brain injury. *Am.J.Psychiatry, 149,* 918-923.

Feil, E. G., Noell, J., Lichtenstein, E., Boles, S. M., & McKay, H. G. (2003). Evaluation of an Internet-based smoking cessation program: lessons learned from a pilot study. *Nicotine.Tob.Res., 5,* 189-194.

Garcia, V., Ahumada, L., Hinkelman, J., Munoz, R. F., & Quezada, J. (2004). Psychology over the Internet: On-Line Experiences. *Cyberpsychol.Behav., 7,* 29-33.

Gega, L., Marks, I., & Mataix-Cols, D. (2004). Computer-aided CBT self-help for anxiety and depressive disorders: experience of a London clinic and future directions. *J.Clin.Psychol., 60,* 147-157.

Glang, A., McLaughlin, K., & Schroeder, S. (2007). Using interactive multimedia to teach parent advocacy skills: an exploratory study. *J.Head Trauma Rehabil., 22,* 198-205.

Gould, K. R., Ponsford, J. L., Johnston, L., & Schonberger, M. (2011). Predictive and Associated Factors of Psychiatric Disorders after Traumatic Brain Injury: A Prospective Study. *J.Neurotrauma..*

Griffiths, K. M., Calear, A. L., Banfield, M., & Tam, A. (2009). Systematic review on Internet Support Groups (ISGs) and depression (2): What is known about depression ISGs? *J.Med.Internet.Res., 11,* e41.

Griffiths, K. M., Farrer, L., & Christensen, H. (2010). The efficacy of internet interventions for depression and anxiety disorders: a review of randomised controlled trials. *Med.J.Aust., 192,* S4-11.

Groom, K. N., Shaw, T. G., O'Connor, M. E., Howard, N. I., & Pickens, A. (1998). Neurobehavioral symptoms and family functioning in traumatically brain-injured adults. *Arch.Clin.Neuropsychol., 13,* 695-711.

Harris, J. K., Godfrey, H. P., Partridge, F. M., & Knight, R. G. (2001). Caregiver depression following traumatic brain injury (TBI): a consequence of adverse effects on family members? *Brain Inj., 15,* 223-238.

Hesdorffer, D. C., Rauch, S. L., & Tamminga, C. A. (2009). Long-term psychiatric outcomes following traumatic brain injury: a review of the literature. *J.Head Trauma Rehabil., 24,* 452-459.

Holsinger, T., Steffens, D. C., Phillips, C., Helms, M. J., Havlik, R. J., Breitner, J. C. et al. (2002). Head injury in early adulthood and the lifetime risk of depression. *Arch.Gen.Psychiatry, 59,* 17-22.

Ipser, J. C., Dewing, S., & Stein, D. J. (2007). A systematic review of the quality of information on the treatment of anxiety disorders on the internet. *Curr.Psychiatry Rep., 9,* 303-309.

Jorge, R. E., Robinson, R. G., Arndt, S. V., Starkstein, S. E., Forrester, A. W., & Geisler, F. (1993). Depression following traumatic brain injury: a 1 year longitudinal study. *J.Affect.Disord., 27,* 233-243.

Kaltenthaler, E., Shackley, P., Stevens, K., Beverley, C., Parry, G., & Chilcott, J. (2002). A systematic review and economic evaluation of computerised cognitive behaviour therapy for depression and anxiety. *Health Technol.Assess., 6,* 1-89.

Kessler, R. C., Berglund, P. A., Bruce, M. L., Koch, J. R., Laska, E. M., Leaf, P. J. et al. (2001). The prevalence and correlates of untreated serious mental illness. *Health Serv.Res., 36,* 987-1007.

Knaevelsrud, C. & Maercker, A. (2007). Internet-based treatment for PTSD reduces distress and facilitates the development of a strong therapeutic alliance: a randomized controlled clinical trial. *BMC.Psychiatry., %19;7:13.,* 13.

Knaevelsrud, C. & Maercker, A. (2009). Long-Term Effects of an Internet-Based Treatment for Posttraumatic Stress. *Cogn Behav.Ther., 12.*

Langlois J.A., Rutland-Brown W., & Thomas K.E. (2006). Traumatic Brain Injury in the United States: Emergency Department Visits, Hospitalizations, and Deaths. *Atlanta, GA: Centers for Disease Control.*

Leach L.R., Frank R.G., Bouman D.E., & Farmer J. (1994). Family functioning, social support, and depression after traumatic brain injury. *Brain Injury, 8,* 599-606.

Linke, S., Brown, A., & Wallace, P. (2004). Down your drink: a web-based intervention for people with excessive alcohol consumption. *Alcohol Alcohol, 39,* 29-32.

Martin, E. M., French, L., & Janos, A. (2010). Home/community monitoring using telephonic follow-up. *NeuroRehabilitation., 26,* 279-283.

McAllister, T. W. & Arciniegas, D. (2002). Evaluation and treatment of postconcussive symptoms. *NeuroRehabilitation., 17,* 265-283.

Meyer, B., Berger, T., Caspar, F., Beevers, C. G., Andersson, G., & Weiss, M. (2009). Effectiveness of a novel integrative online treatment for depression (Deprexis): randomized controlled trial. *J.Med.Internet.Res., 11,* e15.

Mooney, G. & Speed, J. (2001). The association between mild traumatic brain injury and psychiatric conditions. *Brain Inj., 15,* 865-877.

Mooney, G., Speed, J., & Sheppard, S. (2005). Factors related to recovery after mild traumatic brain injury. *Brain Inj., 19,* 975-987.

Nease, D. E., Jr. & Maloin, J. M. (2003). Depression screening: a practical strategy. *J.Fam.Pract., 52,* 118-124.

Patten, S. B. (2003). Prevention of depressive symptoms through the use of distance technologies. *Psychiatr.Serv., 54,* 396-398.

Perini, S., Titov, N., & Andrews, G. (2009). Clinician-assisted Internet-based treatment is effective for depression: randomized controlled trial. *Aust.N.Z.J.Psychiatry., 43,* 571-578.

Proudfoot, J., Goldberg, D., Mann, A., Everitt, B., Marks, I., & Gray, J. A. (2003). Computerized, interactive, multimedia cognitive-behavioural program for anxiety and depression in general practice. *Psychol.Med., 33,* 217-227.

Ricker, J. H., Rosenthal, M., Garay, E., DeLuca, J., Germain, A., Abraham-Fuchs, K. et al. (2002). Telerehabilitation Needs: A Survey of Persons with Acquired Brain Injury. *The Journal of Head Trauma Rehabilitation, 17.*

Ritterband, L. M., Thorndike, F. P., Gonder-Frederick, L. A., Magee, J. C., Bailey, E. T., Saylor, D. K. et al. (2009). Efficacy of an Internet-based behavioral intervention for adults with insomnia. *Arch.Gen.Psychiatry., 66,* 692-698.

Rotondi, A. J., Sinkule, J., & Spring, M. (2005). An interactive Web-based intervention for persons with TBI and their families: use and evaluation by female significant others. *J.Head Trauma Rehabil., 20,* 173-185.

Rutherford, W. H. (1977). Sequelae of concussion caused by minor head injuries. *Lancet., 1,* 1-4.

Schoenhuber, R. & Gentilini, M. (1988). Anxiety and depression after mild head injury: a case control study. *J.Neurol.Neurosurg.Psychiatry., 51,* 722-724.

Spek, V., Nyklicek, I., Smits, N., Cuijpers, P., Riper, H., Keyzer, J. et al. (2007). Internet-based cognitive behavioural therapy for subthreshold depression in people over 50 years old: a randomized controlled clinical trial. *Psychol.Med., 37,* 1797-1806.

Strom, L., Pettersson, R., & Andersson, G. (2004). Internet-based treatment for insomnia: a controlled evaluation. *J.Consult Clin.Psychol., 72,* 113-120.

Szumilas, M. & Kutcher, S. (2009). Teen suicide information on the internet: a systematic analysis of quality. *Can.J.Psychiatry., 54,* 596-604.

Topolovec-Vranic, J., Cullen, N., Michalak, A., Ouchterlony, D., Bhalerao, S., Masanic, C. et al. (2010). Evaluation of an online cognitive behavioural therapy program by patients with traumatic brain injury and depression. *Brain Injury, 24,* 762-772.

van Straten, A., Cuijpers, P., & Smits, N. (2008). Effectiveness of a web-based self-help intervention for symptoms of depression, anxiety, and stress: randomized controlled trial. *J.Med.Internet.Res., 10,* e7.

Wade, S. L., Carey, J., & Wolfe, C. R. (2006). An online family intervention to reduce parental distress following pediatric brain injury. *J.Consult Clin.Psychol., 74,* 445-454.

Wade, S. L., Walz, N. C., Carey, J. C., & Williams, K. M. (2008). Preliminary efficacy of a Web-based family problem-solving treatment program for adolescents with traumatic brain injury. *J.Head Trauma Rehabil., 23,* 369-377.

Wade, S. L., Walz, N. C., Carey, J. C., & Williams, K. M. (2009). Brief report: Description of feasibility and satisfaction findings from an innovative online family problem-solving intervention for adolescents following traumatic brain injury. *J.Pediatr.Psychol., 34,* 517-522.

Wade, S. L., Wolfe, C., Brown, T. M., & Pestian, J. P. (2005). Putting the pieces together: preliminary efficacy of a web-based family intervention for children with traumatic brain injury. *J.Pediatr.Psychol., 30,* 437-442.

Warmerdam, L., van, S. A., Twisk, J., Riper, H., & Cuijpers, P. (2008). Internet-based treatment for adults with depressive symptoms: randomized controlled trial. *J.Med.Internet.Res., 20;10,* e44.

Wilson, J. A., Onorati, K., Mishkind, M., Reger, M. A., & Gahm, G. A. (2008). Soldier attitudes about technology-based approaches to mental health care. *Cyberpsychol.Behav., 11,* 767-769.

Yamagishi, M., Kobayashi, T., Kobayashi, T., Nagami, M., Shimazu, A., & Kageyama, T. (2007). Effect of web-based assertion training for stress management of Japanese nurses. *J.Nurs.Manag., 15,* 603-607.

4

The Case of Hypopituitarism in Traumatic Brain Injury

Klose Marianne and Feldt-Rasmussen Ulla
Copenhagen University Hospital, Rigshospitalet
Denmark

1. Introduction

Traumatic brain injury (TBI) has until recently been considered a rare cause of loss of pituitary function, accounting for less than one percent of all new cases of hypopituitarism. Newer studies have, however, indicated otherwise, and overlooking the condition in case of the life-threatening adrenal insufficiency after brain trauma may be fatal (Schneider et al., 2007a). Thus, chronic anterior pituitary hormone deficits have been described with a higher frequency than previously anticipated and have caused expert panels to propose recommendations for routine assessment of pituitary function after TBI with appropriate replacement of insufficient axes (Ghigo et al., 2005; Ho, 2007; Tanriverdi et al., 2011).

Most populations have a high incidence of TBI of more than 100 in 100,000 inhabitants. On the one hand it is of clinical importance to identify all patients that would benefit from relevant substitution therapy, but on the other hand it is also of major socio-oeconomic interest to ensure a cost-effective strategy. To perform pituitary testing of all TBI patients would be an impossible task both logistically and financially. It is therefore unfortunate that the area despite numerous studies still lacks identification of valid predictors for development of hypopituitarism, and it has also not yet been clarified, which part of the TBI population that should be tested. Additionally, no larger treatment intervention studies have been performed, and it therefore remains quite unclear whether or not patients would benefit from treatment of hypopituitarism at an early or later stage to facilitate neurorehabilitation and improve survival, morbidity and quality of life.

In this chapter, the published clinical studies of posttraumatic hypopituitarism are scrutinized, and current recommendations are discussed in the lines of currently available evidence, with reference to socio-oeconomic aspects.

2. Pathophysiology of hypopituitarism in TBI

The pituitary gland regulates various endocrine organs including the adrenal cortex, the thyroid gland, and the gonads through integration of central and peripheral feedback signals. Hypopituitarism refers to an insufficient secretion of pituitary hormones.

The pathophysiological mechanism of posttraumatic hypopituitarism remains incompletely understood, but may include primary mechanical injury to the hypothalamic-pituitary region, as well as secondary injury from hypotension, hypoxia, anaemia and brain swelling causing restriction of flow in the hypophyseal portal vessels. Support of this pathophysiologic concept comes from autopsy studies of patients with fatal head injury in whom up to one-third had anterior pituitary gland necrosis (Ceballos, 1966; Crompton, 1971; Kornblum & Fisher, 1969). However, whether or not data from fatal cases can be generalised to explain long-term hypopituitarism in TBI survivors is not clear. Two MR studies showed results supportive of such hypothesis. Firstly, an observational case-control study included 41 patients with non-lethal head trauma and demonstrated acute changes such as pituitary enlargement, pituitary haemorrhages, infarctions, signal abnormalities and/or partial stalk transsection in about 30% of adult TBI patients (Maiya et al., 2007). Secondly, other observational data suggested that patients with long-term post-TBI hypopituitarism demonstrated more frequently loss of pituitary volume or virtual empty sella, abnormal pituitary gland signal heterogeneity, perfusion deficits and/or lack of posterior pituitary signal as compared to TBI patients with normal pituitary hormonal function (Schneider et al., 2007b). Accordingly, a higher occurrence of midline lesions or damage to deep brain structures were reported in hypopituitary patients with diffuse axonal injury as compared to those with normal pituitary function (Jeong et al., 2010).

One group suggested an aetiologic role of anti-pituitary and anti-hypothalamic antibodies (Tanriverdi et al., 2010), as well as a genetic predisposition for development of TBI-induced hypopituitarism (Tanriverdi et al., 2008a). This has on the other hand not been confirmed in other populations.

In the acute phase post-TBI, the transient effect of stress from critical illness and medication are important mechanisms to consider. The following medications are very likely to be involved in this patient group in the acute phase, and can by themselves cause life-threatening adrenal insufficiency: Adrenal cortisol synthesis can be impaired by the anaesthetic agent etomidate and the antifungal agent ketokonazol, exogenous corticosteroid therapy may suppress the hypothalamo-pituitary-adrenal (HPA) axis and induce adrenal atrophy that may persist months after cessation, and hepatic metabolism of cortisol may be enhanced by drugs such as phenytoin.

3. Diagnosing insufficient pituitary function

The diagnosis of hypopituitarism relies on basal and stimulated anterior pituitary and peripheral target hormone concentrations, and diagnostic test-panels and criteria suggesting hypopituitarism have been defined (, 1998; Lamberts et al., 1998). Both diagnostic criteria and cut-off points are arbitrary, and grey-zones for each pituitary hormone exist. Thus, test results must be interpreted in the light of pre-test probability and clinical features (Feinstein, 1990). Unfortunately, the clinical symptoms in hypopituitarism are most often vague and unspecific, and the diagnostic decision therefore often relies on the pre-test probability of disease. The diagnostic process is therefore highly challenged by vastly different assays for hormone measurements, all having their own reference range, as well as significantly different cut-off levels between normal persons and patients with pituitary deficiency. Establishment of local diagnostic cut-off points are required, but most often lacking. In most centres hypopituitarism is a rare condition, and ensuring own normative data for all the pituitary tests is cumbersome and expensive, why many physicians rely on 'standard' cut-off limits from the literature. Ideally, assessment of TBI patients should be restricted to few highly specialised collaborative centres using stringent diagnostic criteria for hypopituitarism including obligatory confirmation tests in case of an insufficient test outcome. The latter is highly important partly due to intraindividual test variation in normal people (Bhasin et al., 2010; Vestergaard et al., 1997), partly due to possible transitory changes due to non-pituitary related stress (Fig 1). For logistic reasons such recommendation is often not possible. In the following, assessment of each of the clinically relevant pituitary axes will be scrutinized.

3.1 GH deficiency

Measurement of baseline GH concentrations in serum is rarely informative as the secretion of growth hormone (GH) is pulsatile, and stimulation tests estimating the secretory capacity are mandatory. The pulsatile release of GH is physiologically controlled by stimulation by hypothalamic GH releasing hormone (GHRH) and inhibition by the hypothalamic suppressor, somatostatin. GHRH stimulates both GH synthesis and secretion, whereas somatostatin inhibits only GH secretion (Giustina & Veldhuis, 1998). Multiple neurotransmitter pathways and a variety of peripheral feedback signals modulate GH secretion reflected by the large number of accessible stimulation tests, relying on many different mechanisms. The GH secretory response to insulin induced hypoglycaemia during an insulin tolerance test (ITT) seems to be mediated via stimulated GHRH secretion and a concomitant withdrawal of somatostatin inhibition (Giustina & Veldhuis, 1998). ITT is considered the diagnostic gold standard, as it is the most extensively used and validated test, with very high sensitivity and specificity at standard cut-off limits. It has the advantage of allowing evaluation of the integrated hypothalamic-pituitary function concerning both GH- and adrenocorticotropin (ACTH)- secretions. The disadvantage is related to its contraindications including epilepsy and ischaemic heart disease, and the fact that it is both unpleasant for the patients and labour-intensive. Alternative tests such as the GHRH+arginine and the GHRH-GH releasing peptide (GHRP) -6 test have therefore become increasingly popular for assessment of the somatotroph function. Arginine acts via inhibition of hypothalamic somatostatin release, and GHRP-6 probably antagonizes somatostatin activity, thereby increasing the activity of GHRH-neurons (Giustina & Veldhuis, 1998). Because GHRH stimulates the pituitary directly, and thus circumvents the hypothalamus, tests involving GHRH may give false normal results in the early stage of GHD of hypothalamic origin (Darzy et al., 2003). Taking this into account, the GHRHarg test seems to have similar sensitivity and specificity as compared with the ITT in lean subjects (Biller et al., 2002). However, the GHRHarg is known to depend on the body composition and BMI specific cut-offs are needed (Corneli et al., 2005; Makimura et al., 2008). Obesity (Bonert et al., 2004; Rasmussen et al., 1995) and relative central adiposity (Miller et al., 2005) are generally major confounders by being negative determinants for the stimulated GH concentrations. This makes the distinction between organic GHD and obesity difficult, and poses a major problem in diagnosing isolated GHD, in particular. On the other hand, independent of BMI the likelihood of coexistent severe GHD is more than 90% in patients with two or more additional pituitary deficiencies (Toogood et al., 1994).

3.2 ACTH deficiency

As a consequence of diurnal rhythmicity dynamic testing of the HPA axis is most often required. A basal morning cortisol can be used under certain circumstances, since a concentration less or equal to 100 nmol/L is highly indicative of HPA deficiency (Courtney et al., 2000; Watts & Tindall, 1988), whereas a concentration higher than 400 nmol/L is indicative of HPA sufficiency (Gleeson et al., 2003; Watts & Tindall, 1988). Most commonly basal morning cortisol concentrations are in-between, highly overlapping those of healthy subjects, and dynamic testing is therefore required eventually. At present, the ITT is considered the diagnostic gold standard (Ho, 2007). The test-retest reproducibility is higher than for GH (Vestergaard et al., 1997), but false abnormal results can be seen, in particular, if only borderline attainment of hypoglycaemia is achieved. The 250 μg Synacthen test is often used in clinical practice as it is simple, and without contraindications and unpleasant side effects. It does have limitations, which include a risk of false normal results e.g. in the early phase after hypothalamic or pituitary damage (Klose et al., 2005), as well as in patients with partially degenerated adrenal glands. Irrespective of test preference, there are common problems in interpretation of results and in choice of cut-off level distinguishing normality from HPA deficiency related to the cortisol-assay used (Clark et al., 1998; Klose et al., 2007c), presence of dysproteinaemia and medical treatment with oestrogens (Bonte et al., 1999; Kirschbaum et al., 1999), either as replacement therapy in gonadal insufficiency or as oral contraceptive.

3.3 TSH deficiency

Central hypothyroidism is suspected in patients with low total- (T) or free- (f) T_4 and an inappropriately low TSH. Peripheral thyroid hormone levels have a narrow individual reference range compared with that observed between-individuals (Andersen et al., 2002; Feldt-Rasmussen et al., 1980). The diagnosis therefore depends on the position of the individual's normal set point, which is reflected by TSH in primary hypothyroidism. Whereas measurement of TSH is of major diagnostic importance in primary hypothyroidism, it is of little use in secondary hypothyroidism of hypothalamic or pituitary origin. Most of these patients have a serum TSH within the normal range or even elevated. This apparent contradiction may, to some extent at least, be explained by reduced bioactivity of the circulating TSH (Beck-Peccoz et al., 1985), probably through abnormal glycolysation of the molecule (Oliveira et al., 2001), though the mechanism is not fully understood. The diagnosis of secondary hypothyroidism is thus challenging, as the usual diagnostic criteria based on a normal reference range are not valid. Isolated secondary hypothyroidism is extremely rare and in these patients, samples should be re-analysed by an alternative assay, and low thyroxine binding globulin (TBG) concentrations and non-thyroidal illness have to be excluded before the final diagnosis (Lamberts et al., 1998). Stimulation with thyrotropin releasing hormone (TRH) has given discrepant results (Franklyn, 1997; Hartoft-Nielsen et al., 2004; Lania et al., 2008). The possible confounding by certain antiepileptic drugs is well-described (Cansu et al., 2006; Isojarvi et al., 2001), inducing a biochemical picture mimicking that of secondary hypothyroidism with decreased peripheral thyroid hormone concentrations and a normal TSH.

3.4 LH and FSH deficiency

In postmenopausal women hypogonadotropic hypogonadism is characterised by inappropriately low gonadotropins, and in premenopausal women by amenorrhoea or oligomenorrhoea in addition to low oestradiol and low or normal gonadotropins. Low testosterone and a correspondingly low LH suggest hypogonadotropic hypogonadism in men. Due to the diurnal rhythmicity morning samples are required, and in case of a low or low normal testosterone concentration sampling must be repeated, because 30% of such men may have a normal testosterone level on repeat measurement (Bhasin et al., 2010; Brambilla et al., 2007). Patients with altered sex hormone binding globulin (SHBG) concentrations are a major diagnostic challenge. According to the The Endocrine Society Clinical Practice Guideline, men in whom total testosterone is near the lower limit of normal or in whom SHBG abnormalities are suspected, evaluation should include measurement of free or bioavailable testosterone levels using validated assays(Bhasin et al., 2010). Conditions associated with high SHBG levels are aging, hepatic cirrhosis and hepatitis, hyperthyroidism, use of anticonvulsants, whereas decreased SHBG levels are seen in obesity, hypothyroidism, nephritic syndrome, diabetes mellitus, and use of glucocorticoids and androgenic steroids.

3.5 ADH deficiency

Central ADH deficiency is suspected in patients with polydipsia and polyuria (urine volume > 3 litres/24 hours). Urine analysis demonstrates dilute urine with low specific gravity and low osmolality. A fluid deprivation test may be necessary in case of intermediary results, or in order to determine the type of diabetes insipidus (central versus nephrogenic or dipsogenic).

4. Prevalence of acute hypopituitarism in TBI

A number of studies have assessed the acute neuroendocrine changes following TBI, in order to investigate their correlation to trauma severity, metabolic derangement and variables that may predict outcome (Cernak et al., 1999; Cohan et al., 2005; Della et al., 1998; Feibel et al., 1983; Hackl et al., 1991). The clinical implications of these findings remain unclear.

Four longitudinal studies have been designed to evaluate the relationship between acute and long-term pituitary hormone status after TBI. Agha et al. (Agha et al., 2005a) found secondary gonadotropin-, GH-, ACTH - and TSH deficiency in 80%, 18%, 16% and 2%, respectively of 56 patients with moderate or severe TBI. At one-year follow-up hormonal abnormalities had recovered in most patients, whereas others had developed de novo deficiencies, and although persistent GH and ACTH deficiency was associated with more severe hyposecretion of GH and cortisol during the acute phase, the authors were unable to identify biochemical predictors of long-term hypopituitarism. Tanriverdi et al. (Tanriverdi et al., 2006) reported pituitary hormone deficiency in 50% of 52 evaluated patients, primarily affecting the gonadothroph axis. However, individual data showed no obvious relationship between early and late pituitary dysfunctions. We (Klose et al., 2007b) described acute hormone alterations in 76% of 46 patients, with patients suffering the most severe TBI exhibiting the highest prevalence of alterations mimicking hypogonadotropic hypogonadism, central hypothyroidism, hyperprolactinaemia, and increased HPA-activity, all in agreement with the alterations seen in non-pituitary critical illness (Fig. 1).

We were unable to identify biochemical predictors of persistent hypopituitarism, and did not find any de novo deficiencies from 3 to 12 months post-TBI, whereas late recovery was observed in 1 of the 7 patients that were hypopituitary at 3 months. Kleindienst et al. (Kleindienst et al., 2009) described hormone alterations in 83% of 71 patients, recovering in most within 2 years follow-up. They reported that initial low GH levels predicted persistent deficiency 2 years post-TBI. The existing data, however, relies on rather small cohorts only allowing for case description and therefore clear conclusions and recommendations on this issue are still not possible.

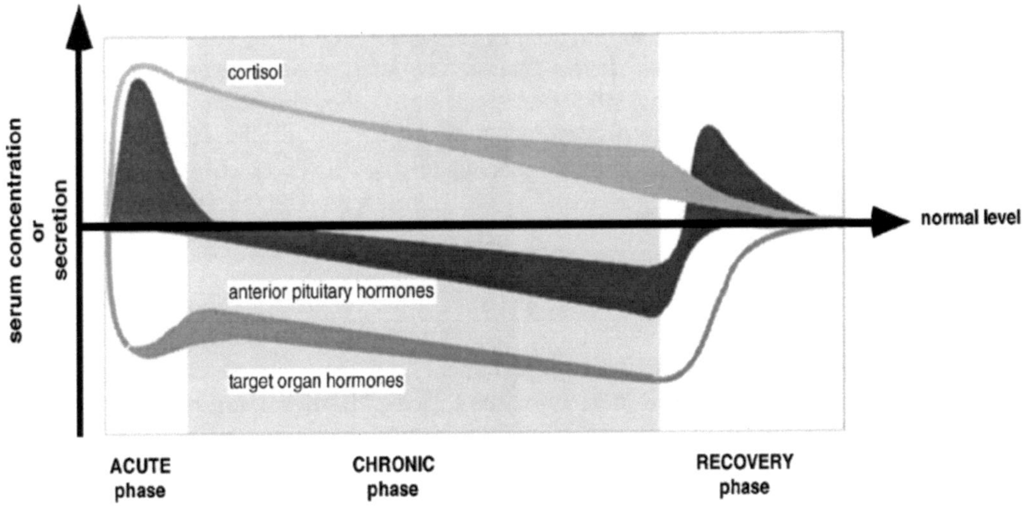

Fig. 1. Simplified concept of the pituitary-dependent changes during the course of critical illness. In the acute phase of illness (first hours to a few days after onset), the secretory activity of the anterior pituitary is essentially maintained or amplified, whereas anabolic target organ hormones are inactivated. Cortisol levels are elevated in concert with ACTH. In the chronic phase of protracted critical illness (intensive care dependent for weeks), the secretory activity of the anterior pituitary appears uniformly suppressed in relation to reduced circulating levels of target organ hormones. Impaired anterior pituitary hormone secretion allows the respective target organ hormones to decrease proportionately over time, with cortisol being a notable exception, the circulating levels of which remain elevated through a peripheral drive, a mechanism that ultimately may also fail. The onset of recovery is characterized by restored sensitivity of the anterior pituitary to reduced feedback control. (Adapted from Van den Berghe, G (1998) Clinical review 95: Acute and prolonged critical illness as different neuroendocrine paradigms. *Journal of Clinical Endocrinology and Metabolism*, 83 (6), pp. 1827-1834).

Case reports have provided clinical data to justify an increased attention towards potential occurrence of secondary hypoadrenalism from the acute phase in TBI patients. In order to illustrate the possible pitfall in diagnosing the causes of hyponatraemia in TBI patients, Agha et al. (Agha et al., 2007) reported data from 3 patients with severe TBI, who were initially misdiagnosed as syndrome of inappropriate ADH secretion (SIADH). In two of the cases hypoadrenalism was subsequently suspected due to the combination of hyponatraemia, hypoglycaemia and hypotension, and in the third case because plasma sodium did not correct with fluid restriction. All three patients had extremely low baseline cortisol concentrations of 33 - 110 nmol/L, and undetectable ACTH levels. The condition ameliorated in all upon glucocorticoid replacement. It should be emphasized that patients may present with more subtle signs and symptoms, and still be life-threatened by undiagnosed hypoadrenalism.

5. Prevalence of chronic hypopituitarism in TBI

Anterior pituitary hormone deficiency following TBI has traditionally been considered very rare, and mainly reported as single cases or series of cases. Over the last 10 years, the field has received increased attention and chronic anterior pituitary hormone deficiency has been reported with a prevalence ranging from 1% and up to 83% (Table 1). The results from most studies have suggested that persistent posttraumatic hypopituitarism might be a more common complication in TBI than previously believed, although some studies have failed to show such high occurrence rates (Kokshoorn et al., 2011; van der Eerden et al., 2010).

The diversity of the reported prevalences of chronic anterior pituitary hormone deficiency is likely to be explained by differences in study populations, study designs, and diagnostic procedures. Trauma severity varied considerably among the studies (Table 1). In general, a lower prevalence of posttraumatic hypopituitarism tended to be recorded in studies recruiting less severely injured patients (Kokshoorn et al., 2011; van der Eerden et al., 2010), and indicators of increased trauma severity was also suggested to be associated with development of hypopituitarism by some (Bavisetty et al., 2008; Bondanelli et al., 2004; Kelly et al., 2000; Klose et al., 2007a; Schneider et al., 2008), while not by others (Agha et al., 2004; Aimaretti et al., 2005; Leal-Cerro et al., 2005). In 22 TBI patients Kelly et al.(Kelly et al., 2000) identified injury severity in terms of an initial Glasgow Coma Scale score (GCS) of less than 10, diffuse brain swelling and hypoxia/hypotension as risk factors of posttraumatic hypopituitarism. Bavisetty et al. (Bavisetty et al., 2008) found that the degree of injury as defined by acute cerebral CT was the strongest predictor for long-term pituitary deficiencies, and in the cohort examined by us (Klose et al., 2007a), a normal CT excluded development of long-term deficiencies. On the other hand, the role of acute CT was recently contradicted by Kleindienst el al (Kleindienst et al., 2009) who found no relationship between acute or late CT findings and development of hypopituitarism. Other surrogate measures of trauma severity have been suggested to predict post-TBI hypopituitarism, including increased intracranial pressure (Klose et al., 2007a), diffuse axonal injury and basal skull fractures (Schneider et al., 2008).

Recently, Kokshoorn et al. (Kokshoorn et al., 2010) questioned the considerable variation of the reported prevalence, and assessed the impact of methodological differences among the present studies. They confirmed that part of the variation indeed seemed to be caused by differences in study design, diagnostic procedures, and other confounding factors such as BMI, prohibiting simple generalization from the original studies. In general, a lower prevalence of posttraumatic hypopituitarism tended to be recorded in studies using the ITT for the evaluation of the GH reserve (Kelly et al., 2000; Klose et al., 2007a; Kokshoorn et al., 2011), and in the studies using confirmatory tests (Agha et al., 2004; Klose et al., 2007a; Leal-Cerro et al., 2005; van der Eerden et al., 2010).

Table 2 a-d illustrates the relationship between diagnostic stringency and reported prevalence of GH, ACTH, LH/FSH and TSH deficiencies. Diagnostic stringency was rated according to information in the publications on pituitary tests, comparison with own and sufficient normative data and performance of confirmatory testing, There was an apparent association between diagnostic stringency and reported prevalence of GH deficiency (Table 2a). The diagnostic cut-offs have varied considerably between studies, and as suspected, the reported prevalence of GH deficiency increased with increasing test related cut-off limits. Furthermore, some studies only reported severe GH deficiency, whereas others reported both severe and partial cases.

			Anterior Pituitary Hormone deficiency (%)					
Authors	*n*	GCS<13	Total	Multiple deficiencies	GH deficiency*	ACTH deficiency	LH/FSH deficiency	TSH deficiency
Kelly et al., 2000	22	NS	36	23	18^	5	23	5
Lieberman et al., 2001	70	NS	69	18	15	46	1	22
Agha et al., 2004	102	100%	29	6	8 (3)	13	12	1
Bondanelli et al., 2004	50	86%	54	12	8 (20)	0	14	10
Popovic et al., 2004	67	100%	34	10	15 (15)	7	9	4
Aimaretti et al., 2005	70	45%	23	10	20 (16)	7	11	6
Leal-Cerro et al., 2005	170[b]	100%	25	9	6	6	17	6
Schneider et al., 2006	70	78%	36	4	10	9	20	3
Tanriverdi et al., 2006	52	40%	51	10	33	19	8	6
Herrmann et al., 2006	76	100%	24	7	8	2	17	2
Klose et al., 2007	104	58%	15	6	11 (5)	5	2	2
Bavisetty et al., 2008	70	NS	21	4	16	0	10	0
Wachter et al., 2009	53	61%	25	2	2	4	15	6
Kleindienst et al., 2009	23	78%	83	30	39	48	0	0
v der Eerden et al., 2010	107	28%	< 1	0	0	< 1	0	0
Krahulik et al., 2010	87	NS	21	-	14	0	6	0
Park et al., 2010	45	100%	31	13	20	13	18	7
Kokshoorn et al., 2011	112	43%	5	1	3	4	1	0

GCS: Glasgow Coma Scale score; NS: nor specified; *Severe (partial) when reported as such; ^GHD+GHI; [b] only 99 patients tested

Table 1. Present publications on the prevalence of chronic posttraumatic anterior pituitary dysfunction.

A	Diagnostic tests and cut-offs used for the diagnosis of GH deficiency				
Authors	**Test**	**Cut-offs**	**Confirmatory test**	**Prevalence of GH deficiency**	**Diagnostic stringency**
van der Eerden et al., 2010	GHRH-arg; if GHRH-arg response low then ITT or GHRH-arg	GHRHarg: peak GH < 3.5ug/l ITT: peak GH < 3,4 ug/l	Yes	0	
Kokshoorn et al., 2011	ITT; if contraindicated then GHRH-arg	ITT: peak GH < 3 ug/l GHRHarg:: BMI<25; peakGH < 11 ug/l BMI25-30: peakGH <8 ug/l BMI>30: peak GH < 4 ug/l	No	3	
Herrmann et al., 2006	GHRH-arg; if GHRH-arg & IGF-1 low, then additional ITT	GHRH-arg: peak GH < 9 ug/l ITT: peak GH < 3 ug/l	Yes	8	
Klose et al., 2007	ITT; if contraindicated then GHRH-arg	ITT: peak GH < 3 ug/l GHRHarg: peak GH < 9 ug/l	Yes	11	
Leal-Cerro et al., 2005	If IGF-1 low or pituitary deficiency other than GHD, then GHRH-GHRP-6 & ITT &. GST	GHRH-GHRP-6: peak GH ≤ 10 ug/l; If peak GH 10-20 ug/l then confirmed by ITT: peak GH < 3 ug/l GST: peak GH < 3 ug/l	Yes	6	
Agha et al., 2004	GST; if sub-normal then ITT: if ITT contra-indicated then GHRH-arg	GST: peak GH <5 ug/l ITT: peak GH < 5 ug/l GHRH-arg: peak GH < 9 ug/l	Yes	8	
Kleindienst et al., 2009	GHRH-arg	peak GH <9 ug/l	No	39	
Schneider et al., 2006	GHRH-arg	peak GH ≤9 ug/l	No	10	
Aimaretti et al., 2005	GHRH-arg	peak GH <9 ug/l	No	20	
Bondanelli et al., 2004	GHRH-arg	peak GH <9 ug/l	No	8	
Lieberman et al., 2001	Glucagon test in a NS subset of patients	peak GH <3 ug/l	No	15	
Popovic et al., 2004	GHRH-GHRP6	peak GH <10 ug/l	No	15	
Tanriverdi et al., 2006	GHRH-GHRP6	peak GH <10 ug/l	No	33	
Kelly et al., 2000	ITT	NS; <5th percentile from 18 HC	No	18	
Bavisetty et al., 2008	GHRH-arg	peak GH < 12 ug/l	No	16	
Park et al., 2010	ITT	peak GH < 10 ug/l	No	20	
Krahulik et al., 2010	Arginine or GHRH	Arginine: < 10th percentile of HC Glucagon: NS	No	14	-
Wachter et al., 2009	GHRH*	NS	No	2	-

Table 2. a.

B	Diagnostic tests and cut-offs used for the diagnosis of ACTH deficiency				
Authors	**Test**	**Cut-offs**	**Confirmatory test**	**Prevalence of ACTH deficiency**	**Diagnostic stringency**
Kelly et al., 2000	ITT	peak cort below 283 nmol/l^; pt diagnosed on clinical picture	No	5	
Bavisetty et al., 2008	LDST	peak cort < 331 nmol/l^^	No	0	
Klose et al., 2007	ITT; if contraindicated then SST	peak cort < 500 nmol/l	Yes	5	
Kokshoorn et al., 2011	ITT; if contraindicated then LDST or SST	peak cort < 500 nmol/l	No	4	
Herrmann et al., 2006	Baseline or ITT, selection criteria for ITT NS	baseline cort < 180 nmol/l peak cort < 500 nmol/l	No	2	
Agha et al., 2004	GST; if subnormal then ITT; if ITT contraindicated then SST	GST: peak cort < 450 nmol/l ITT: peak cort < 500 nmol/l SST: peak cort < 500 nmol/l	Yes	13	
Leal-Cerro et al., 2005	Basal cortisol; if low then ITT	Basal cort: < 200 nmol/l ITT: peak cort < 550 nmol/l + peak ACTH < 6.6 pmol/l	Yes	6	
van der Eerden et al., 2010	Basal cortisol; if low then ITT	basal cort < 200 nmol/l peak cort < 550 nmol/l	Yes	< 1	
Schneider et al., 2006	SST	peak cort < 500 nmol/l	No	9	
Tanriverdi et al., 2006	Basal cortisol; if low then LDST	basal cort: < 193 nmol/l LDST: peak cort < 550 nmol/l	No	19	
Park et al., 2010	ITT	peak cort: < 550 nmol/l	No	13	
Kleindienst et al., 2009	SST	peak cort: < 550 nmol/l	No	48	
Aimaretti et al., 2005	Basal morning cortisol and UFC	9.00 h cort: < 220 nmol/l (evt. low 24-h UFC)	No	7	
Bondanelli et al., 2004	Basal morning cortisol	basal cort: < 220 nmol/l	No	0	
Lieberman et al., 2001	Basal cortisol	basal cort: < 193 nmol/l	No	46*	
Krahulik et al., 2010	If basal cortisol < 500 nmol/l, then ACTH test	peak cort: < 5th percentile of HC, NS	No	0	
Wachter et al., 2009	CRH	NS	No	4	-
Popovic et al., 2004	Basal morning cortisol	NS	No	7	-

Table 2. b.

C	Diagnostic tests and cut-offs used for the diagnosis of LH/FSH deficiency				
Authors	**Test**	**Cut-offs**	**Confirmatory test**	**Prevalence of LH/FSH deficiency**	**Diagnostic stringency**
Kleindienst et al., 2009	Baseline	[**M**: T < 3,1 nmol/dl **preF**: E < 60 pg/dl **postF**: E < 10 pg/dl] + inapp low LH&FSH	No	0	
Tanriverdi et al., 2006	Baseline	**M**: T < 4,6 nmol/l + low/norm LH/FSH **preF**: E < 40 pmol/l+inapp low LH/FSH **post F**: LH&FSH in premenopausal range	No	8	
Klose et al., 2007	Baseline	**M**: T < 10 nmol/l & inapp low LH **preF**: a-/oligomenorrhea + low E & inapp low LH&FSH **postF**: LH&FSH in premenopausal range	Yes	2	
van der Eerden et al., 2010	Baseline	**M**: T < 11 nmol/l & low fT & low/norm LH&FSH **preF**: amenorrhea, low E & low/norm LH&FSH **postF**: low gonadotropins	Yes	0	
Leal-Cerro et al., 2005	Baseline; if low then GnRH test	**M**: fT below age dependant ref & low /norm LH&FSH **F**: menstrual distb.+ low E+low/norm LH&FSH **GnRH:** peak LH<10 fold increment above base-line & peak LH > 10 U/l	Yes	17	
Herrmann et al., 2006	Baseline	**M**: T < 9,5 nmol/l + low/normal LH/FSH **preF**: amenorrhea + low E **postF**: LH&FSH in premenopausal range	No	17	
Agha et al., 2004	Baseline	**M**: T < 10.3 nmol/l + low/normal LH&FSH **preF**: amenorrhea + low E **postF**: LH/FSH in premenopausal range	No	12	
Aimaretti et al., 2005	Baseline	**M**: T < 10 nmol/l + low/normal LH/FSH **preF**: menstrual disturb. + E < 20pg/ml	No	11	
Bondanelli et al., 2004	Baseline	**M**: T < 10 nmol/l + low/normal LH/FSH **F**: NS	No	14	
Bavisetty et al., 2008	Baseline	**M:** T < 10 nmol/l ^ **F**: E < 27.6 pg/ml + menstrual disturb.	No	10	
Schneider et al., 2006	Baseline	**M**: T < 12 nmol/l + low/norm LH&FSH **preF**: amenorea after TBI **postF:** inapp low LH&FSH	No	20	
Kelly et al., 2000	M. GnRH F: Baseline	NS	No	23	
Lieberman et al., 2001	Baseline; if low then GnRH	M: low T (NOS) F: menstrual history	No	1	
Popovic et al., 2004	Baseline	**M**: NS **F**: menstrual history	No	9	
Wachter et al., 2009	Baseline / TRH	NS	No	15	
Krahulik et al., 2010	Baseline	M: T<5th perc form HC F: menstrual history; low E	No	6	
Park et al., 2010	Baseline	(M: low T; Pre F: low E with inapp low gonadotropins. Post F: LH/FSH in premenopausal range	No	18	

Table 2. c.

D	**Diagnostic tests and cut-offs used for the diagnosis of TSH deficiency**				
Authors	**Test**	**Cut-offs**	**Confirmatory test**	**Prevalence of TSH deficiency**	**Diagnostic stringency**
van der Eerden et al., 2010	Baseline	fT4 < 8 pmol/l & norm/low TSH	Yes	0	
Leal-Cerro et al., 20051.	Baseline; if low then TRH	fT4 < 7,7 pmol/l & norm/low TSH TRH: TSH peak < 7 mU/ml	Yes	6	
Agha et al., 20041.	Baseline	fT4 < 8 pmol/l & norm/low TSH	No	1	
Bondanelli et al., 2004.	Baseline	fT4 < 10,3 pmol/l & norm/low TSH	No	10	
Aimaretti et al., 2005.	Baseline	fT4 < 10,3 pmol/l & norm/low TSH	No	6	
Tanriverdi et al., 2006.	Baseline	fT4 < 10,3 pmol/l & norm/low TSH	No	6	
Kleindienst et al., 2009.	Baseline	fT4 < 10 pmol/l or TT3 < 0,8 ng/dl & TSH < 0,45 U/L	No	0	
Herrmann et al., 2006.	Baseline	fT4 < 10 pmol/l & norm/low TSH	No	2	
Bavisetty et al., 2008.	Baseline	Low TT4 (NS) and fT4 < 10 pmol/l^	No	0	
Klose et al., 2007.	Baseline	fT4 < 12 pmol/l & norm/low TSH	Yes	2	
Schneider et al., 2006	Baseline	fT4 < 12 pmol/l & norm/low TSH	No	3	
Lieberman et al., 2001	Baseline; TRH in some (NS)	Low fT4 and normal/low TSH; or normal fT4 and low TSH TRH: TSH < 5mU/l	No	22	
Wachter et al., 2009	Baseline TRH	NS	No	6	
Popovic et al., 2004	Baseline	NS	No	4	
Kelly et al., 2000.	TRH	NS^^	No	5	
Krahulik et al., 2010.	Baseline	FT4 and TSH (NOS)	No	0	
Park et al., 20101.	Baseline	Low FT4 & norm/low TSH; NOS	No	7	
Kokshoorn et al., 2011.	Baseline	NS	No	0	

BMI: body mass index; cort: cortisol level; disturb: disturbances; E: estradiol; F: females; fT$_4$: free thyroxine; ftest: free testosterone; GHD: GH deficiency; GHRHarg: GHRH-arginine test; GHRH-GHRP-6: GHRH-GHRP-6 test; GnRH: GnRH-test; GST: glucagon stimulation test; HC: healthy control; inapp: inappropriately; ITT: insulin tolerance test; LDST: low-dose synacthen test; M: males; norm: normal i.e. within the normal range; NOS: not otherwise specified; NS: not specified; preF: premenopausal women; postF: postmenopausal women; pt: patient; SST: short synacthen test; test: total testosterone level; TBG: thyroid binding globulin; TRH: TRH-test; tT$_4$: total thyroxine; UFC: urine free cortisol; ^5th percentile from 18 HC; ^^5th percentile from 39 HC; * 7,1 % of the total cohort had a peak cortisol < 500 nmol/l in response to the SST.

Table 2. a-d. Overview of diagnostic procedures and reported prevalence in previous studies on chronic posttraumatic hypopituitarism. Studies are ranged according to diagnostic stringency based on stimulation tests, cut-off criteria, as well as performance of confirmatory tests or not.

GH deficiency, being the most frequently observed deficiency in the studies, was often found to be positively associated with BMI, which was not surprising as obesity (Bonert et al., 2004; Rasmussen et al., 1995) and relative central adiposity (Miller et al., 2005) are major confounders, and negative determinants for the stimulated GH concentrations in persons without hypothalamo-pituitary disturbances. This makes the distinction between organic GH deficiency and obesity difficult or even impossible, and poses a major diagnostic problem in isolated GH deficiency, in particular. The earliest TBI studies using the GHRH+arg test used a fixed cut-off independent on BMI of the subjects, and only later studies adjusted for the known confounding from BMI, by application of BMI related cut-offs that were then available. Many of the studies should in fact reanalyse their data with this information in hand in order to clarify the 'true' number of individuals with GHD, or at least less emphasis should be paid on these study results in meta-analyses, reviews and recommendations.

The association between diagnostic stringency and reported prevalence is not as clear when it comes to secondary hypoadrenalism. However, the two studies reporting the lowest prevalence also applied the most stringent criteria. Kelly et al. defined their cut-off limit for the ITT as the 5th percentile of peak GH derived from 18 healthy control subjects. It was not further specified, but was somewhat below 283 nmol/l, which is striking. Establishment of local diagnostic cut-off points are generally recommended, due to assays dependency. However, cut-offs limits, based on 5th percentiles from normative data from such small populations, may be heavily influenced by outliers, which may explain the low cut-off limit used in this study. This hypothesis seems reinforced by the fact that although passing the biochemical definition having peak cortisol of 286 nmol/l, one patient was diagnosed with secondary hypoadrenalism on clinical manifestations (Kelly et al., 2000). In the other end of the spectrum, Libermann et al. reported a total prevalence of anterior pituitary hormone deficiency of 69%, including 46% with secondary hypoadrenalism. The occurrence of secondary hypoadrenalism would, however, be reduced to 7%, if data had relied on the results from dynamic testing.

The definition of gonadotropin deficiency mostly differed as concern the chosen cut-off of testosterone in men (Table 1c). Not unanticipated, those studies applying the lowest cut-offs tended to report lower prevalences of gonadotropin deficiency. Furthermore, studies following the general recommendation of repeated sampling in case of a low or low normal testosterone concentration, reported lower prevalences of gonadotropin deficiency (Klose et al., 2007a; van der Eerden et al., 2010), which is probably due to the low test-retest reproducibility (Bhasin et al., 2010; Brambilla et al., 2007) of testosterone measurements.

Although the diagnosis of secondary hypothyroidism is challenging, the studies used very similar definitions, with cut-offs mostly differing according to the local reference ranges applied (Table 1d). Only one study differed significantly, reporting a prevalence of 22%, explained by a much wider definition (Lieberman et al., 2001). Applying the general definition (low fT4 and low/normal TSH) to this study, the prevalence would have been lowered to 12%.

Certain antiepileptic drugs may have various side effects on the endocrine function. Given the relatively high incidence of posttraumatic epilepsy in TBI survivors, biochemical alterations induced by epilepsy in itself or the antiepileptic drugs may have confounded the estimated prevalence in the present TBI studies. There are, however, insufficient data to enable a proper evaluation of the impact of such confounder.

Thus, diagnostic uncertainties are likely to have affected the published prevalences, and although plentiful in general, it is of special interest in post-TBI hypopituitarism, given that the large majority of these patients were reported with isolated GHD or with only one additional deficit. This is in contrast to patients with objective evidence of hypothalamic-pituitary damage, and thus a high pre-test probability of hypopituitarism, where isolated GHD is less frequent.

6. Outcome studies on hypopituitarism in TBI

Concerns have been raised whether undiagnosed and thus untreated hypopituitarism may contribute to the mortality and severe morbidity seen in TBI. The magnitude of such contribution has still not been defined, and again data are conflicting.

Increased disability, decreased QoL and a greater likelihood of depression has been described in patients with posttraumatic GH deficiency (Bavisetty et al., 2008; Kelly et al., 2006), although others have suggested that neuropsychological and QoL deficits are more closely associated to presence of haemorrhagic lesions on CT, than to hypopituitarism per se (Wachter et al., 2009). Although not taking presence of cerebral lesions into account, we described that when adjusted for confounders such as trauma severity, posttraumatic hypopituitarism remained an independent predictor of the classical phoenotypic features of hypopituitarism, including an unfavourable lipid and body-composition profile, as well as worsened QoL (Klose et al., 2007d), which could point to an association. Bondanelli et al. (Bondanelli et al., 2007) found that peak GH was an independent predictor of poorer outcome as measured by rehabilitation scales evaluating cognition, disability and functional dependency. Such association between cognitive function impairment and GH axis integrity was recently questioned by Pavlovic et al. (Pavlovic et al., 2010) who applied a very extensive neuropsychological battery, selected for high sensitivity for subtle brain dysfunction. No differences were found comparing patients with GH deficiency and those with normal GH function, and no correlation was found between neuropsychological variables and stimulated peak GH or insulinlike growth factor-I (IGF-I) levels.

A recent study focused on another outcome measure, and found reduced aerobic- and endurance capacity in patients with posttraumatic isolated GHD as compared to those with normal pituitary function (Mossberg et al., 2008).

Discrepancies in the reported outcome data, are likely to be explained by lack of power, variable diagnostic validity questioning the grouping of patients, and problems to correct for the enormous heterogeneity of co-morbidities in TBI patients. Furthermore, use of different patient reported outcome questionnaires complicates direct comparison.

7. Treatment of pituitary insufficiency

7.1 Acute phase

Although pituitary hormone alterations are a very common phenomenon in the acute phase after TBI, the diagnosis entails plenty of problems, and currently there are no reliable diagnostic cut-offs for anterior pituitary hormone deficiency in critically ill patients. Furthermore, there is no evidence to support a clinical benefit from hormonal replacement therapy with GH, thyroid hormone, nor reproductive hormones in the critically ill. Treatment with pharmacological doses of GH has been shown to increase morbidity and mortality (Takala et al., 1999), whether or not administration of thyroid hormone is beneficial or harmful remains controversial (De Groot, 2006; Stathatos et al., 2001), and no conclusive clinical benefit has been demonstrated for androgen treatment in prolonged critical illness (Angele et al., 1998). The diagnosis of adrenal failure and management of this disorder also remains controversial, with poor agreement among the experts. The threshold that best describes the patients at need for acute or chronic glucocorticoid replacement is still to be defined and is likely to depend on the underlying illness. The evidence of a clinical benefit from glucocorticoid replacement therapy in the acute phase of TBI relies on case reports (Agha et al., 2005b; Webster & Bell, 1997). At present time, recommendations are pragmatic and mainly rely on the clinical evaluation of the patient, where a combination of hyponatraemia, hypoglycaemia, and hypotension is highly suggestive (Agha et al., 2005b; Cooper & Stewart, 2003), but not prerequisite, of secondary hypoadrenalism, and should elicit an immediate therapeutic trial of glucocorticoid replacement. The subsequent treatment response should guide the decision of further treatment and follow-up.

7.2 Chronic phase

The negative effects of chronic glucocorticoid-, thyroid- and gonadal hormone deficiencies are well recognised, as is the beneficial effect from appropriate replacement therapy. Yet randomised clinical trials have never been performed in such classical endocrine deficiencies, and neither are randomised studies available to document such effect in TBI patients. These deficiencies and their treatment, however, have more distinct clinical features, than e.g. GH deficiency, which is the most frequently reported deficiency in TBI patients. It is associated with impaired linear growth and attainment of normal body composition in children, but in adults the features are less specific with reduced lean body mass, decreased exercise capacity, reduced bone mineral density, unfavourable changes in the lipid profile and decreased QoL.

There are limited data on treatment effect in this specific subpopulation of patients with anterior pituitary hormone deficiency. Two studies have compared clinical and other outcome variables measured at baseline and after one year of hGH replacement in TBI patients and in patients with non-functioning pituitary adenoma (NFPA) from Pfizer International Metabolic (KIMS) database(Casanueva et al., 2005; Kreitschmann-Andermahr et al., 2008). At one-year follow-up, IGF-I SDS levels had increased to the normal range, and improved QoL was observed, in TBI as in NFPA patients, suggesting that TBI patients with GH deficiency benefit from hGH replacement in terms of improved QoL in a similar fashion as do NFPA patients. Worth mentioning, however, is the fact that this registry study was biased in having included only patients diagnosed with GHD, and this cohort is therefore not representative for a general cohort of TBI patients. Recently, data was published from a study including 23 patients with posttraumatic GH deficiency/insufficiency randomised to either a year of placebo or GH replacement therapy (High, Jr. et al., 2010). Data suggested that some of the cognitive impairments observed in these patients might be partially reversible with appropriate replacement therapy. Similar observations were recorded by Maric et al. (Maric et al., 2010). Reimunde et al. (Reimunde et al., 2011) compared the effect of daily neurocognitive rehabilitation plus GH replacement, with neurocognitive rehabilitation alone and reported larger scale improvements in the GH deficient TBI patients on combined treatment schedule. Although encouraging, there is still inadequate evidence to demonstrate that pituitary replacement therapy improves the metabolic profile, neuro-cognitive symptoms, psychosocial problems, and work-related activities in TBI patients, and larger randomised placebo-controlled studies are much awaited, and crucial for proper evidence based clinical decisions.

8. When should testing and treatment be considered in patients with TBI?

Currently no evidence exists to suggest introduction of anterior pituitary hormone screening in the acute phase, due to both the aforementioned diagnostic difficulties and lack of evidence of the beneficial effects from hormonal substitution. Adrenal insufficiency should be treated upon clinical suspicion.

The temporal relationship between TBI and hypopituitarism is poorly understood. Longitudinal studies examining TBI patients at variable time points from the acute phase to years after the trauma, have reported transient, permanent, and de novo deficiencies all through the time span (Agha et al., 2005a; Kleindienst et al., 2009; Klose et al., 2007b; Tanriverdi et al., 2006). Part of this variation may be ascribed to diagnostic difficulties, including those caused by the stress of severe illness, but may also in some cases be related to medication effects, and lack of test re-test reproducibility. It is therefore often recommended that neuroendocrine evaluation should be performed no earlier than one year post trauma unless the clinical picture indicates otherwise (Ghigo et al., 2005; Ho, 2007; Tanriverdi et al., 2011).

Another important issue is which patients that should be considered for neuroendocrine evaluation. This is particularly important considering the high incidence of TBI (> 100 in 100,000 inhabitants). On the one hand it is of clinical importance to identify all patients that would benefit from relevant substitution therapy, but on the other hand it is of major socio-oeconomic interest to ensure a cost-effective strategy. To perform pituitary testing in all TBI patients would be an impossible task both logistically and financially. Unfortunately, the area lacks valid clinical, biochemical or other predictors and it has not yet been clarified, which part of the TBI population that should be tested (Klose & Feldt-Rasmussen, 2008). Symptoms of hypopituitarism are usually very unspecific and highly overlap those of TBI patients in general, and can thus rarely be used for patient selection. Different markers of increased trauma severity, and injury location have been proposed as predictive (Bavisetty et al., 2008; Kelly et al., 2000; Klose et al., 2007a; Schneider et al., 2007b; Schneider et al., 2008), but unfortunately data are very inconsistent.

Finally, data are still awaited to document the effect of hormone replacement therapy in this patient category, and until such data are available, one should be cautious to introduce uncritical routine anterior pituitary testing and replacement therapy. Certain categories of patients with TBI may be at a greater risk, including those with increased ICP (Klose et al., 2007a), CT abnormalities (Bavisetty et al., 2008), diffuse axonal injury, and those with basal skull fractures (Schneider et al., 2008), and should probably be regarded with a higher priority for pituitary assessment.

9. Conclusion

Anterior pituitary hormone alterations are frequently encountered in the acute phase after TBI. The relevance and therapeutic implications of such endocrine changes are still debated. Acute phase assessment of the growth hormone, thyroid, and gonadal axis is not recommended, as there is no evidence of a clinical benefit from replacement therapy at this stage. Untreated adrenal insufficiency can be life threatening. As biochemical assessment is difficult in the acute phase, the diagnosis should mainly be based on the clinical picture, and immediate treatment instituted on suspicion.

Chronic anterior pituitary hormone deficits are reported with a much higher frequency than previously thought, and this has caused expert panels to propose recommendations for hormone assessment of pituitary insufficiency and consequent appropriate replacement after TBI. Which subgroups of patients that should be considered for assessment, and at what time-point is, however, still debated.

Introduction of a routine screening program at this stage would be tempting, but remains problematic. The annual incidence rate of TBI leading to hospitalisation is roughly 100 in 100,000 inhabitants (Engberg & Teasdale, 2001), and it is thus of major socio-oeconomic interest to ensure a cost-effective screening strategy, as pituitary testing in all TBI patients would be an impossible task both logistically and economically. Much larger cohorts are needed for further evaluation and confirmation of reliable screening markers. Future studies should be designed to ensure a high diagnostic robustness for proper identification of reliable predictors, and to ensure that data can be generalised to an every-day TBI population, as the results may be highly dependent on selection criteria, confirmation of abnormal test results or not, and use of different diagnostic tests and criteria. Coexisting morbidities such as obesity and epilepsy, may also confound the results of neuroendocrine testing, and thus render the diagnostic process as well as the decision-making regarding replacement therapy difficult. Had the patients with high BMI had additional hormone deficiencies to GHD, and all patients diagnosed with isolated GHD been lean many of the reported results would have been more convincing. Finally, properly designed randomised intervention studies are awaited to document an effect of hormone replacement therapy in this patient category, and until such data are available, one should be cautious to introduce uncritical routine anterior pituitary testing and replacement therapy in TBI patients.

10. Acknowledgement

Present and previous work within this subject was supported by unrestricted grants from: Copenhagen University, The Danish Agency for Science, Technology and Innovation, The Reseach Council of the Capital Region of Denmark, The Lundbeck Foundation, Novo Nordisk, The A.P. Møller Foundation for the Advancement of Medical Science, Arvid Nielssons Foundation, Chistenson-Cesons Foundation, Axel-Muusfeldts Foundation and Else and Mogens Wedell-Wedellsborgs Foundation.

11. Reference list

(1998) Consensus guidelines for the diagnosis and treatment of adults with growth hormone deficiency: summary statement of the Growth Hormone Research Society Workshop on Adult Growth Hormone Deficiency. *Journal of Clinical Endocrinology and Metabolism*, 83 (2), pp. 379-381.

Agha, A., Phillips, J., O'Kelly, P., Tormey, W., & Thompson, C.J. (2005a) The natural history of post-traumatic hypopituitarism: implications for assessment and treatment. *The American Journal of Medicine*, 118 (12), pp. 1416-

Agha, A., Rogers, B., Sherlock, M., O'Kelly, P., Tormey, W., Phillips, J., & Thompson, C.J. (2004) Anterior pituitary dysfunction in survivors of traumatic brain injury. *Journal of Clinical Endocrinology and Metabolism*, 89 (10), pp. 4929-4936.

Agha, A., Sherlock, M., & Thompson, C.J. (2005b) Post-traumatic hyponatraemia due to acute hypopituitarism. *Monthly Journal of the Association of Physicians*, 98 (6), pp. 463-464.

Agha, A., Walker, D., Perry, L., Drake, W.M., Chew, S.L., Jenkins, P.J., Grossman, A.B., & Monson, J.P. (2007) Unmasking of central hypothyroidism following growth hormone replacement in adult hypopituitary patients. *Clinical Endocrinology*, 66 (1), pp. 72-77.

Aimaretti, G., Ambrosio, M.R., Di Somma, C., Gasperi, M., Cannavo, S., Scaroni, C., Fusco, A., Del Monte, P., De Menis, E., Faustini-Fustini, M., Grimaldi, F., Logoluso, F., Razzore, P., Rovere, S., Benvenga, S., Uberti, E.C., De Marinis, L., Lombardi, G., Mantero, F., Martino, E., Giordano, G., & Ghigo, E. (2005) Residual pituitary function after brain injury-induced hypopituitarism: a prospective 12-month study. *Journal of Clinical Endocrinology and Metabolism,*

Andersen, S., Pedersen, K.M., Bruun, N.H., & Laurberg, P. (2002) Narrow individual variations in serum T(4) and T(3) in normal subjects: a clue to the understanding of subclinical thyroid disease. *Journal of Clinical Endocrinology and Metabolism*, 87 (3), pp. 1068-1072.

Angele, M.K., Ayala, A., Cioffi, W.G., Bland, K.I., & Chaudry, I.H. (1998) Testosterone: the culprit for producing splenocyte immune depression after trauma hemorrhage. *American Journal of Physiology*, 274 (6 Pt 1), pp. C1530-C1536.

Bavisetty, S., Bavisetty, S., McArthur, D.L., Dusick, J.R., Wang, C., Cohan, P., Boscardin, W.J., Swerdloff, R., Levin, H., Chang, D.J., Muizelaar, J.P., & Kelly, D.F. (2008) Chronic hypopituitarism after traumatic brain injury: risk assessment and relationship to outcome. *Neurosurgery*, 62 (5), pp. 1080-1093.

Beck-Peccoz, P., Amr, S., Menezes-Ferreira, M.M., Faglia, G., & Weintraub, B.D. (1985) Decreased receptor binding of biologically inactive thyrotropin in central hypothyroidism. Effect of treatment with thyrotropin-releasing hormone. *The New England Journal of Medicine*, 312 (17), pp. 1085-1090.

Bhasin, S., Cunningham, G.R., Hayes, F.J., Matsumoto, A.M., Snyder, P.J., Swerdloff, R.S., & Montori, V.M. (2010) Testosterone therapy in men with androgen deficiency syndromes: an Endocrine Society clinical practice guideline. *Journal of Clinical Endocrinology and Metabolism*, 95 (6), pp. 2536-2559.

Biller, B.M., Samuels, M.H., Zagar, A., Cook, D.M., Arafah, B.M., Bonert, V., Stavrou, S., Kleinberg, D.L., Chipman, J.J., & Hartman, M.L. (2002) Sensitivity and specificity of six tests for the diagnosis of adult GH deficiency. *Journal of Clinical Endocrinology and Metabolism*, 87 (5), pp. 2067-2079.

Bondanelli, M., Ambrosio, M.R., Cavazzini, L., Bertocchi, A., Zatelli, M.C., Carli, A., Valle, D., Basaglia, N., & Uberti, E.C. (2007) Anterior pituitary function may predict functional and cognitive outcome in patients with traumatic brain injury undergoing rehabilitation. *Journal of Neurotrauma*, 24 (11), pp. 1687-1697.

Bondanelli, M., De Marinis, L., Ambrosio, M.R., Monesi, M., Valle, D., Zatelli, M.C., Fusco, A., Bianchi, A., Farneti, M., & degli Uberti, E.C. (2004) Occurrence of pituitary dysfunction following traumatic brain injury. *Journal of Neurotrauma*, 21 (6), pp. 685-696.

Bonert, V.S., Elashoff, J.D., Barnett, P., & Melmed, S. (2004) Body mass index determines evoked growth hormone (GH) responsiveness in normal healthy male subjects: diagnostic caveat for adult GH deficiency. *Journal of Clinical Endocrinology and Metabolism*, 89 (7), pp. 3397-3401.

Bonte, H.A., van den Hoven, R.J., van, d.S., V, & Vermes, I. (1999) The use of free cortisol index for laboratory assessment of pituitary-adrenal function. *Clinical Chemistry and Laboratory Medicine*, 37 (2), pp. 127-132.

Brambilla, D.J., O'Donnell, A.B., Matsumoto, A.M., & McKinlay, J.B. (2007) Intraindividual variation in levels of serum testosterone and other reproductive and adrenal hormones in men. *Clinical Endocrinology*, 67 (6), pp. 853-862.

Cansu, A., Serdaroglu, A., Camurdan, O., Hirfanoglu, T., Bideci, A., & Gucuyener, K. (2006) The evaluation of thyroid functions, thyroid antibodies, and thyroid volumes in children with epilepsy during short-term administration of oxcarbazepine and valproate. *Epilepsia*, 47 (11), pp. 1855-1859.

Casanueva, F.F., Leal, A., Koltowska-Haggstrom, M., Jonsson, P., & Goth, M.I. (2005) Traumatic brain injury as a relevant cause of growth hormone deficiency in adults: A KIMS-based study. *Archives of Physical Medicine and Rehabilitation*, 86 (3), pp. 463-468.

Ceballos, R. (1966) Pituitary changes in head trauma (analysis of 102 consecutive cases of head injury). *The Alabama Journal of Medical Sciences*, 3 (2), pp. 185-198.

Cernak, I., Savic, V.J., Lazarov, A., Joksimovic, M., & Markovic, S. (1999) Neuroendocrine responses following graded traumatic brain injury in male adults. *Brain Injury*, 13 (12), pp. 1005-1015.

Clark, P.M., Neylon, I., Raggatt, P.R., Sheppard, M.C., & Stewart, P.M. (1998) Defining the normal cortisol response to the short Synacthen test: implications for the investigation of hypothalamic-pituitary disorders. *Clinical Endocrinology*, 49 (3), pp. 287-292.

Cohan, P., Wang, C., McArthur, D.L., Cook, S.W., Dusick, J.R., Armin, B., Swerdloff, R., Vespa, P., Muizelaar, J.P., Cryer, H.G., Christenson, P.D., & Kelly, D.F. (2005) Acute secondary adrenal insufficiency after traumatic brain injury: A prospective study. *Critical Care Medicine*, 33 (10), pp. 2358-2366.

Cooper, M.S. & Stewart, P.M. (2003) Corticosteroid insufficiency in acutely ill patients. *The New England Journal of Medicine*, 348 (8), pp. 727-734.

Corneli, G., Di Somma, C., Baldelli, R., Rovere, S., Gasco, V., Croce, C.G., Grottoli, S., Maccario, M., Colao, A., Lombardi, G., Ghigo, E., Camanni, F., & Aimaretti, G. (2005) The cut-off limits of the GH response to GH-releasing hormone-arginine test related to body mass index. *European Journal of Endocrinology*, 153 (2), pp. 257-264.

Courtney, C.H., McAllister, A.S., McCance, D.R., Bell, P.M., Hadden, D.R., Leslie, H., Sheridan, B., & Atkinson, A.B. (2000) Comparison of one week 0900 h serum cortisol, low and standard dose synacthen tests with a 4 to 6 week insulin hypoglycaemia test after pituitary surgery in assessing HPA axis. *Clinical Endocrinology*, 53 (4), pp. 431-436.

Crompton, M.R. (1971) Hypothalamic lesions following closed head injury. *Brain*, 94 (1), pp. 165-172.

Darzy, K.H., Aimaretti, G., Wieringa, G., Gattamaneni, H.R., Ghigo, E., & Shalet, S.M. (2003) The usefulness of the combined growth hormone (GH)-releasing hormone and arginine stimulation test in the diagnosis of radiation-induced GH deficiency is dependent on the post-irradiation time interval. *Journal of Clinical Endocrinology and Metabolism*, 88 (1), pp. 95-102.

De Groot, L.J. (2006) Non-thyroidal illness syndrome is a manifestation of hypothalamic-pituitary dysfunction, and in view of current evidence, should be treated with appropriate replacement therapies. *Critical Care Clinics*, 22 (1), pp. 57-86, vi.

Della, C.F., Mancini, A., Valle, D., Gallizzi, F., Carducci, P., Mignani, V., & De, M.L. (1998) Provocative hypothalamopituitary axis tests in severe head injury: correlations with severity and prognosis. *Critical Care Medicine*, 26 (8), pp. 1419-1426.

Einaudi, S., Matarazzo, P., Peretta, P., Grossetti, R., Giordano, F., Altare, F., Bondone, C., Andreo, M., Ivani, G., Genitori, L., & de, S.C. (2006) Hypothalamo-hypophysial dysfunction after traumatic brain injury in children and adolescents: a preliminary retrospective and prospective study. *Journal of Pediatric Endocrinology and Metabolism*, 19 (5), pp. 691-703.

Engberg, A.W. & Teasdale, T.W. (2001) Traumatic brain injury in Denmark 1979-1996. A national study of incidence and mortality. *European Journal of Epidemiology*, 17 (5), pp. 437-442.

Feibel, J., Kelly, M., Lee, L., & Woolf, P. (1983) Loss of adrenocortical suppression after acute brain injury: role of increased intracranial pressure and brain stem function. *Journal of Clinical Endocrinology and Metabolism*, 57 (6), pp. 1245-1250.

Feinstein, A.R. (1990) The inadequacy of binary models for the clinical reality of three-zone diagnostic decisions. *Journal of Clinical Epidemiology*, 43 (1), pp. 109-113.

Feldt-Rasmussen, U., Hyltoft, P.P., Blaabjerg, O., & Horder, M. (1980) Long-term variability in serum thyroglobulin and thyroid related hormones in healthy subjects. *Acta Endocrinologica (Copenh)*, 95 (3), pp. 328-334.

Franklyn, J. (1997) Diagnosis and treatment of thyrotrophin deficiency. pp. 99-109.

Ghigo, E., Masel, B., Aimaretti, G., Leon-Carrion, J., Casanueva, F.F., Dominguez-Morales, M.R., Elovic, E., Perrone, K., Stalla, G., Thompson, C., & Urban, R. (2005) Consensus guidelines on screening for hypopituitarism following traumatic brain injury. *Brain Injury*, 19 (9), pp. 711-724.

Giustina, A. & Veldhuis, J.D. (1998) Pathophysiology of the neuroregulation of growth hormone secretion in experimental animals and the human. *Endocrine Reviews*, 19 (6), pp. 717-797.

Gleeson, H.K., Walker, B.R., Seckl, J.R., & Padfield, P.L. (2003) Ten years on: Safety of short synacthen tests in assessing adrenocorticotropin deficiency in clinical practice. *The Journal of Clinical Endocrinology and Metabolism*, 88 (5), pp. 2106-2111.

Hackl, J.M., Gottardis, M., Wieser, C., Rumpl, E., Stadler, C., Schwarz, S., & Monkayo, R. (1991) Endocrine abnormalities in severe traumatic brain injury--a cue to prognosis in severe craniocerebral trauma? *Intensive Care Medicine*, 17 (1), pp. 25-29.

Hartoft-Nielsen, M.L., Lange, M., Rasmussen, A.K., Scherer, S., Zimmermann-Belsing, T., & Feldt-Rasmussen, U. (2004) Thyrotropin-releasing hormone stimulation test in patients with pituitary pathology. *Hormone Research*, 61 (2), pp. 53-57.

Herrmann, B.L., Rehder, J., Kahlke, S., Wiedemayer, H., Doerfler, A., Ischebeck, W., Laumer, R., Forsting, M., Stolke, D., & Mann, K. (2006) Hypopituitarism following severe traumatic brain injury. *Experimental and Clinical Endocrinology & Diabetes*, 114 (6), pp. 316-321.

High, W.M., Jr., Briones-Galang, M., Clark, J.A., Gilkison, C., Mossberg, K.A., Zgaljardic, D.J., Masel, B.E., & Urban, R.J. (2010) Effect of growth hormone replacement therapy on cognition after traumatic brain injury. *Journal of Neurotrauma*, 27 (9), pp. 1565-1575.

Ho, K.K. (2007) Consensus guidelines for the diagnosis and treatment of adults with GH deficiency II: a statement of the GH Research Society in association with the European Society for Pediatric Endocrinology, Lawson Wilkins Society, European

Society of Endocrinology, Japan Endocrine Society, and Endocrine Society of Australia. *European Journal of Endocrinology*, 157 (6), pp. 695-700.

Isojarvi, J.I., Turkka, J., Pakarinen, A.J., Kotila, M., Rattya, J., & Myllyla, V.V. (2001) Thyroid function in men taking carbamazepine, oxcarbazepine, or valproate for epilepsy. *Epilepsia*, 42 (7), pp. 930-934.

Jeong, J.H., Kim, Y.Z., Cho, Y.W., & Kim, J.S. (2010) Negative effect of hypopituitarism following brain trauma in patients with diffuse axonal injury. *Journal of Neurosurgery*, 113 (3), pp. 532-538.

Kelly, D.F., Gonzalo, I.T., Cohan, P., Berman, N., Swerdloff, R., & Wang, C. (2000) Hypopituitarism following traumatic brain injury and aneurysmal subarachnoid hemorrhage: a preliminary report. *Journal of Neurosurgery*, 93 (5), pp. 743-752.

Kelly, D.F., McArthur, D.L., Levin, H., Swimmer, S., Dusick, J.R., Cohan, P., Wang, C., & Swerdloff, R. (2006) Neurobehavioral and quality of life changes associated with growth hormone insufficiency after complicated mild, moderate, or severe traumatic brain injury. *Journal of Neurotrauma*, 23 (6), pp. 928-942.

Khadr, S.N., Crofton, P.M., Jones, P.A., Wardhaugh, B., Roach, J., Drake, A.J., Minns, R.A., & Kelnar, C.J. (2010) Evaluation of pituitary function after traumatic brain injury in childhood. *Clinical Endocrinology*, 73 (5), pp. 637-643.

Kirschbaum, C., Kudielka, B.M., Gaab, J., Schommer, N.C., & Hellhammer, D.H. (1999) Impact of gender, menstrual cycle phase, and oral contraceptives on the activity of the hypothalamus-pituitary-adrenal axis. *Psychosomatic Medicine*, 61 (2), pp. 154-162.

Kleindienst, A., Brabant, G., Bock, C., Maser-Gluth, C., & Buchfelder, M. (2009) Neuroendocrine function following traumatic brain injury and subsequent intensive care treatment: a prospective longitudinal evaluation. *Journal of Neurotrauma*, 26 (9), pp. 1435-1446.

Klose, M. & Feldt-Rasmussen, U. (2008) Does the type and severity of brain injury predict hypothalamo-pituitary dysfunction? Does post-traumatic hypopituitarism predict worse outcome? *Pituitary.*, 11 (3), pp. 255-261.

Klose, M., Juul, A., Poulsgaard, L., Kosteljanetz, M., Brennum, J., & Feldt-Rasmussen, U. (2007a) Prevalence and predictive factors of post-traumatic hypopituitarism. *Clinical Endocrinology*, 67 (2), pp. 193-201.

Klose, M., Juul, A., Struck, J., Morgenthaler, N.G., Kosteljanetz, M., & Feldt-Rasmussen, U. (2007b) Acute and long-term pituitary insufficiency in traumatic brain injury: a prospective single-centre study. *Clinical Endocrinology*, 67 (4), pp. 598-606.

Klose, M., Lange, M., Kosteljanetz, M., Poulsgaard, L., & Feldt-Rasmussen, U. (2005) Adrenocortical insufficiency after pituitary surgery: an audit of the reliability of the conventional short synacthen test. *Clinical Endocrinology*, 63 (5), pp. 499-505.

Klose, M., Lange, M., Rasmussen, A.K., Skakkebaek, N.E., Hilsted, L., Haug, E., Andersen, M., & Feldt-Rasmussen, U. (2007c) Factors influencing the adrenocorticotropin test: role of contemporary cortisol assays, body composition, and oral contraceptive agents. *Journal of Clinical Endocrinology and Metabolism*, 92 (4), pp. 1326-1333.

Klose, M., Watt, T., Brennum, J., & Feldt-Rasmussen, U. (2007d) Posttraumatic hypopituitarism is associated with an unfavorable body composition and lipid profile, and decreased quality of life 12 months after injury. *Journal of Clinical Endocrinology and Metabolism*, 92 (10), pp. 3861-3868.

Moon, R.J., Sutton, T., Wilson, P.M., Kirkham, F.J., & Davies, J.H. (2010) Pituitary function at long-term follow-up of childhood traumatic brain injury. *Journal of Neurotrauma*, 27 (10), pp. 1827-1835.

Mossberg, K.A., Masel, B.E., Gilkison, C.R., & Urban, R.J. (2008) Aerobic capacity and growth hormone deficiency after traumatic brain injury. *Journal of Clinical Endocrinology and Metabolism*, 93 (7), pp. 2581-2587.

Niederland, T., Makovi, H., Gal, V., Andreka, B., Abraham, C.S., & Kovacs, J. (2007) Abnormalities of pituitary function after traumatic brain injury in children. *Journal of Neurotrauma*, 24 (1), pp. 119-127.

Oliveira, J.H., Persani, L., Beck-Peccoz, P., & Abucham, J. (2001) Investigating the paradox of hypothyroidism and increased serum thyrotropin (TSH) levels in Sheehan's syndrome: characterization of TSH carbohydrate content and bioactivity. *Journal of Clinical Endocrinology and Metabolism*, 86 (4), pp. 1694-1699.

Park, K.D., Kim, D.Y., Lee, J.K., Nam, H.S., & Park, Y.G. (2010) Anterior pituitary dysfunction in moderate-to-severe chronic traumatic brain injury patients and the influence on functional outcome. *Brain Injury*, 24 (11), pp. 1330-1335.

Pavlovic, D., Pekic, S., Stojanovic, M., Zivkovic, V., Djurovic, B., Jovanovic, V., Miljic, N., Medic-Stojanoska, M., Doknic, M., Miljic, D., Djurovic, M., Casanueva, F., & Popovic, V. (2010) Chronic cognitive sequelae after traumatic brain injury are not related to growth hormone deficiency in adults. *European Journal of Neurology*, 17 (5), pp. 696-702.

Poomthavorn, P., Maixner, W., & Zacharin, M. (2008) Pituitary function in paediatric survivors of severe traumatic brain injury. *Archives of Disease in Childhood*, 93 (2), pp. 133-137.

Popovic, V., Pekic, S., Pavlovic, D., Maric, N., Jasovic-Gasic, M., Djurovic, B., Medic, S.M., Zivkovic, V., Stojanovic, M., Doknic, M., Milic, N., Djurovic, M., Dieguez, C., & Casanueva, F.F. (2004) Hypopituitarism as a consequence of traumatic brain injury (TBI) and its possible relation with cognitive disabilities and mental distress. *Journal of Endocrinological Investigation*, 27 (11), pp. 1048-1054.

Rasmussen, M.H., Hvidberg, A., Juul, A., Main, K.M., Gotfredsen, A., Skakkebaek, N.E., Hilsted, J., & Skakkebae, N.E. (1995) Massive weight loss restores 24-hour growth hormone release profiles and serum insulin-like growth factor-I levels in obese subjects. *Journal of Clinical Endocrinology and Metabolism*, 80 (4), pp. 1407-1415.

Reimunde, P., Quintana, A., Castanon, B., Casteleiro, N., Vilarnovo, Z., Otero, A., Devesa, A., Otero-Cepeda, X.L., & Devesa, J. (2011) Effects of growth hormone (GH) replacement and cognitive rehabilitation in patients with cognitive disorders after traumatic brain injury. *Brain Injury*, 25 (1), pp. 65-73.

Schneider, H.J., Kreitschmann-Andermahr, I., Ghigo, E., Stalla, G.K., & Agha, A. (2007a) Hypothalamopituitary dysfunction following traumatic brain injury and aneurysmal subarachnoid hemorrhage: a systematic review. *The Journal of the American Medical Association*, 298 (12), pp. 1429-1438.

Schneider, H.J., Samann, P.G., Schneider, M., Croce, C.G., Corneli, G., Sievers, C., Ghigo, E., Stalla, G.K., & Aimaretti, G. (2007b) Pituitary imaging abnormalities in patients with and without hypopituitarism after traumatic brain injury. *Journal of Endocrinological Investigation*, 30 (4), pp. RC9-RC12.

Schneider, H.J., Schneider, M., Saller, B., Petersenn, S., Uhr, M., Husemann, B., von Rosen, F., & Stalla, G.K. (2006) Prevalence of anterior pituitary insufficiency 3 and 12 months after traumatic brain injury. *European Journal of Endocrinology*, 154 (2), pp. 259-265.

Schneider, M., Schneider, H.J., Yassouridis, A., Saller, B., von Rosen, F., & Stalla, G.K. (2008) Predictors of anterior pituitary insufficiency after traumatic brain injury. *Clinical Endocrinology*, 68 (2), pp. 206-212.

Stathatos, N., Levetan, C., Burman, K.D., & Wartofsky, L. (2001) The controversy of the treatment of critically ill patients with thyroid hormone. *Best Practice and Research.Clinical Endocrinology & Metabolism*, 15 (4), pp. 465-478.

Takala, J., Ruokonen, E., Webster, N.R., Nielsen, M.S., Zandstra, D.F., Vundelinckx, G., & Hinds, C.J. (1999) Increased mortality associated with growth hormone treatment in critically ill adults. *New England Journal of Medicine*, 341 (11), pp. 785-792.

Tanriverdi, F., Agha, A., Aimaretti, G., Casanueva, F.F., Kelestimur, F., Klose, M., Masel, B.E., Pereira, A.M., Popovic, V., & Schneider, H.J. (2011) Manifesto for the current understanding and management of traumatic brain injury (TBI) induced hypopituitarism. *Journal of Endocrinological Investigation*,

Tanriverdi, F., De, B.A., Battaglia, M., Bellastella, G., Bizzarro, A., Sinisi, A.A., Bellastella, A., Unluhizarci, K., Selcuklu, A., Casanueva, F.F., & Kelestimur, F. (2010) Investigation of antihypothalamus and antipituitary antibodies in amateur boxers: is chronic repetitive head trauma-induced pituitary dysfunction associated with autoimmunity? *European Journal of Endocrinology*, 162 (5), pp. 861-867.

Tanriverdi, F., Senyurek, H., Unluhizarci, K., Selcuklu, A., Casanueva, F.F., & Kelestimur, F. (2006) High risk of hypopituitarism after traumatic brain injury: a prospective investigation of anterior pituitary function in the acute phase and 12 months after trauma. *Journal of Clinical Endocrinology and Metabolism*, 91 (6), pp. 2105-2111.

Tanriverdi, F., Taheri, S., Ulutabanca, H., Caglayan, A.O., Ozkul, Y., Dundar, M., Selcuklu, A., Unluhizarci, K., Casanueva, F.F., & Kelestimur, F. (2008a) Apolipoprotein E3/E3 genotype decreases the risk of pituitary dysfunction after traumatic brain injury due to various causes: preliminary data. *Journal of Neurotrauma*, 25 (9), pp. 1071-1077.

Tanriverdi, F., Ulutabanca, H., Unluhizarci, K., Selcuklu, A., Casanueva, F.F., & Kelestimur, F. (2008b) Three years prospective investigation of anterior pituitary function after traumatic brain injury: a pilot study. *Clinical Endocrinology*, 68 (4), pp. 573-579.

Toogood, A.A., Beardwell, C.G., & Shalet, S.M. (1994) The severity of growth hormone deficiency in adults with pituitary disease is related to the degree of hypopituitarism. *Clinical Endocrinology*, 41 (4), pp. 511-516.

van der Eerden, A.W., Twickler, M.T., Sweep, F.C., Beems, T., Hendricks, H.T., Hermus, A.R., & Vos, P.E. (2010) Should anterior pituitary function be tested during follow-up of all patients presenting at the emergency department because of traumatic brain injury? *European Journal of Endocrinology*, 162 (1), pp. 19-28.

Vestergaard, P., Hoeck, H.C., Jakobsen, P.E., & Laurberg, P. (1997) Reproducibility of growth hormone and cortisol responses to the insulin tolerance test and the short ACTH test in normal adults. *Hormone and Metabolic Research*, 29 (3), pp. 106-110.

Wachter, D., Gundling, K., Oertel, M.F., Stracke, H., & Boker, D.K. (2009) Pituitary insufficiency after traumatic brain injury. *Journal of Clinical Neuroscience*, 16 (2), pp. 202-208.

Watts, N.B. & Tindall, G.T. (1988) Rapid assessment of corticotropin reserve after pituitary surgery. *The Journal of the American Medical Association*, 259 (5), pp. 708-711.

Webster, J.B. & Bell, K.R. (1997) Primary adrenal insufficiency following traumatic brain injury: a case report and review of the literature. *Archives of Physical Medicine and Rehabilitation*, 78 (3), pp. 314-318.

Part 2

Rehabilitation

5

Use of the International Classification of Functioning, Disability and Health in Brain Injury Rehabilitation

Pavel Ptyushkin, Gaj Vidmar, Helena Burger and Crt Marincek
MURINET project (Multidisciplinary Network on Health and Disability in Europe)
University Rehabilitation Institute, Republic of Slovenia, Ljubljana
Slovenia

1. Introduction

In 1887 a book titled "The International Language" was published by Dr. Ludwig Zamenhof in Warsaw. In the introductory part the famous inventor of Esperanto stated: "How much time, labour, and money are wasted in translating the literary productions of one nation into the language of another, and yet, if we rely on translations alone, we can only become acquainted with a tiny part of foreign literature. If an international language existed, all the translations would have been made into it alone, as into a tongue intelligible to everybody, and works of an international character would be written directly in it. The Chinese wall dividing literatures would disappear, and the works of other nations would be as readily intelligible to us as those of our own authors. Books being the same for everyone, education, ideals, convictions, aims, would be the same too" (Zamenhof, 1887).
Decades after with the development of rehabilitation medicine as an independent discipline it turned out that it faced virtually the same problems and hopes: "Chinese walls" in the communication among professionals of different specialties involved in rehabilitation of the same person, the possibility to "become acquainted with a tiny part of foreign literature" due to the language barriers and different national standards in different countries and even within the same country. All this resulting in "much time, labour, and money wasted" that could have been used more efficiently for a good cause of the patient.
The situation changed in 2001 with the unanimous approval by the World Health Assembly of the International Classification of Functioning, Disability and Health (ICF) (WHO, 2001). The main purpose of the classification is exactly to provide a common language for professionals working in health-related areas and establish an international standard for description of health-related states including brain injury rehabilitation. The ICF model and classification are briefly introduced below.

2. The integrative model of functioning, disability and health

The ICF is a comprehensive classification of health-related domains containing 1424 categories that can exhaustively describe the functional status of a person or simply functioning. WHO proposed to use the term functioning when referring to the real impact of a health condition on the day to day life of a person. When the term "health" can be interpreted in many different and sometimes contradictory ways "functioning" is clearly defined within the ICF. Namely, in the ICF *functioning* refers to body functions, body structures, activities and participation, and disability refers to impairments in body functions and body structures, limitations in activities and restrictions in participation. Most importantly, although functioning and disability are associated with a health condition (diseases, disorders, natural processes of aging), they are not conceptualized as direct consequences of health conditions but rather the result of interactions between health conditions and contextual factors (environmental and personal factors).

The ICF complements the widely used International Classification of Diseases (ICD) allowing to describe the full lived experience of people with a health condition coded by the ICD. ICF captures multiple dimensions of functioning, related to a health condition in order to amplify the ICD predominantly biomedical perspective. It would be therefore beneficial to use ICD and ICF jointly because of their synergy and additional information advantages (Kostanjsek, 2010). This understanding is represented in Figure 1 which depicts the ICF model.

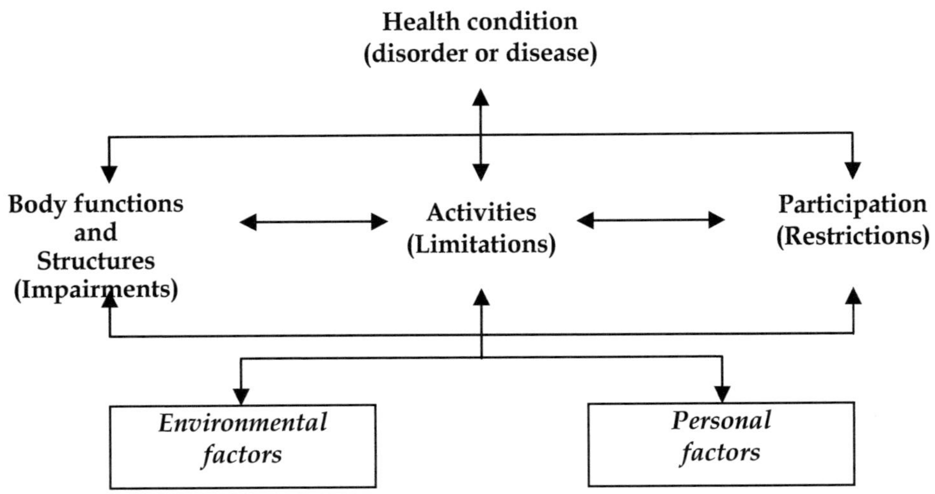

Fig. 1. The bio-psycho-social model of functioning, disability and health

As one can see there is a dynamic and bidirectional interaction among all the components of this model. Changes in one component may influence one or more of the other components. These modifications can always work in all directions. This model illustrates also the essential role of environmental and personal factors for the individual's functioning. Environmental factors can act as *barriers* (producing or increasing the severity of a disability, or as *facilitators* (improving or eliminating a disability). For this reason, environmental factors must always be taken into account in when assessing functioning before and after the rehabilitation.

2.1 The structure and codes of the ICF

Overall, the classification consists of two parts - *functioning and disability* and *contextual factors,* each with two *components.* Part 1 includes the lists of Body Functions and Structures and Activities and Participation. Part 2 integrates Environmental and Personal Factors. Although personal factors have an impact on functioning and they are included in the ICF model they are not yet classified. In all other components, *chapters* represent the 1st level of the classification which is the broadest. Each chapter is subdivided into the specific elements of the classification, called *categories,* which are also organized in a hierarchical structure of 2nd, 3rd or 4th levels.

For all categories, except those in body structures, definitions with inclusion and exclusion criteria are provided as shown in the following example:

d520 Caring for body parts

Looking after those parts of the body, such as skin, face, teeth, scalp, nails and genitals, that require more than washing and drying. *Inclusions: caring for skin, teeth, hair, finger and toe nails*

*Exclusions: washing oneself (**d510**); toileting (**d530**)*

The definitions and inclusion criteria provided for each category give a detailed description of the meaning of the category and help practitioners to correctly use the ICF codes. The exclusion criteria help to differentiate among related and seemingly similar ICF categories.

ICF codes are composed of a prefix (**b** for body functions, **s** for body structure, **d** for activity and participation, and **e** for environmental factors) followed by a numeric code that consists of one digit for the first or chapter level, three digits for the second, four for the third, and five for the fourth level (see example below).

The hierarchical organization of the classification allows users to choose a broader (e.g. by using a 1st level chapter or a 2nd level category) or a more specific (e.g. by using a 3rd or 4th level category) description of an aspect of functioning. The level of specificity increases with each level as it is shown in the above example. The hierarchical organization allows users to choose the level of specificity that is required for the description of functioning for their purpose and information need. Although personal factors are not classified, users may assess and describe them in a manner that is suitable for their purposes.

2.2 ICF qualifiers

ICF qualifiers allow to describe the extent of a problem in functioning (impairment, limitation, restriction) and the impact of the environment on functioning and disability. To be meaningful, an ICF code requires at least one qualifier. Hence, a complete ICF code (composed of the letter and numeric code) is completed by at least the first qualifier placed after a dot following the numeric code, e.g. b280.**3**. For all components (body functions, body structures, activities and participation and environmental factors), the description of the extent of a problem uses the following *generic scale:*

xxx.**0** NO problem	(none, absent, negligible,...)	0-4%
xxx.**1** MILD problem	(slight, low,...)	5-24%
xxx.**2** MODERATE problem	(medium, fair,...)	25-49%
xxx.**3** SEVERE problem	(high, extreme,...)	50-95%
xxx.**4** COMPETE problem	(total,...)	96-100%
xxx.**8** not specified (if only insufficient information for the description of the extent of the problem is available)		
xxx.**9** not applicable (if the description of a problem is inappropriate, e.g. in 'b650 Menstruation functions' in men)		

A different number of qualifiers is available for each of the four component (see Table 1). While there is only one qualifier (extent of impairment) for Body Functions, Body

Structures may be denoted with three qualifiers (first qualifier = extent of impairment, second qualifier = nature of impairment, third qualifier = location of impairment). For example, the ICF code **s7302.412** describes a complete impairment (**4**) due to total absence (**1**) of the left (**2**) hand (s7302).

For Activities and Participation, two qualifiers are used. The first qualifier is to describe *performance*, the second qualifier to describe *capacity*. Performance is understood as what an individual actually does in his or her current environment in light of the positive or negative impact of the environmental factors (including all aspects of the physical, social and attitudinal environment). Capacity, by contrast, describes an individual's intrinsic ability to perform a task or an action independently of the impact of the environment, including the particular personal assistance or assistive devices. Hence, when describing both performance and capacity for the same category the difference between them reflects the extent of the impact of environmental factors on an individual's functional state resulting in the experienced level of disability. For example, the ICF code d450**.04** describes a person whose ability to walk is completely impaired (**4** = complete problem in capacity) but totally compensated by a prosthesis which is reflected with no limitations in walking in the performance (**0** = no problem with performance).

Environmental factors are quantified by only one qualifier. However, the impact on the level of disability can be positive (facilitator) or negative (barrier). To denote this, a facilitator is marked with a plus sign instead the dot (+X) and a barrier follows the dot (.X), as in the following examples: e310**+2** (= Moderate facilitator 'Immediate family'), e310**.2** (=Moderate barrier 'Immediate family').

Qualifiers complement an ICF code and provide the complete description of a person's level of functioning or disability. If assessment instruments or other standards are used to measure the level of disability of a specific aspect of functioning, the results of such measurement can be 'translated' into a qualifier. Using qualifiers for the description of disability facilitates a common understanding of the description of a person's level of disability. Furthermore, the use of qualifiers makes it possible to develop functioning profile of a patient.

3. ICF core sets

With its 1424 categories, the ICF is an exhaustive classification. It allows to create a very detailed and highly individualized functional profile of a person when used as a whole. However, with exhaustiveness can be associated complexity and in some cases even impracticability. ICF is often considered too comprehensive and too complicated for daily practice. The obvious requirement of practicability was the primary reason for the WHO to develop user-friendly tools that would include a purpose-tailored selection of the ICF categories relevant for describing functioning and disability in various contexts related to health conditions (Stucki et al., 2008). These tools are called ICF Core Sets. An ICF Core Set is a selection of categories from the full ICF that correspond to a health condition as coded by the ICD or a particular purpose. There are two main types of the ICF Core Sets, namely, Comprehensive ICF Core Set and Brief ICF Core set.

The Comprehensive ICF Core Set includes categories that reflect the whole spectrum of typical problems a patient may face. The Comprehensive ICF Core Set can guide practitioners through the assessment and helps to *avoid overlooking* aspects of functioning *that are likely to present a problem* in a patient. Due to its comprehensive amount of categories it is a tool that allows a thorough and multidisciplinary assessment of functioning of a person with a health

Component	1st Qualifier	2nd qualifier	3rd qualifier
Body functions	**Extent of impairment** 0 = NO impairment 1 = MILD impairment 2 = MODERATE impairment 3 = SEVERE impairment 4 = COMPLETE impairment 8 = not specified 9 = not applicable	-	-
Body structures	**Extent of impairment** 0 = NO impairment 1 = MILD impairment 2 = MODERATE impairment 3 = SEVERE impairment 4 = COMPLETE impairment 8 = not specified 9 = not applicable	**Nature of impairment** 0 = no change in structure 1 = total absence 2 = partial absence 3 = additional part 4 = aberrant dimension 5 = discontinuity 6 = deviating position 7 = qualitative changes in structure, including accumulation of fluid 8 = not specified 9 = not applicable	**Location of impairment** 0 = more than one region 1 = right 2 = left 3 = both sides 4 = front 5 = back 6 = proximal 7 = distal 8 = not specified 9 = not applicable
Activities and Participation	**Extent of difficulty in performance** 0 = NO difficulty 1 = MILD difficulty 2 = MODERATE difficulty 3 = SEVERE difficulty 4 = COMPLETE difficulty 8 = not specified 9 = not applicable	**Extent of difficulty in capacity** 0 = NO difficulty 1 = MILD difficulty 2 = MODERATE difficulty 3 = SEVERE difficulty 4 = COMPLETE difficulty 8 = not specified 9 = not applicable	-
Environmental factors	**Extend of the impact of the environment** 0 = NO barrier 1 = MILD barrier 2 = MODERATE barrier 3 = SEVERE barrier 4 = COMPLETE barrier 8 = barrier, not specified 9 = not applicable or +0 = NO facilitator +1 = MILD facilitator +2 = MODERATE facilitator +3 = SUBSTANTIAL facilitator +4 = COMPLETE facilitator +8 = facilitator, not specified 9 = not applicable	-	-

Table 1. Overview of qualifiers for different components of the ICF

condition. *The Brief ICF Core Set* is derived from the Comprehensive ICF Core Set and is composed of categories that should be taken into account for any patient with a health condition or in any setting for which the ICF Core Set was developed, and captures the *essence of person's experience.* Hence, the *Brief ICF Core Set* is used when a brief assessment of functioning of a patient is necessary and sufficient. It therefore serves as the starting point for condition- or setting- specific description of functioning and creation of the basic clinical documentation.

3.1 ICF Core Sets for traumatic brain injury

Any ICF Core Set including the one for traumatic brain injury (TBI) is a result of a structured international scientific process. 139 ICF categories were selected for inclusion into the Comprehensive ICF Core Set for traumatic brain injury. These categories should be taken into account when conducting a comprehensive, multidisciplinary assessment. Out of these 139 categories, 23 ICF categories were selected for inclusion into the Brief ICF Core for TBI. Brief ICF Core Set for traumatic brain injury is presented below (ICF Research Branch, 2010).

ICF Code	ICF Category Title
Body Functions (8)	
b164	Higher-level cognitive functions
b152	Emotional functions
b130	Energy and drive functions
b760	Control of voluntary movement functions
b144	Memory functions
b280	Sensation of pain
b140	Attention functions
b110	Consciousness functions
Body Structures (1)	
s110	Structure of brain
Activities & Participation (8)	
d230	Carrying out daily routine
d350	Conversation
d450	Walking
d720	Complex interpersonal interactions
d845	Acquiring, keeping and terminating a job
d5	Self care
d920	Recreation and leisure
d760	Family relationships
Environmental Factors (6)	
e310	Immediate family
e580	Health services, systems and policies
e115	Products and technology for personal use in daily living
e320	Friends
e570	Social security services, systems and policies
e120	Products and technology for personal indoor and outdoor mobility and transportation

Table 2. ICF Brief Core Set for traumatic brain injury

4. ICF in brain injury rehabilitation. An overview

From the ICF perspective, rehabilitation medicine can be defined as the interdisciplinary management of a person's functioning and health. Rehabilitation therefore aims to enable people experiencing or likely to experience disability to *achieve and maintain optimal functioning*. At the same time, functioning is not considered as the consequence of a disease, but rather as the human experience that is the result of the *dynamic interaction* between a health condition and both personal and environmental factors (contextual factors). Assessment of functioning is the starting point of a patient and goal oriented, evidence-based and iterative rehabilitation process (Stucki et al., 2007).

The ICF as a conceptual model and ICF-based tools, such as ICF Core Sets, as practical instruments may contribute to a more holistic and structured description of functioning of persons after brain injury (BI). For example, the current data indicate that ICF can be useful in classifying the currently used assessment scales in traumatic brain injury (Cameron et al., 2009). It also allows a standardised and comprehensive analysis of health and health-related consequences, fully applicable to the rehabilitation after BI. Particularly in the area of neurorehabilitation, it may contribute to the evaluation of deficits and identification of treatment goals and targets for intervention (Bilbao et al., 2003). A special additional value of the ICF is seen in its capacity to describe and categorise the environmental factors relevant for rehabilitation (Fries et al., 2008). The rehabilitation programmes designed for patients with BI have to include assessment and treatment of the contextual factors and there is a need for development of the instruments that can quantify these factors. The information about functioning collected using the ICF could be also used to identify needs, match patients to interventions, track functioning over time, measure clinical outcomes and monitor treatment effectiveness.

The applicability of the ICF in brain injured patients was explored in at least fourteen articles published from 2002 to 2010. One article from 2003 generally discusses the applicability of the ICF model to brain injury concluding that it is a potentially useful tool to adequately classify and assess functioning and disability, related to TBI. Two articles are related to the development of the ICF Core Set for traumatic brain injury (TBI) discussing the need for having a practical ICF-based tool to describe functioning of TBI patients which would at the same time allow clinicians to adopt a comprehensive and holistic approach. The Italian clinical perspective on the potential of ICF core set for TBI argues that ICF makes it possible to describe in a systematic way not only body functions and structures, but also the activities and participation and the influence of the environmental factors. Another study tested the applicability of the ICF checklist for the description of patients with TBI. The authors concluded that although the checklist can be practical for clinical work, an ICF core set for TBI would be more adequate. Two other articles discuss the application of the ICF model for treatment of communication and cognitive disorders following the TBI. Larkins suggests that the ICF supports a systematic approach for understanding cognitive-communication disorders in persons with TBI and presents an example of the application of the ICF in such patients. Worral and associates, however, point out that the WHO classification scheme simplifies the real-life communication and can be more useful for a generic description of communicational functioning rather than a individualized one. One study analyzed the possible benefits of the ICF for the description of functioning of returning war veterans who frequently suffer from the consequences of a traumatic brain injury. The author argues that ICF can help to refine the understanding of the challenges the veterans have to confront after coming back. This can assist in making more appropriate decisions for allocation of resources, and for the development and implementation of therapies and rehabilitation interventions. One study summarized the available evidence on the use of the ICF to describe the functioning of severely brain injured persons and concluded that in light of available evidence, the ICF is a useful tool that describes the functioning and needs of patients with TBI. The authors point out that a wider utilization of the ICF can help to allocate resources in order to reach the improvement of the quality of life of patients with TBI. Quality of life is also a concern in another article by Pierce and Hanks. They tested whether the description of functioning based on the ICF can predict life satisfaction, concluding that a combination of ICF components and demographic factors significantly predicted life satisfaction. The study performed by Ehrenfors and associates examined the widely used assessment instruments for description of functioning of school-aged children with traumatic brain injury through the ICF lens. In their opinion widely used assessment instruments do not cover essential aspects of functioning and disability. An ICF-based questionnaire was developed for TBI patients by a group of Dutch researchers to assess activities and participation (Ptyushkin et al., 2010).

An important additional value of the ICF is seen in its capacity to describe and categorize environmental factors relevant for rehabilitation. Current rehabilitation programs designed for patients with TBI, it has been suggested, have to include assessment and response to contextual factors and there is a need for the development of instruments that can quantify these factors. The role of the ICF in this conceptual shift is discussed.

Finally, Whyte suggests that the direction brain injury research will take depends on a variety of factors and is guided in part by underlying theory and in part depends on the location of the target of treatment and how it is classified in the ICF. Recent data also indicate that ICF can be useful in classifying the currently used assessment scales for traumatic brain injury (Whyte, 2009).

5. Linking medical records of a patient with brain injury to the ICF. A case study

ICF allows to create individual functional profiles of persons with any health condition. Such profiles can be especially valuable when dealing with the complicated and multifaceted health conditions like brain injury. Depending on the purpose when applying ICF in brain injury rehabilitation one can create an ICF profile of a patient either from the start or by linking the already existing medical records to the ICF. An example of the latter is presented below (Ptyushkin et al., 2009).

Medical records of a patient after brain injury caused by a traffic accident that took place in April, 2008, who was admitted to the University Rehabilitation Institute (URI) of the Republic of Slovenia in July, 2008, were linked to the ICF. The patient was male, 31 years old at the time of admission, and his Glasgow Coma Scale score after the accident was 6. He was admitted to our Institute after the acute treatment with 8 different diagnoses, all of them corresponding to the ICD section "S" ("Injury, poisoning and certain other consequences of external causes"). Information about functioning at admission and discharge was entered separately. Medical records comprised the admission and discharge form and the reports from physiotherapist, occupational therapist, speech therapist and psychologist.

The medical records, which were mostly in text format, were linked to the ICF using the so-called linking rules. The process was divided into the following stages:

- identification of the meaning unit - a short phrase or sentence that describes one concrete aspect of functioning;
- linking of the meaning unit to the ICF code; and
- selection of the appropriate qualifier.

An example of the linking process is shown in Table 3. Additionally, the Functional Independence Measure (FIM), which had been previously linked to the ICF by a group of experts at the level of code in the current study (4, 5, 6), was linked to the level of qualifier. The correspondence of the FIM scores to the ICF qualifiers is presented in Table 4. For practical purposes, it was assumed that the higher level of dependence by FIM, the higher the level of the problem.

Source	Report from psychologist
Meaning unit	…"marked decrease in attention"…
Correspondent ICF Code	**b140** Attention functions
Correspondent qualifier	3 (serious problem - "marked")

Table 3. Identification of a meaning unit and linking it to the ICF code and qualifier.

FIM score	**ICF qualifier**
1	4
2	3
3	3
4	2
5	1
6	1
7	0

Table 4. Correspondence of FIM scores to the ICF qualifiers.

Obtained ICF-based functional profile of a patient is presented in Table 5. The profile describes functioning of the patient at the admission and at the discharge. The majority of functional problems of a patient at the level of "body functions" were found in the domains of mental functions and movement-related functions. Within the list of "activities and participation", the patient experienced more difficulties with acquiring skills, communication and activities, related to mobility and self-care. Several relevant environmental factors were identified as well.

In this particular example ICF did not provide any additional information about functioning of a patient, as all the information was taken from the existing medical records. Nevertheless, ICF provided structure to the large amount of diverse information and gave a clear, easy and holistic view of all the different aspects of functioning reflected in different reports and documents.

This case study also demonstrates some weak points of the medical documentation. For example, almost no information was found in the medical records regarding activities, related to the daily life (chapter 6 - Domestic life, which includes preparing meals, caring for

Code	Description	Admission ICF qualifier	Discharge ICF qualifier
b1	**MENTAL FUNCTIONS**		
b110	**Consciousness functions** General mental functions of the state of awareness and alertness, including the clarity and continuity of the wakeful state.	0	0
b114	**Orientation functions** General mental functions of knowing and ascertaining one's relation to self, to others, to time and to one's surroundings.	3	1
b140	**Attention functions** Specific mental functions of focusing on an external stimulus or internal experience for the required period of time.	3	3
b144	**Memory functions** Specific mental functions of registering and storing information and retrieving it as needed.	3	1
b156	**Perceptual functions** Specific mental functions of recognizing and interpreting sensory stimuli.	0	0
b167	**Mental functions of language** Specific mental functions of recognizing and using signs, symbols and other components of a language.	3	1
b2	**SENSORY FUNCTIONS AND PAIN**		
b230	**Hearing functions** Sensory functions relating to sensing the presence of sounds and discriminating the location, pitch, loudness and quality of sounds.	8	8
b5	**FUNCTIONS OF THE DIGESTIVE, METABOLIC AND ENDOCRINE SYSTEMS**		
b510	**Ingestion functions** Functions related to taking in and manipulating solids or liquids through the mouth into the body.	1	0
b525	**Defecation functions** Functions of elimination of wastes and undigested food as faeces and related functions.	0	0
b6	**GENITOURINARY AND REPRODUCTIVE FUNCTIONS**		
b620	**Urination functions** Functions of discharge of urine from the urinary bladder.	0	0
b7	**NEUROMUSCULOSKELETAL AND MOVEMENT RELATED FUNCTIONS**		
b710	**Mobility of joint functions** Functions of the range and ease of movement of a joint.	1	1
b730	**Muscle power functions** Functions related to the force generated by the contraction of a muscle or muscle groups.	8	8
b750	**Motor reflex functions** Functions of involuntary contraction of muscles automatically induced by specific stimuli.	2	1
s	**BODY STRUCTURES**		
s2	**THE EYE, EAR AND RELATED STRUCTURES**	8	8
s610	**Structure of urinary system**	8	8
s750	**Structure of lower extremity**	8	8
s550	**Structure of pancreas**	8	8
s420	**Structure of immune system**	8	8
d	**ACTIVITIES AND PARTICIPATION**		
d155	**Acquiring skills** Developing basic and complex competencies in integrated sets of actions or tasks so as to initiate and follow through with the acquisition of a skill, such as manipulating tools or playing games like chess.	Cap 3	Cap 1
d166	**Reading** Performing activities involved in the comprehension and interpretation of written language (e.g. books, instructions or newspapers in text or Braille), for the purpose of obtaining general knowledge or specific information.	Cap 0 Per 0	Cap 0 Per 0
d175	**Solving problems** Finding solutions to questions or situations by identifying and analysing issues, developing options and solutions, evaluating potential effects of solutions, and executing a chosen solution, such as in resolving a dispute between two people.	Cap 3	Cap 1
d3	**COMMUNICATION**		
d310	**Communicating with – receiving – spoken messages** Comprehending literal and implied meanings of messages in spoken language, such as understanding that a statement asserts a fact or is an idiomatic expression.	Cap 3	Cap 1
d350	**Conversation** Starting, sustaining and ending an interchange of thoughts and ideas, carried out by means of spoken, written, sign or other forms of language, with one or more people one knows or who are strangers, in formal or casual settings.	Cap 1 Per 1	Cap 1 Per 1
d4	**MOBILITY**		

d410	**Changing basic body position** Getting into and out of a body position and moving from one location to another, such as getting up out of a chair to lie down on a bed, and getting into and out of positions of kneeling or squatting.	Cap 1 Per 1	Cap 1 Per 1
d420	**Transferring oneself** Moving from one surface to another, such as sliding along a bench or moving from a bed to a chair, without changing body position.	Cap 1 Per 1	Cap 1 Per 1
d440	**Fine hand use** Performing the coordinated actions of handling objects, picking up, manipulating and releasing them using one's hand, fingers and thumb, such as required to lift coins off a table or turn a dial or knob.	Cap 1 Per 1	Cap 0 Per 0
d450	**Walking** Moving along a surface on foot, step by step, so that one foot is always on the ground, such as when strolling, sauntering, walking forwards, backwards, or sideways.	Cap 3 Per 2	Cap 1 Per 1
d455	**Moving around** Moving the whole body from one place to another by means other than walking, such as climbing over a rock or running down a stree, skippin, scapering, jumping, somersaulting or running around obstacles.	Cap 1 Per 1	Cap 1 Per 1
d460	**Moving around in different locations** Walking and moving around in various places and situations, such as walking between rooms in a house, within a building, or down the street of a town.	Cap 1 Per 1	Cap 1 Per 1
d465	**Moving around using equipment** Moving the whole body from place to place, on any surface or space, by using specific devices designed to facilitate moving or create other ways of moving around, such as with skates, skis, or scuba equipment, or moving down the street in a wheelchair or a walker.	Cap 9	Cap 0
d5	SELF-CARE		
d510	**Washing oneself** Washing and drying one's whole body, or body parts, using water and appropriate cleaning and drying materials or methods, such as bathing, showering, washing hands and feet, face and hair, and drying with a towel.	Cap 1 Per 1	Cap 1 Per 1
d520	**Caring for body parts** Looking afer those parts of the body, such as skin, face, teeth, scalp, nails and genitals, that require more than washing and drying.	Cap 1 Per 1	Cap 1 Per 1
d530	**Toileting** Planning and carrying out the elimination of human waste (menstruation, urination and defecation), and cleaning oneself afterwards.	Cap 1 Per 1	Cap 1 Per 1
d540	**Dressing** Carrying out the coordinated actions and tasks of putting on and taking off clothes and footwear in sequence and in keeping with climatic and social conditions, such as by putting on, adjusting and removing shirts, skirts, blouses, pants, undergarments, saris, kimono, tights, hats, gloves, coats, shoes, boots, sandals and slippers.	Cap 1 Per 1	Cap 1 Per 1
d550	**Eating** Carrying out the coordinated tasks and actions of eating food that has been served, bringing it to the mouth and consuming it in culturally acceptable ways, cutting or breaking food into pieces, opening bottles and cans, using eating implements, having meals, feasting or dining.	Cap 1 Per 1	Cap 0 Per 0
d560	**Drinking** Taking hold of a drink, bringing it to the mouth, and consuming the drink in culturally acceptable ways, mixing, stirring and pouring liquids for drinking, opening bottles and cans, drinking through a straw or drinking running water such as from a tap or a spring; feeding from the breast.	Cap 1 Per 1	Cap 0 Per 0
d7	INTERPERSONAL INTERACTIONS AND RELATIONSHIPS	Cap 3 Per 3	Cap 1 Per 1
e1	PRODUCTS AND TECHNOLOGY		
e120	**Products and technology for personal indoor and outdoor mobility and transportation** Equipment, products and technologies used by people in activities of moving inside and outside buildings, including those adapted or specially designed, located in, on or near the person using them.	9	+3
e3	SUPPORT AND RELATIONSHIPS		
e310	**Immediate family** Individuals related by birth, marriage or other relationship recognized by the culture as immediate family, such as spouses, partners, parents, siblings, children, foster parents, adoptive parents and grandparents.	+8	+8
e355	**Health professionals** All service providers working within the context of the health system, such as doctors, nurses, physiotherapists, occupational therapists, speech therapists, audiologists, orthotist-prosthetists, medical social workers.	+8	+8
e5	SERVICES, SYSTEMS AND POLICIES		
e580	**Health services, systems and policies** Services, systems and policies for preventing and treating health problems, providing medical rehabilitation and promoting a healthy lifestyle.	+8	+8

Table 5. ICF-based functional profile of the patient (Cap=capacity, Per=performance).

household objects, doing housework etc.), interpersonal interactions and relationships, major life areas (which include education, work and employment, and economic life) and community, social and civic life (which includes recreation and leisure, religion and spirituality).

Little information was also found concerning the relevant environmental factors. Those that were identified correspond to "products and technology for daily use" and "support and relationships". Health professionals and "health services, systems and policies" were also found to be the facilitating environmental factors. Rehabilitation had a positive influence mostly on functions of language and memory and activities that are related to mobility and self-care. Some of these are difficult to assess in a rehabilitation hospital, since the patient has to stay at home for some time in order to comprehend the extent of problems with these activities. The impact of the environment is also difficult to assess before the patient has been living at home for a while. Before finishing the rehabilitation, patients usually go home for a weekend to face the reality. After such visits, clinicians should describe the problems that the patients had at home better and be able to suggest feasible solutions. The later should also be written in the medical records.

Many areas could not be assessed specifically. The qualifier "8" (standing for "not specified") was used due to the fact that particular aspects of functioning are not described sufficiently enough to determine the scale of the problem or the role of an environmental factor. In these areas, it was also not possible to demonstrate any improvement. Clinicians will have to find appropriate outcome measures for assessing these categories.

Another advantage of the ICF lies in its easy and language-independent format that is especially important in the united Europe and the globalised world of today. Being neutral, ICF also underlines the strong sides of an individual that are important for rehabilitation and further functioning. However, little information was found in relation with the environmental factors.

Therefore even in cases when conventional medical records have been already created ICF may help to structure the information about functioning in a clear, easy and holistic way. The study revealed that some aspects of functioning are currently not sufficiently described in the medical records. In the future, ICF could help professionals to draw more attention to the important aspects of functioning and the environmental factors relevant for functioning.

6. ICF as a tool to organize clinical information and evaluate the outcome of rehabilitation

Another retrospective study conducted in Slovenia involved analysis of the medical records of 100 patients with brain injury admitted to the URI. Its goal was to explore to what extend the ICF can be a useful tool to organize existing clinical information and to retrospectively evaluate the effect of interventions in patients with BI (Ptyushkin et al. 2010).

Overall (i.e., for all the patients included in the study, at admission and/or at discharge), 51 codes for body functions, 22 for body structures, 62 for activities and participation, and 35 relevant environmental factors were identified. They are presented in the Tables 6-9 below.

As it can be seen from Table 6, three major groups of functional problems corresponding to the list of *body functions* were identified: related to mental functions (15 out of 51 codes or nearly 30%), related to sensory functions (12 out of 51 codes or nearly 24%), and related to mobility (8 out of 51 codes or nearly 16%). Functional problems were also frequently found for speech (b310, b320 and b330). Major improvements were found regarding *orientation functions* (b114), *energy and drive functions* (b130), *memory functions* (b144), *mental functions of language* (b167), *vestibular functions* (b235), *sensation of pain* (b280), *voice and articulation functions* (b310 and b320), *ingestion functions* (b510), *defecation and urination functions* (b525 and b620), *mobility and muscle power functions* (b710 and b730), and *control of voluntary movement functions* (b760). Little or no changes were observed for most of the mental functions. Worsening of a body function was detected in three patients - one in *perceptual functions* (b156), one in *sensation of pain* (b280), and one in *control of voluntary movement functions* (b760).

ICF code	Description	Described at admission	Described at admission as a problem	At discharge			
				Improvement	Worsening	No change	Unclear
Mental functions							
b110	Consciousness functions	100	0	0	0	100	0
b114	Orientation functions	89	63	22	0	66	1
b117	Intellectual functions	23	18	3	0	20	0
b126	Temperament and personality functions	44	38	2	0	42	0
b130	Energy and drive functions	61	22	10	0	51	0
b134	Sleep functions	6	5	0	0	5	1
b140	Attention functions	77	75	4	0	72	1
b144	Memory functions	97	93	33	0	64	0
b147	Psychomotor functions	18	16	2	0	10	6
b152	Emotional functions	48	39	5	0	42	1
b156	Perceptual functions	26	18	1	1	23	1
b160	Thought functions	32	30	0	0	31	1
b164	Higher-level cognitive functions	59	46	2	0	57	0
b167	Mental functions of language	95	79	34	0	61	0
b172	Calculation functions	3	3	0	0	2	1
Sensory functions							
b210	Seeing functions	32	32	2	0	26	4
b215	Functions of structures adjoining the eye	4	4	0	0	4	0
b230	Hearing functions	19	18	0	0	18	1
b235	Vestibular functions	55	53	23	0	21	11
b240	Sensations associated with hearing and vestibular function	16	16	1	0	13	2
b250	Taste function	5	4	1	0	4	0
b255	Smell function	7	6	0	0	7	0
b265	Touch function	2	2	1	0	1	0
b280	Sensation of pain	49	45	10	1	31	7
Voice and speech							
b310	Voice functions	12	12	6	0	6	0
b320	Articulation functions	28	21	9	0	19	0

b330	**Fluency and rhythm of speech functions**	26	23	4	0	22	0
Different organs functions							
b410	**Heart functions**	11	3	1	0	9	1
b415	**Blood vessel functions**	1	1	0	0	1	0
b420	**Blood pressure functions**	20	14	0	0	20	0
b430	**Hematological system functions**	2	1	0	0	2	0
b440	**Respiration functions**	7	5	0	0	7	0
b510	**Ingestion functions**	100	83	43	0	57	0
b525	**Defecation functions**	100	54	29	0	71	0
b530	**Weight maintenance functions**	3	3	0	0	3	0
b540	**General metabolic functions**	1	1	1	0	0	0
b550	**Thermoregulatory functions**	1	0	0	0	1	0
b555	**Endocrine gland functions**	5	5	0	0	5	0
b620	**Urination functions**	100	57	33	0	67	0
Mobility-related functions							
b710	**Mobility of joint functions**	69	50	19	0	43	7
b730	**Muscle power functions**	80	72	29	0	38	13
b735	**Muscle tone functions**	33	16	3	1	23	6
b750	**Motor reflex functions**	32	16	3	0	26	3
b755	**Involuntary movement reaction functions**	11	11	2	0	5	4
b760	**Control of voluntary movement functions**	20	16	9	1	8	2
b765	**Involuntary movement functions**	1	1	1	0	0	0
b770	**Gait pattern functions**	1	1	1	0	0	0
b8	**FUNCTIONS OF THE SKIN AND RELATED STRUCTURES**	1	1	0	0	1	0

Table 6. Body Functions (all values are no. of cases, which equal percentages since n=100).

Table 7 shows that the general profile of the patients regarding body structures corresponds to the diagnoses according to the ICD-10. Some of the structures are related to the TBI itself or concomitant injuries (structure of the brain and spinal cord, structure of head and neck region and extremities). Others (like structure of cardiovascular or respiratory system) reflect the comorbidities of the patient.

Restrictions in activities and participation (Table 8) were frequently found in *acquiring skills* (d155), *reading* and *writing* (d166 and d170), *solving problems* (d175) and *undertaking a task* (d210 and d220). Another group of common restrictions is related to communication - *receiving messages* (d310 and d315), *speaking* (d330), *writing messages* (d345) and *conversation* (d350). Frequently there were also disturbed activities related to mobility (*changing and maintaining a body position, transferring oneself, walking and moving around*) and very

ICF code	Description	Described at admission	Described at admission as a problem	At discharge			
				Improvement	Worsening	No change	Unclear
s110	Structure of brain	100	100	1	0	87	12
s120	Spinal cord and related structures	2	2	0	0	2	0
S2	THE EYE, EAR AND RELATED STRUCTURES	7	7	0	0	7	0
s3200	Teeth	1	1	0	0	1	0
s410	Structure of cardiovascular system	11	11	0	0	10	1
s420	Structure of immune system	1	1	0	0	1	0
s430	Structure of respiratory system	7	7	0	0	7	0
s550	Structure of pancreas	1	1	0	0	1	0
s610	Structure of urinary system	2	2	0	0	2	0
s630	Structure of reproductive system	1	1	0	0	1	0
s710	Structure of head and neck region	26	26	0	0	25	1
s720	Structure of shoulder region	4	4	0	0	4	0
s730	Structure of upper extremity	10	10	0	0	10	0
s740	Structure of pelvic region	1	1	0	0	1	0
s750	Structure of lower extremity	20	20	3	1	15	1
s760	Structure of trunk	9	9	0	0	9	0
S8	SKIN AND RELATED STRUCTURES	32	32	0	0	27	5

Table 7. Body Structures (all values are no. of cases, which equal percentages since n=100).

frequently those related to self-care (d510-d570). Finally problems were found frequently in the areas of interpersonal relationships (d710 - d770), *in acquiring, keeping and terminating a job* (d845) and *recreation and leisure* (d920).

Considerable improvements at the discharge were detected in the following areas: acquiring skills, solving problems and receiving spoken messages, mobility (d410-d460) and self-care (d510 - d560). Improvement was also found for general interpersonal interactions (d7). Worsening was frequently found for *driving* (d475). Worsening was also found once for *complex interpersonal interactions* (d720), *formal relationships* (d740) and *acquiring, keeping and terminating of a job* (d845).

Based on the medical records, 35 environmental factors were identified in the 100 studied individuals. Twenty of them, which are presented in Table 9, were present in the majority of patients. Some of those environmental factors may act both as facilitators and barriers in different patients. For example, the role of the *immediate family* (e310) may be either a strong facilitator of equally strong barrier for rehabilitation.

ICF code	Description	Described at admission	Described at admission as a problem	At discharge			
				Improvement	Worsening	No change	Unclear
d110	Watching	4	3	1	0	3	0
d115	Listening	5	4	2	0	3	0
d155	Acquiring skills	96	91	34	0	62	0
d166	Reading	27	20	3	0	22	2
d170	Writing	34	26	5	0	27	2
d172	Calculating	10	9	1	0	9	0
d175	Solving problems	96	91	34	0	60	2
d210	Undertaking a single task	24	14	4	0	19	1
d220	Undertaking multiple tasks	24	18	3	0	19	2
d230	Carrying out daily routine	26	19	11	0	13	2
d310	Communicating with - receiving - spoken messages	96	80	33	0	63	0
d315	Communicating with - receiving - nonverbal messages	23	19	9	0	14	0
d330	Speaking	26	15	7	0	19	0
d335	Producing nonverbal messages	2	1	2	0	0	0
d345	Writing messages	31	28	2	0	26	3
d350	Conversation	36	29	6	0	28	2
d360	Using communication devices and techniques	2	2	0	0	1	1
d410	Changing basic body position	100	88	40	0	60	0
d415	Maintaining a body position	26	17	10	0	15	1
d420	Transferring oneself	100	80	43	0	57	0
d430	Lifting and carrying objects	1	1	0	0	1	0
d440	Fine hand use	100	83	43	0	57	0
d450	Walking	81	60	45	1	34	1
d455	Moving around	89	75	41	0	48	0
d460	Moving around in different locations	88	72	51	0	37	0
d465	Moving around using equipment	14	11	5	0	5	4
d475	Driving	34	33	0	14	19	1
d510	Washing oneself	100	93	52	0	48	0
d520	Caring for body parts	100	88	45	0	55	0
d530	Toileting	100	82	41	0	59	0
d540	Dressing	100	89	49	0	51	0
d550	Eating	100	83	43	0	57	0
d560	Drinking	100	83	43	0	57	0
d570	Looking after one's health	11	6	3	0	8	0
d630	Preparing meals	1	1	1	0	0	0
d640	Doing housework	6	5	2	0	3	1
d660	Assisting others	1	0	1	0	0	0

D7	INTERPERSONAL INTERACTIONS AND RELATIONSHIPS	95	86	34	0	60	1
d710	Basic interpersonal interactions	15	6	3	0	11	1
d720	Complex interpersonal interactions	15	10	4	1	10	0
d730	Relating with strangers	4	1	0	0	4	0
d740	Formal relationships	26	7	3	1	22	0
d750	Informal social relationships	5	0	0	0	5	0
d760	Family relationships	6	2	0	0	6	0
d770	Intimate relationships	1	1	0	0	1	0
d810	Informal education	1	1	0	0	1	0
d820	School education	5	4	1	0	3	1
d830	Higher education	4	4	0	0	4	0
d845	Acquiring, keeping and terminating a job	39	35	0	1	28	10
d850	Remunerative employment	1	1	0	0	1	0
d920	Recreation and leisure	13	10	1	0	10	2
d950	Political life and citizenship	1	1	0	0	1	0

Table 8. Activities and Participation – Performance (all values are no. of cases, which equal percentages since n=100).

After linking, it became clear that the three major groups of functional problems regarding *body functions* in patients after TBI are related to mental functions, sensory functions and mobility. Another important group is related to speech. The improvements found at the end of rehabilitation for mobility-related functions (b710-b770), and in some patients for speech functions, can be explained by the fact that the current rehabilitation program is mainly focused on these particular aspects of functioning. At the same time much less improvement was observed for mental functions with the exception of orientation, energy and drive functions and memory, although the patients were assessed and advised by a psychologist. This important difference in the evolution of mental and physical consequences is very common in patients after the TBI. It can be also related to the fact that the time of rehabilitation is usually too short to produce and detect substantial changes at the level of mental functions.

The general profile of patients regarding *body structures* corresponded to the diagnoses according to the ICD-10. Some of the structures are related to the TBI itself or concomitant injuries (structure of the brain and spinal cord, structure of head and neck region and extremities). Others (like structure of cardiovascular or respiratory system) reflect the comorbidities of the patient.

Restrictions in *activities and participation* found in the study were frequently caused by or related to the disturbances in *mental functions* (like *acquiring skills, reading* and *writing, solving problems* and *undertaking a task)* and generally show little to moderate changes from the admission to the discharge. Another large group of restricted *activities and participation* which showed considerable improvement was related to mobility functions (11 out of 62 codes or nearly 18%). Notable improvements were also found in activities related to self-care and this can be explained by the fact that the work of nurses and occupational therapists involved in the process of rehabilitation is mainly focused on these aspects of

Environmental factors			
Barriers		**Facilitators**	
e155	**Design, construction and building products and technology of buildings for private use**	**e110**	**Products or substances for personal consumption**
e165	**Assets**	**e115**	**Products and technology for personal use in daily living**
e210	**Physical geography**	**e120**	**Products and technology for personal indoor and outdoor mobility and transportation**
e310	**Immediate family**	**e310**	**Immediate family**
e460	**Societal attitudes**	**e320**	**Friends**
e525	**Housing services, systems and policies**	**e330**	**People in positions of authority**
e570	**Social security services, systems and policies**	**e355**	**Health professionals**
e575	**General social support services, systems and policies**	**e410**	**Individual attitudes of immediate family members**
		e570	**Social security services, systems and policies**
		e575	**General social support services, systems and policies**
		e580	**Health services, systems and policies**
		e585	**Education and training services, systems and policies**

Table 9. The Environmental Factors found to be relevant for the majority of patients.

functioning. More serious problems described for *driving* at the discharge were not because at the admission the driving abilities of the patients were necessarily better, but because during the rehabilitation they were found insufficient, often after being tested on the driving simulator and this was clearly stated at the time of the discharge.

Some of the relevant environmental factors identified in the study may act both as facilitators and barriers in different patients. For example, the role of the immediate family (e310) may be either a strong facilitator of equally strong barrier for rehabilitation. The potential of the ICF to describe the impact of the environmental factors is an important strength of the classification and ICF-based tools. However, it should be mentioned that the study also revealed that insufficient attention is still drawn to the role of environmental factors for rehabilitation and after rehabilitation life of an individual. This can be due to the lack of suitable instruments for describing the environment. Gathering information about the environmental factors in a systematic and internationally standardized way can help take the influences of the environment more into consideration at all levels, and the ICF may be helpful in this respect.

The ICF also structures the large amount of information and provides a clear, easy and holistic view of all different aspects of functioning, reflected in different reports and documents. Another advantage of the ICF is in its easy and language-independent format that is especially important in a united Europe and globalized world of today. Being neutral, ICF can also underline the strong sides of an individual important for rehabilitation and further functioning. Frequent use of the qualifier "8" ("not specified") is mainly related to the fact that particular aspects of functioning are not described sufficiently enough to determine the scale of the problem or the role of an environmental factor. At the same time, the value of the qualifier "not specified" should not be underestimated as it draws attention to a particular aspect of functioning where based on the available information the level of the problem cannot be clearly defined. Activities and participation related with the daily life that are especially important for functioning after discharge (like Chapter 6, Domestic life, and Chapter 9, Community, social and civic life) were poorly described in the medical records. This indicates that still not enough attention is drawn to these aspects of human functioning during rehabilitation. We assume that in some cases it is very difficult if not impossible to assess these aspects of functioning during the hospitalization and it is only possible to predict that difficulties will be there when a person is back in his or her common environment.

A strength of the ICF is also in its capacity to describe the consequences of the comorbidities, i.e., conditions that are not related to the main condition (TBI).

In general it can be said that substantial improvement was found for those functions, activities and participation, the current rehabilitation program is focused on. Therefore the ICF may help in modifying the existing programs or adapting them to the individual cases.

7. Conclusions

Use of the ICF in brain injury rehabilitation interactively models functioning and disability associated with this health condition. The appropriate tools for daily practice such as ICF Core Sets for Traumatic Brain Injury allow to apply this interactive holistic approach into practice. ICF-based rehabilitation of the persons after brain injury facilitates truly interdisciplinary work by providing a common framework for all professionals involved in rehabilitation of such a patient. Practical ICF tools can allow specialists to speak the common professional language and extend the boundaries of rehabilitation making the whole process highly individualized on solving problems of a concrete patient thou rigorously standard.

8. Acknowledges

The authors are grateful to Michaela Coenen, Heinrich Gall and Alarcos Cieza, ICF Research Branch, WHO FIC Collaborating Center, Institute for Health and Rehabilitation Sciences, Ludwig-Maximilian University in Munich, for technical help. The studies described in this chapter were conducted within the MURINET project (Multidisciplinary Research Network on Health and Disability in Europe).

9. References

Andelic N, Sigurdardottir S, Schanke AK, Sandvik L, Sveen U, Roe C. Disability, physical health and mental health 1 year after traumatic brain injury. Disabil Rehabil 2010;32:1122–1131.

Bilbao A, Kennedy C, Chatterji S, Ustün B, Barquero JL, Barth JT. The ICF: Applications of the WHO model of
functioning, disability and health to brain injury rehabilitation. NeuroRehabilitation 2003;18:239–250.

Cameron ID, Tate RL, Leibbrandt L. Applying the ICF to assessment scales in acquired brain injury [Presentation]. Canberra: Australian Institute of Health and Welfare; 2009. Available online at: http://www.docstoc.com/docs/3825602/Applying-the-ICF-to-assessment-scales-in-acquired-brain-injury, accessed 24 April 2010.

Kokshoorn, N., Smit, J.W., Nieuwlaat, W.A., Tiemensma, J., Bisschop, P., Groote, V.R., Roelfsema, F., Franken, A.A., Wassenaar, M., Biermasz, N.R., Romijn, J.A., & Pereira, A.M. (2011) Low prevalence of hypopituitarism after traumatic brain injury - a multi-center study. *European Journal of Endocrinology,*

Kokshoorn, N.E., Wassenaar, M.J., Biermasz, N.R., Roelfsema, F., Smit, J.W., Romijn, J.A., & Pereira, A.M. (2010) Hypopituitarism following traumatic brain injury: prevalence is affected by the use of different dynamic tests and different normal values. *European Journal of Endocrinology,* 162 (1), pp. 11-18.

Kornblum, R.N. & Fisher, R.S. (1969) Pituitary lesions in craniocerebral injuries. *Archives of pathology,* 88 (3), pp. 242-248.

Krahulik, D., Zapletalova, J., Frysak, Z., & Vaverka, M. (2010) Dysfunction of hypothalamic-hypophysial axis after traumatic brain injury in adults. *Journal of Neurosurgery,* 113 (3), pp. 581-584.

Kreitschmann-Andermahr, I., Poll, E.M., Reineke, A., Gilsbach, J.M., Brabant, G., Buchfelder, M., Fassbender, W., Faust, M., Kann, P.H., & Wallaschofski, H. (2008) Growth hormone deficient patients after traumatic brain injury--baseline characteristics and benefits after growth hormone replacement--an analysis of the German KIMS database. *Growth Hormone & IGF Research,* 18 (6), pp. 472-478.

Lamberts, S.W., de Herder, W.W., & van der Lely, A.J. (1998) Pituitary insufficiency. *Lancet,* 352 (9122), pp. 127-134.

Lania, A., Persani, L., & Beck-Peccoz, P. (2008) Central hypothyroidism. *Pituitary.,* 11 (2), pp. 181-186.

Leal-Cerro, A., Flores, J.M., Rincon, M., Murillo, F., Pujol, M., Garcia-Pesquera, F., Dieguez, C., & Casanueva, F.F. (2005) Prevalence of hypopituitarism and growth hormone deficiency in adults long-term after severe traumatic brain injury. *Clinical Endocrinology,* 62 (5), pp. 525-532.

Lieberman, S.A., Oberoi, A.L., Gilkison, C.R., Masel, B.E., & Urban, R.J. (2001) Prevalence of neuroendocrine dysfunction in patients recovering from traumatic brain injury. *Journal of Clinical Endocrinology and Metabolism,* 86 (6), pp. 2752-2756.

Maiya, B., Newcombe, V., Nortje, J., Bradley, P., Bernard, F., Chatfield, D., Outtrim, J., Hutchinson, P., Matta, B., Antoun, N., & Menon, D. (2007) Magnetic resonance imaging changes in the pituitary gland following acute traumatic brain injury. *Intensive Care Medicine,*

Makimura, H., Stanley, T., Mun, D., You, S.M., & Grinspoon, S. (2008) The effects of central adiposity on growth hormone (GH) response to GH-releasing hormone-arginine stimulation testing in men. *Journal of Clinical Endocrinology and Metabolism,* 93 (11), pp. 4254-4260.

Maric, N.P., Doknic, M., Pavlovic, D., Pekic, S., Stojanovic, M., Jasovic-Gasic, M., & Popovic, V. (2010) Psychiatric and neuropsychological changes in growth hormone-deficient patients after traumatic brain injury in response to growth hormone therapy. *Journal of Endocrinological Investigation,* 33 (11), pp. 770-775.

Miller, K.K., Biller, B.M., Lipman, J.G., Bradwin, G., Rifai, N., & Klibanski, A. (2005) Truncal adiposity, relative growth hormone deficiency, and cardiovascular risk. *Journal of Clinical Endocrinology and Metabolism,* 90 (2), pp. 768-774.

Cerniauskaite M, Quintas R, Boldt C, et al. Systematic literature review on ICF from 2001 to 2009: its use, implementation and operationalisation. Disabil Rehabil 2010.

Cieza A, Geyh S, Chatterji S, Kostanjsek N, Ustün B, Stucki G. ICF linking rules: an update based on lessons learned. J Rehabil Med. 2005 Jul;37(4):212-8.

Cieza A, Ewert T, Ustun TB, Chatterji S, Kostanjsek N, Stucki G. Development of ICF Core Sets for patients with chronic conditions. J Rehabil Med 2004:9-11.

ICF Research Branch. ICF Core Set for Traumatic Brain Injury. http://www.icf-research-branch.org/icf-core-sets-projects/neurological-conditions/development-of-icf-core-sets-for-traumatic-brain-injury-tbi.html Last accessed June 2011

Jelsma J. Use of the International Classification of Functioning, Disability and Health: a literature survey. J Rehabil Med 2009;41:1-12.

Fries W, Fischer S. Participation limitations following acquired brain damage: A pilot study on the relationship

among functional disorders as well as personal and environmental context factors. Rehabilitation (Stuttg) 2008;47:265–274.

Kostanjsek N, Rubinelli S, Escorpizo R, Cieza A, Kennedy C, Selb M, Stucki G, Ustün TB. Assessing the impact of health conditions using the ICF. Disabil Rehabil. 2011;33(15-16):1475-82. Epub 2010 Oct 14

Ptyushkin P, Vidmar G, Burger H, Marincek C. Linking Medical Records and Assessment Instruments to the ICF. Presentation of a Case. Rehabilitacija - VIII, 2 (2009)

Ptyushkin P, Vidmar G, Burger H, Marincek C. Use of the International Classification of Functioning, Disability and Health (ICF) in patients with traumatic brain injury. Brain Inj. 2010;24(13-14):1519-27. Epub 2010 Oct 25.

Rauch A., Cieza A., Stucki G. How to apply the ICF for Rehabilitation management in clinical practice, Eur J Phys Rehabil Med 2008; 44:329-42

Rentsch HP, Bucher P, Dommen Nyffeler I, et al. The implementation of the 'International Classification of Functioning, Disability and Health' (ICF) in daily practice of neurorehabilitation: an interdisciplinary project at the Kantonsspital of Lucerne, Switzerland. Disabil Rehabil 2003;25:411-21.

Stucki G., Ewert T., Cieza A. Value and application of the ICF in rehabilitation medicine. Disabil Rehabil. 2003 Jun 3-17;25(11-12):628-34.

Stucki G, Cieza A, Melvin J. The ICF: A unifying model for the conceptual description of the rehabilitation strategy. J Rehabil Med 2007; 39: 279-285

Stucki G, Kostanjsek N, Ustun B, Cieza A. ICF-based classification and measurement of functioning. European journal of physical and rehabilitation medicine 2008; 44:315-28.

Schweizer Paraplegiker Forschung, Implementation of the International Classification of Functioning, Disability and Health (ICF) in rehabilitation practice. (Accessed 18. November 2010), at www.icf-casestudies.org.

Svestkova O, Angerova Y, Sladkova P, Bickenbach JE, Raggi A. Functioning and disability in traumatic brain injury. Disabil Rehabil. 2010;32 Suppl 1:S68-77. Epub 2010 Oct 7.

Svestkova O, Angerova Y. ICF Model in Neurorehabilitation (MHADIE) International Journal of Rehabilitation Research. 32():S48-S49, Aug 2009.

Whyte J. Directions in brain injury research: From concept to clinical implementation. Neuropsychol Rehabil. 2009 Dec;19(6):807-23. Epub 2009 Jun 19.

World Health Organization. ICF: International classification of functioning, disability and health. Geneva, Switzerland: WHO Publishing; 2001

Zamenhof L. Dr. Esperanto's International Language. Introduction and complete grammar. http://www.genekeyes.com/Dr_Esperanto.html Last accessed June 2011

6

The Impact of Intensive Community Based Rehabilitation on Community Participation and Life Satisfaction Following Severe Traumatic Brain Injury

Steven Wheeler
West Virginia University School of Medicine, Occupational Therapy Division
Morgantown, West Virginia
USA

1. Introduction

Brain injury represents the leading cause of death and disability worldwide (International Brain Injury Association [IBIA], 2011). While a small percentage of traumatic brain injury (TBI) survivors continue in a persistent state of coma, the vast majority return to the community with some residual cognitive, psychosocial, behavioral, or physical impairment (Kersel et al., 2001). These impairments contribute to a dramatic change in the individual's life course, profound disruption of the family, enormous loss of income or earning potential and large expenses over a lifetime (McKinlay and Watkiss, 2001).

The need for effective post-acute rehabilitation for traumatic brain injuries has emerged out of both the limited effectiveness of inpatient models (Department of Health and Human Services [DHHS], 2001) and health care system changes that support reduced average length of inpatient stay (Canadian Institute for Health Information, 2008). Within a traditional inpatient model, interventions generally center around medications, surgery, and therapeutic exercises / activities. While this approach is recognized as a necessary component of TBI treatment, it has been argued that by fostering the 'patient' role, the inpatient setting has been inadequate for facilitating improvement in important life roles (Willer, et al., 1992). Roles such as parent, spouse, student, employee, and friend are considered essential to successful and satisfying performance in community settings yet are rarely specifically addressed in traditional brain injury rehabilitation models.

Determining what constitutes "successful" rehabilitation following traumatic brain injury has received considerable attention among brain injury clinicians and researchers. Many researchers view community integration as the goal of rehabilitation professionals and the rehabilitation programs (Doig, et al., 2001; McColl, et al., 1998). Successful community integration has been described as settling clients into communities where they are both happy and productive (McColl et al., 1998). Life satisfaction has also been considered an important health indicator and measure of rehabilitation outcome (Department of Health and Human Services [DHHS], 2001).

This study examined community integration and life satisfaction over a one-year period among persons with severe traumatic brain injury who are participated in a residential, interdisciplinary, community based rehabilitation program. It is an extension of the work of Wheeler, et al., (2007) who studied the effectiveness of intensive, life skills training with individuals with severe TBI. Findings from that research supported the treatment approach to improve community integration. However, no change was observed in self-reported life satisfaction at 90-day follow-up.

2. Literature review

In *Healthy People 2010*, a list of objectives designed to serve as a framework for improving the health of people in the United States, both societal participation and life satisfaction are highlighted in the discussion of health related goals for persons with disabilities in the United States (Department of Health and Human Services [DHHS], 2001). Participation is also the core construct of the World Health Organization's *International Classification of Functioning, Disability, and Health* (ICF) (World Health Organization [WHO], 2001). Within the ICF, a disability is considered to be the consequence of thwarted efforts to interact and participate in a variety of environments (Scherer, 2002).

Problems with community participation and life satisfaction are commonly reported in outcomes based research with persons with TBI. Persons with TBI have been found to be less likely to live independently, be fully employed, and participate successfully in housekeeping, parenting, or leisure activities. Additionally, TBI is often associated with profound social isolation. Several studies have shown that persons with TBI experience reductions in the size of their social networks as well as the loss of pre-injury friends (Morton & Wehman, 1995; Kersel, et al., 2001; Siebert, et al., 2002). Hoofien and colleagues (2001) reported that 30% of participants endorsed having no social contacts outside the family system 10-20 years after TBI. Other studies have supported limited social contacts post injury with accompanying feelings of loneliness (Lezak, 1988; Harrick, et al., 1994).

2.1 Community participation following TBI

Gordon, Hibbard, Brown, et al. (1999) used the Community Integration Questionnaire (CIQ) to evaluate differences in community functioning between TBI and non-disabled samples. The CIQ is a measure designed to assess reintegration into the community after TBI (Willer, et al., 1993). Findings of this study were consistent with similar studies (Corrigan & Deming, 1995; Willer, et al., 1993) in that the TBI group had a lower CIQ total score and lower scores on each of the instrument's three subscales than the non-disabled samples. Subscales of the CIQ represent the individual's degree of integration in the home, in social networks, and into productive activities. By focusing on an individual's societal participation as the end objective of rehabilitation, as opposed to more discrete deficit measurement of impairment and activities, treatment planning and programming becomes more sensitive to the interplay among intra-individual and extra-individual factors that characterize the disablement process (Verbrugge & Jette, 1994). Societal participation hence represents the defining characteristic of a life with a disability.

A commonly used indicator of successful rehabilitation and participation following TBI is return to work. Considerable variability exists in return to work rates, ranging from 20% to 66% across studies (Levin, et al., 1979; Brooks, et al., 1987; Olver, et al., 1996). Commonly cited variables affecting study outcome include age, time since injury, and severity of injury among participants studied identified in the literature. Asikainen, et al. (1998) indicate that the critical age for successful return to work to be 45 years of age, with TBI survivors over that age less likely to return to work. While return to work rates have been found to be affected by time since injury, cross sectional work rates of 23%, 17%, and 25% over a three year period following injury suggest that the nature of this relationship is not clearly established. In a longitudinal study, Olver et al., (1996) found that only 32% of persons with TBI employed at two years post injury were still employed at five years. Analyzing a large (n=208) heterogeneous data set, Doig, et al. (2001) found poor overall community integration and return to work success for persons with severe TBI 2-5 years post-discharge from brain injury rehabilitation.

The importance of environmental consideration in the assessment and treatment of TBI continues to gain importance as clinical outcomes research recognizes the dangers in assuming that treatment gains from the protected medical setting to the more external world is fraught with risks (Varney & Menefee, 1993; Hayden et al., 2000). Barriers to successful community living and quality of life for many following TBI reflect a complex mix of chronic physical, cognitive, and social challenges together with a variety of unmet needs (Gordon et al., 1999). Barriers also include issues of access to needed services within a managed healthcare system. Gordon et al. (1999) indicate that managed care approaches limits access to services, which in turn, "threatens to restrict community integration and quality of life, while increasing the likelihood of secondary disabilities and long-term institutionalization" (p.323). Willer and Corrigan (1994) note that professional and bureaucratic barriers are created when funding sources imposes limitations to type or availability of health services. They summarize the negative impact of the current managed care system on community based rehabilitation services for TBI as follows:

If the payer refuses to reimburse for certain services that may be the most useful, but will reimburse for services that are less useful or even unnecessary, professionals and family members are forced to encourage inappropriate services. Payer requirements often dictate that services be provided in a hospital setting, thus making community based programs inaccessible (p.656).

2.2 Satisfaction with life following TBI

Significant personal and social costs often accompany traumatic brain injury, each contributing to reduced self-respect, dignity, autonomy, and participation in the community (Rowlands, 2001). Evidence from long term follow-up studies indicate that interpersonal relations, employment, and psychological well-being remain problematic long after injury to the brain, and may persist over an individual's lifetime (Thomsen, 1987). Central to the difficulties experienced by persons with TBI in resuming interpersonal relationships is personality change (Bond, 1984). The interaction of unemployment, behavior change and motor and sensory impairment combine to contribute to dissatisfying social relationships. With the passing of time following TBI, studies have found that social relationships increase in number but tend to be superficial, contributing to the common complaint of loneliness (Rowlands, 2001; Willer, et al., 1990). Opportunities to develop new relationships are limited, further reducing self-esteem and contributing to a sense of isolation and depression. New relationships take on a transient quality, lacking many of the features of durable, supportive relationships (Rowlands, 2001).

Life satisfaction is a subjective measure of quality of life according to Dijkers (1999). Flanagan (1982) recognizes the complex issues associated with defining quality of life and categorizes the concept into five groups: (a) physical and material well-being, (b) relations with other people, (c) social, community, and civic activities, (d) personal development and (e) fulfillment and recreation. Given the previously described long-term sequelae that commonly follow TBI, the impact of the condition on quality of life would seem considerable. Using items from the Bigelow Quality of Life Questionnaire (BQOL), Gordon et al. (1999) discovered differences between TBI and non-disabled subjects in the areas of psychological distress, basic need satisfaction, independence, social support, work at home, employability, and leisure time. In all instances, the direction of difference was in favor of the non-disabled group.

Research examining life satisfaction within the TBI population has received increasing attention over the past decade. Burleigh, et al. (1998) examined the relationship between community integration, as measured by the Community Integration Questionnaire (CIQ), and life satisfaction among 30 persons with TBI ranging in age from 26-60 and at least eight years post injury. Findings indicated a significant relationship between life satisfaction and social integration (a component of community integration), such as social interactions with friends and family, leisure pursuits with others, and community activities, but no such relationship between life-satisfaction and total community integration score. The CIQ total community integration score encompasses home integration (meal preparation, home management, etc.) and productivity (work, volunteering, and educational activities) in addition to social integration. Additionally, research looking at life satisfaction among persons with TBI one year after hospital discharge found a positive association between life satisfaction and employment, functional memory capacity, bowel independence, marital status, perceived responsibility for the injury, and family satisfaction (Warren, et al., 1996).

Corrigan, Smith-Knapp, and Granger (1998) evaluated a cross sectional sample of persons with TBI who were six months to five years post-discharge from acute rehabilitation. Findings indicated that functional status (as measured by items on the Functional Independence Measure [FIM]) was not correlated with life satisfaction but that time since injury was correlated with lower life satisfaction for persons one to two years post-discharge. Mood, income, age, race/ethnicity, and degree of impairment also correlated with life satisfaction. These findings are consistent with those obtained by Corrigan, Bogner, Mysiw, Clinchot, and Fugate (2001). These researchers used the Satisfaction with Life Scale (SWLS) with 218 consecutive patients admitted for rehabilitation one and/or two years after injury. Motor independence at rehabilitation discharge, not having a pre-injury history of substance abuse, absence of depressed mood, social integration, and having gainful employment at the time of follow-up were associated with higher self-reported life satisfaction. It was concluded that life satisfaction is an important aspect of a person's quality of life that seems related to one's reestablishing a healthy and productive lifestyle (Corrigan et al., 2001).

Research has shown that depression is a factor in lower life satisfaction among survivors of TBI (Corrigan et al., 2001). A longitudinal study of 324 survivors of TBI showed that persons acknowledging a diagnosis of depression at some point during the first 24 months post-injury showed lower scores on the Life Satisfaction Index at 24, 48, and 60 months post injury than persons surveyed without the depression diagnosis (Underhill et al., 2003). The prevalence of the depression among persons post TBI has been difficult to assess from the literature because of varying definitions of the condition and varying periods of post-injury follow-up (Underhill et al., 2003). However, it appears that it occurs in somewhere between 22-50% of all TBI survivors (McCleary et al., 1998). Depression complicates the process of recovery and rehabilitation because it contributes to increased cognitive effort in information processing and by creating general apathy toward rehabilitation (Jean-Bay, 2000). As a result, treatment goals to reestablish meaningful social and occupational roles are compromised. Theories attempting to explain the nature of the relationship between TBI and depression include pre-existing depression, pre-injury personality type, social integration after injury, family support, neurochemical imbalances, and site of anatomical damage (Jean-Bay, 2000; Rosenthal, et al., 1998; Ownsworth and Oei, 1998).

A review of the research by Rice, et al. (1980) indicated that people who are satisfied with work also tend to be satisfied with other domains of life and with life as a whole. Among the 324 persons surveyed by Underhill et al. (2003), persons with TBI that were employed reported higher life satisfaction than those unemployed. Similarly, Melamed, et al. (1992) concluded that work involvement significantly contributes to subjective satisfaction with rehabilitation outcome. Positive relationships between perceived quality of life and employment with the TBI population were also found by O'Neill et al. (1998) and Webb, et al. (1995). Unfortunately, returning to meaningful work is a frequently cited problem after TBI. In a study of adults with TBI and role changes, more than 85% of the subjects reported a worker role loss (Hallett, Zasler, Maurer, & Cash, 1994). While such findings of a positive relationship between work status and life satisfaction represent the majority of outcomes in this area, Lindberg (1995) and Johansson and Bernspang (2001) found low self reported life satisfaction following TBI regardless of whether an individual working at the time of evaluation.

Several studies have reported generally low self-reported life satisfaction among persons following TBI (Johansson & Bernspang, 2001; Viitanen, et al., 1988). However, a study of 275 persons with TBI reported high self-rated quality of life (Steadman-Pare, et, al., 2001). In addition, a Finnish study of quality of life in 17 persons with very severe TBI found that 70% of the participants were satisfied or rather satisfied with life as a whole 10 years after injury (Koskinen, 1998). Such discrepancies may be attributable in part to differences in severity of injury and the time post injury at which evaluations were conducted (Johansson & Bernspang, 2001).

2.3 Community based rehabilitation approaches

Community based models of TBI rehabilitation vary greatly, ranging from traditional residential programs to home based therapies occurring within an individual's natural environment. O'Hara and Harrell (1991) describe the goals and objectives of TBI rehabilitation in the community setting as seeking to address the following: improved motivation; improved self-control; understanding brain injury and its effects; skill development in problem solving ability, stress management, and socialization; and internal acceptance and redefinition of the self. Community based TBI program models are generally grounded in the philosophy that skills are most likely to generalize when taught in the environment where they are to be used, that environmental manipulations and assistive devices may be needed to function in the community, and that empowerment, self determination and self-respect are important aspects of rehabilitation (Willer & Corrigan, 1994). Many community-based models are designed to serve as a bridge between the structure of the hospital setting and independent life in the community.

Efforts to enhance services for persons with TBI have resulted in the emergence of treatment approaches attempting to address the complexity of problems that has impeded successful rehabilitation (Corrigan, 2001). It is commonly suggested that a more client centered approach is needed whereby treatment environments match information processing and executive abilities of the individual at admission and then are modified as the patient can tolerate increased distractions and decreased structure (Hayden et al., 2000). Personally meaningful settings, activities, themes, and interactions in rehabilitation have also been postulated as critical to overcoming problems of transferring clinical gains in hospital based environments to the community (Feeney, et al, 2001).

Willer and Corrigan (1994) suggest that in order to be successful, TBI rehabilitation programs must give careful consideration to the environmental barriers that an individual may face as well as any needed natural supports that may be necessary for long-term community integration. Their proposed 'Whatever it Takes' model of community based TBI rehabilitation reflects a practical approach to fostering improved community integration outcomes. The model seeks to achieve a maximal level of self-determination for persons with TBI through the development of rehabilitation programs that are based upon the following principles:

1. No two individuals with acquired brain injury are alike
2. Skills are more likely to generalize when taught in the environment where they can be used
3. Environments are easier to change than people
4. Community integration should be holistic
5. Life is a place-and-train venture
6. Natural supports last longer than professionals
7. Interventions must not do more harm than good
8. The service system presents many barriers to community integration
9. Respect for the individual is paramount
10. Needs of individuals last a lifetime; so should their resources

While emphasizing that natural community settings are the ideal setting to foster independence amid the complications commonly associated with living with TBI, the authors acknowledge the challenge of implementing such a model within the context of current healthcare and reimbursement systems that continue to emphasize acute care (Willer & Corrigan, 1994).

Successful community re-entry following TBI has rarely been quantified or measured yet is the primary objective of rehabilitation. In its 1998 *Consensus Statement,* pertaining to the rehabilitation of persons with traumatic brain injury, the National Institutes of Health (NIH) identified investigation into the effectiveness of community based rehabilitation programs as a research priority (NIH, 1998). Willer et al. (1999) point out weaknesses in existing TBI rehabilitation effectiveness research and suggest the need for studies utilizing any form of comparison group, clarity on type and descriptors of program being evaluated, and research evaluating the effectiveness of rehabilitation on both disabilities and handicap.

Willer et al. (1999) compared outcomes of individuals with severe TBI treated in a post-acute residential rehabilitation program with a matched sample of individuals receiving limited services in their homes or on an outpatient basis. Employing the Health and Activity Limitations Survey (HALS) and the Community Integration Questionnaire (CIQ), the researchers concluded that the residential based services appeared to produce greater functional improvement, whereas home-based services were more effective at maintaining community integration. Warden et al. (2000), employing a qualitative analysis, concluded that a home based rehabilitation program, consisting of home program activities and weekly telephone calls in addition to multidisciplinary evaluation and medical treatment, "may provide effective care at a lower cost" (p.1101). Additionally, Hayden et al. (2000) reported significant gains in levels of independence for mild head injured patients participating in a "simulated" natural setting. Both studies indicated the need for further research looking at the effectiveness of home and community based models of rehabilitation following TBI.

Seale et al. (2002) used the CIQ to investigate community integration for persons discharged from a post-acute rehabilitation program. Participants of the rehabilitation program resided at a facility during treatment which included an individualized plan of medical care, case management, occupational therapy, physical therapy, speech therapy, residential services, therapeutic recreation, vocational services, and neuropsychology. Two groups, one comprised of individuals admitted for treatment less than one year post-injury and another comprised of persons admitted for treatment 1-5 years post-injury, were evaluated after discharge using a phone interview. Results of the study indicated that the rehabilitation program was beneficial for both groups of individuals, although those admitted less than one year post injury demonstrated more pronounced positive change based upon CIQ scores.

After examining the relationship between community integration and life satisfaction, Burleigh et al. (1998) recommended the need for rehabilitation programs to provide long-term assistance with community-based social integration. In their study, participants receiving home based rehabilitation demonstrated improvements in the performance of home management but did not develop a greater level of social participation over the course of treatment. These authors emphasized the need to discover more effective treatment strategies to develop the social skills and improve social participation among persons with TBI.

Using a design similar to that of the current study, Prigatano et al. (1984) studied a sample of 18 patients with severe TBI ranging from 6 months to 54 months after injury and participating in a comprehensive post-acute community integration program. A control group of 17 patients never enrolled in the program were matched to the treatment sample on gender, age, education, and severity of injury. After six months in the rehabilitation program, 50% of the treatment sample was employed versus 36% of persons in the control group.

Malec, et al. (1993) reviewed outcomes from post-acute rehabilitation program for 29 individuals with mixed medical conditions, 20 of which were TBI. The researchers concluded that the program effectively met its objective of improved community integration based on the fact that 90% of participants were living independently at discharge versus 48% at admission. In addition, improvements in work status were noted, with 61% of persons completing the program being employed at discharge (including competitive employment and employment with temporary supports). However, as with the majority of outcome based TBI studies, the lack of comparison group makes it impossible to fully dissociate the effect of treatment from spontaneous recovery.

2.4 Research study overview

This study assessed the impact of an intensive, residential transitional program for persons with traumatic on both community participation and life satisfaction. It was hypothesized that the intervention program would have a positive impact on both variables.

3. Methods

3.1 Sample

Rehabilitation outcome scores were reviewed for a convenience sample of 41 consecutive admissions (meeting study inclusion criteria) to Radical Rehab Solutions (RRS), LLC, a community based, residential rehabilitation program in West Virginia and Kentucky. The program, located in West Virginia and Kentucky, utilizes both intensive life skills and group therapy to facilitate community integration. Like many post-acute brain injury treatment models, the program is grounded in the philosophy that skills are most likely to generalize when taught in the environment where they are to be used. RRS is designed to serve as a bridge between the structure of the hospital setting and independent life in the community. All participants in RRS received similar individualized life skills training, daily group therapy, and services from an interdisciplinary team of rehabilitation professionals including occupational therapy, speech therapy, and psychology. A detailed description of the program is provided in section 3.2.

Due to the retrospective data collection technique used in the study (medical record review and program evaluation data review), individuals were not aware that they would be involved in a research study at the time the intervention was provided. The scores used in the study were part of the RRS program evaluation model.

Individuals whose cognitive deficits prevented competent completion of the Satisfaction with Life Scale were not included in the study. Determination of competence was established by an RRS licensed clinical psychologist. RRS participants included in the study were those who:

- Were between the ages of 18 and 55 years;
- Were considered to have suffered a moderate to severe TBI as determined by duration of coma of one hour or longer;
- Had the ability to self-complete baseline and follow-up evaluation measures;
- Had no history of severe neurological or psychiatric illness, e.g., previous severe TBI, stroke, multiple sclerosis, or psychosis; and
- Were full time participants in RRS based on full-time, residential status.

Additionally, the researchers limited eligibility for the treatment group to those RRS participants receiving training for a minimum 10 week consecutive period.

3.2 Intervention

Radical Rehab Solutions (RRS), LLC is a provider of community-based transitional living programs for individuals with brain injury in West Virginia and Kentucky. Transitional living programs serve as a "bridge" between the brain-injured individual's discharge from the hospital-based rehabilitation and their return to independent living in the community. The following program description is reprinted with permission based upon the information provided in the RRS policy and procedure manual and summarized in RRS print (Implement Neurorehabilitation, 2000) and online resources (www.radicalrehab.com).

The RRS transitional living program provides intensive social learning via four avenues: I) intensive one-on-one **Life Skills Training**; II) participation in a **therapeutic community/milieu**; III) daily process-oriented **cognitive re-training group**, and IV) weekly group **goal-setting sessions**.

1. **Intensive Life Skills Training**: Each program incorporates the services of a one-on-one Life Skills Trainer (LST) to maximize the client's level of personal accountability, to

provide immediate and consistent feedback regarding the social appropriateness of the client's behavior, and to provide ongoing training in the use of compensatory cognitive strategies. The LST provides continual intervention to facilitate and enhance the client's independent living skills via verbal cuing, training in compensatory skills, structuring of daily activities, redirection, assistance with problem-solving, encouragement of targeted behaviors, and cuing for safety awareness. LST's are from varied educational and employment backgrounds but all receive a minimum of 40 hours of training in brain injury and life skills coaching prior to interacting with clients.

2. **Therapeutic Community/Milieu**: All RRS clients participate in daily group activities, including a process-oriented, cognitive re-training group, a structured day treatment program, and community outings that utilize the power of the relationships in the group to reinforce desirable behavior and extinguish undesirable behavior. These group activities provide the opportunity for interpersonal learning - for the client to learn how they are perceived by others and for the client to practice new behaviors in a supportive environment. Within the context of these group activities, clients are provided with immediate feedback from their co-clients regarding the appropriateness of their behavior. Further, clients set weekly attainable goals in the presence of the community and receive positive or negative feedback from the group when progress toward goals is reviewed each week.
   One of the most important therapeutic elements of the RRS program is that, on an ongoing and frequent basis, clients are provided with social feedback - both positive and negative - from their co-clients. This feedback occurs during the daily cognitive retraining group, during weekly goal-setting sessions, during the weekday day treatment program, and on community outings. For example, if a client makes an inappropriate verbalization (e.g., sexual or rude remark, repetitive or irrelevant statement), the activity will be temporarily halted and the leader will query the group as to their response to the verbalization (e.g., , "What does the rest of the group think about what <client> said?). Similarly, if a client achieves a goal or experiences a success (e.g., ambulating into class with a walker, responding to orientation questions correctly), the group will provide positive feedback (cheers, applause).
3. Clients participate in a daily, process-oriented, **Cognitive Re-Training Group** that a) provides intensive education regarding cognitive, neurobehavioral, and psychological issues related to brain injury, b) intensive training in compensatory techniques for managing cognitive and behavioral changes, and c) provides daily opportunities to utilize the power of the relationships in the group to reinforce desirable behavior and extinguish undesirable behavior. Each week the daily cognitive retraining group focuses on a different theme. Therapists from each of the treatment modalities - occupational therapy, speech therapy, physical therapy, and psychology - focus their therapy sessions on the same theme to provide repetition of the concepts associated with the weekly theme.
4. Weekly **Goal-Setting Groups** are conducted as part of the daily Cognitive Re-Training Group. Each Friday morning, all clients, LST's and therapy staff gather so that clients may set attainable goals (typically 3-5 specific objectives) for the following week and receive positive or negative feedback - depending on their success at meeting their weekly goals - from the remainder of the group when progress toward goals is reviewed. Setting weekly attainable goals provides the individual with a brain injury with the very important feedback that they are continuing to recover - thereby

increasing their self-efficacy, i.e., their belief in their ability to do what is necessary to cope with their brain injury.

3.3 Instruments

The instruments used in the study were consistent with current state of the research pertaining to TBI outcomes in regards to community integration and life satisfaction. The measures were among those being used by RRS for the purpose of program evaluation and quality assurance. The study measures are administered by RRS staff as components of neuropsychological and occupational therapy initial evaluation and follow-up. The use of patient self-evaluation was consistent with a client-centered approach that emphasizes the inherent worth of individuals and their experience of problems (Law & Mills, 1998). Subjective measures, as used in this study, also reflect the importance of evaluating the unique person who is influenced by cultural and social factors.

3.3.1 Measure of community participation

The Community Integration Questionnaire (CIQ) is a 15-item self-report inventory that was developed within the context of the WHO model of disablement to measure level of handicap of individuals with TBI after discharge from hospital (Willer, Ottenbacher, & Coad, 1994). Willer and Corrigan (1994) note that the CIQ was developed for program evaluation purposes and, although not its original intent, recommend its use for individual assessments. The measure considers community integration to be made up of three areas of community functioning: control over one's home environment, integration into a social support network, and integration into productive and meaningful daytime activities (Willer and Corrigan, 1994). The items on the CIQ produce a total score that reflect three subscales: the extent of an individual's integration within the home, in social networks, and into productive activities. The range for total CIQ score is 0-29. The larger the score, the more integrated the individual.

Evidence for the instruments validity and reliability with the TBI population is well established by the test developers and by other researchers in subsequent investigations (Sander et al., 1999). Test-retest reliability coefficients have ranged from .83 to .97, and concurrent and discriminant validity have been established (Willer, Rosenthal et al., 1993; Willer et al., 1994; Corrigan & Deming, 1995; Sander et al., 1997). A three-factor structure was confirmed by a factor analysis based upon a sample of 312 subjects (Sander et al., 1999). The three factors are represented in the instrument's three subscales: home integration, productivity, and social integration.

Subscale scores for home integration, productive activities, and social integration have demonstrated predictable relationships with measures of functional independence and severity of injury (Heinemann & Whiteneck, 1995). CIQ subscales and total score have been found to correlate with degree of impairment and disability, time since injury, and subjective quality of life (Heinemann and Whiteneck, 1995). Additionally, the available research shows that the CIQ can validly distinguish between persons with TBI and non-disabled controls (Gordon et al., 1999; Corrigan and Deming, 1995; Willer et al., 1994). Gordon et al. (1999) found that a group of 298 individuals living in the community following TBI had a lower CIQ total score (16.1 vs. 19.5) and had lower scores on each of three CIQ subscales than a non-disabled comparison group. Furthermore, in the Willer et al. (1994) study, CIQ scores distinguished between three groups of persons with TBI living in settings differentiated by supervision/support level: independent in the community, in the community with some (natural) support, and in an institution such as a nursing home, rehabilitation facility, etc.

Contrasting findings to those noted above were found in a comparison between individuals with mild TBI and normal controls (Paniak, et al., 1999). In this study, individuals with mild TBI scored significantly lower on the productivity subscale but there were no differences between the two groups in the home and social integration subscales. Gordon et al. (1999), in comparing differences in scores among studies using the CIQ suggest that time since injury may affect scoring related to community participation, particularly in regard to participation in vocational activities. Differences in severity of injury may also play a factor in the measures sensitivity given the fact that functional outcomes for mild brain injuries tend to be more favorable than those for more severe injuries.

The CIQ represents the current standard for measuring community integration in the area of brain injury rehabilitation (McColl, et al., 2001). It represents one of the main outcome measures of the TBI Model Systems National Data Base and is the most commonly used comprehensive measure of community integration following TBI (Dijkers, 1997). While frequently used in research to quantify functional status, studies using the CIQ to measure change over time following rehabilitation are rare. Employment rates and independent living status (both included among CIQ questions) have historically served as variables for measuring the effectiveness of rehabilitation programs focusing on community integration (Prigatano et al., 1984; Johnston & Lewis, 1991; Cope, et al., 1991; Ben-Yishay, et al., 1987). Sander et al. (2001) used the CIQ as part of a longitudinal cohort study that sought to investigate maintenance of gains after discharge from a post-acute rehabilitation program. The researchers describe reliability in CIQ scores across evaluation periods based upon high correlations (greater than .60) at rehabilitation program discharge and one year and four-year post discharge follow-up periods.

In the current study, CIQ scores were obtained through structured interview by RRS rehabilitation program staff who collect CIQ scores as part of initial evaluation and follow-up. Community integration has been traditionally recognized as a difficult to measure construct. The validity and reliability data supporting the psychometric properties of the CIQ along with the instruments easy to administer format made a suitable measure of community participation for this study.

3.3.2 Measure of life satisfaction

Self reported life satisfaction was measured in this study using the Satisfaction with Life Scale (SWLS) (Diener, Emmons, Larsen & Griffin, 1985). The SWLS is a measure of general life satisfaction, a factor of the more general construct of subjective well-being. By design, items of the SWLS measure general life satisfaction as opposed to satisfaction with specific life areas for the purpose of avoiding assumptions about the importance each individual ascribes to satisfaction with particular domains of their life (Bogner, et al., 2001). The SWLS has five items with a 7-point Likert-type response format that are added to create a total score ranging from 5 to 35. Scoring criteria range from "strongly disagree" to "strongly agree" in response to five statements that include:

- In most ways my life is close to my ideal
- The conditions of my life are excellent
- I am satisfied with my life

- So far I have gotten the important things I want in life
- If I could live my life over again, I would change almost nothing

A score of 20 represents a neutral point at which the respondent is equally satisfied and dissatisfied. Most non-clinical populations obtain scores between 23 and 28 (Pavot & Diener, 1993). By design, items of the SWLS measure general life satisfaction as opposed to satisfaction with specific life areas for the purpose of avoiding assumptions about the importance each individual ascribes to satisfaction with particular domains of their life (Bogner, et al., 2001).

The validity and reliability of the SWLS are well established (Pavot, et al., 1991; Shevlin, et al., 1998; Pavot & Diener, 1993). The initial item selection for the SWLS included 48 items that all had face validity as indicators of one's appraisal of life. Construct validity of the SWLS can be drawn from a number of investigations. For instance, test-retest stability has been found to decline as time between testing increases, suggesting that the instrument is sensitive to changes that occur with life and not just a direct effect of stable personality traits (Pavot, et al., 1991). The SWLS has also been found to change in the expected directions in response to major life events, such as elderly caregivers who had a spouse diagnosed with primary degenerative dementia (Vitaliano, et al., 1991), and patients receiving psychotherapy (Pavot & Diener, 1993).

Criterion validity studies correlated the SWLS with ten other measures of subjective well being (Pavot et al., 1991). Most measures correlated at an $r = .50$ or higher for each of the two samples from the original work. Subsequent studies have found comparable or higher correlations with other populations when interviewer ratings, informant reports, or other objective measures are used (Shevlin, et al., 1998; Neto, 1993; Arrinddell, et al., 1991). The SWLS has been administered in conjunction with measures of positive and negative affective appraisal. The SWLS tends to correlate with scales measuring both constructs even though the two are unrelated. The absolute values of these correlations range from .26 to .47, indicating that the SWLS taps a dimension of subjective well-being different from either positive or negative affectivity. Also consistent with theoretical postulations about subjective well being, SWLS scores have been positively correlated with extroversion and inversely correlated with neuroticism (Diener et al., 1985; Pavot & Diener, 1993, Pavot et al., 1991). The SWLS has consistently shown good internal consistency with alpha coefficients consistently exceeding .80 (Pavot & Diener, 1993). Test-retest reliabilities have ranged from .54 for a four-year interval to .84 for a two-month interval. Additionally, Pavot and Diener (1993) reported a test-retest correlation coefficient of .89 for subjects tested after two weeks.

3.4 Data collection and data management

CIQ and SWLS scores for 41 consecutive subjects meeting study criteria were reviewed by the researcher. Information on severity of injury (duration of coma), time since injury, gender, and age was obtained through medical record review. Permission to complete the program evaluation was obtained by both Radical Rehab Solutions and the West Virginia University Institutional Review Board.

To investigate changes between baseline and follow-up periods, the Wilcoxon matched pairs test was used. This test is the nonparametric alternative to the dependent *t* test (Munro, 1997). The test is used to compare two groups of matched subjects designs or to compare one group when one group of subjects us evaluated in two or more conditions (Munro, 1997). Nonparametric tests were used for the analysis of both community integration and satisfaction with life due to the fact that both CIQ and SWLS are ordinal data scales and to the fact that general assumptions necessary for the use of parametric measures (large sample size, normal sample distribution) could not be met (Berg and Latin, 2004). The significance level was set to $p = .05$. SPSS version 19.0 was used for all statistical calculations.

4. Results

Analysis of each variable at baseline, 90 day, and one year follow-up periods, along with an analysis of the relationships between variables, is detailed below.

4.1 Community participation / integration

Overall community participation is summarized in figure 1. While mean overall CIQ scores improved at each evaluation period, only scores from baseline (x=9.78) to 90-day follow-up (x=13.19) and baseline to 1 year follow-up (x=14.57) increased to a level of statistically significance (p<.05). Overall mean CIQ scores did not improve significantly after the 90-day evaluation period.

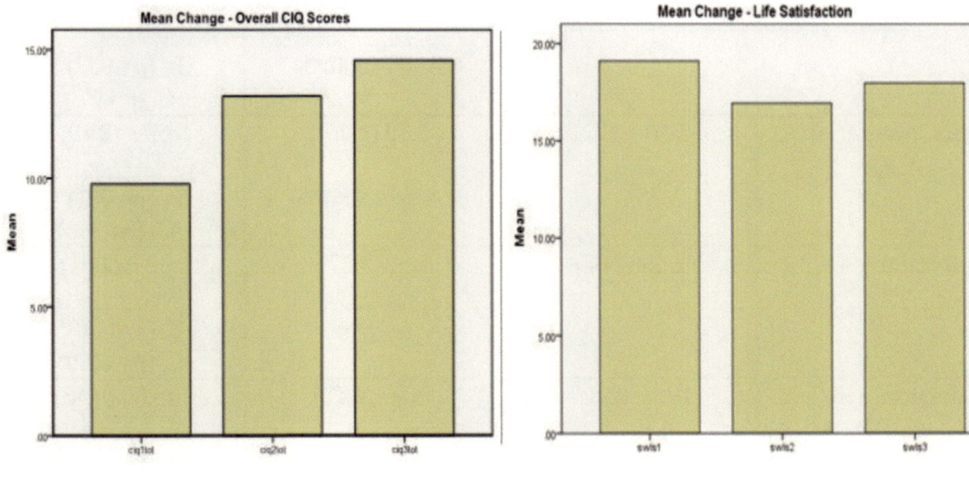

Fig. I. Mean changes in CIQ and SWLS scores from baseline to 90 day and one year follow-up.

These findings were consistent with those from the CIQ home integration subscale and social integration subscales (see table 1). On the CIQ productivity subscales, statistically significant gains were noted at both follow-up periods. Mean baseline productivity levels increased from 1.61 to 2.80 at 90 day follow-up. At one year, productivity levels had increased to a mean of 3.90. Analysis of individual scores showed that 82.9% (34/41) of the subjects had increased their level of community integration at 90 day follow-up while two others scores indicated no change. Five subjects had a lower overall CIQ score at the first follow-up period. At one-year follow-up, 18 of the 34 subjects showing initial gains, made additional gains while three others had an equal overall score. 90% (37/41) of subjects had a higher CIQ score at one year follow-up while 4 subjects had a lower total CIQ at one year follow-up compared to baseline.

4.2 Satisfaction with life

Mean SWLS scores and standard deviations for baseline and follow-up periods are summarized in table 1 and figure 1. Mean SWLS scores showed a statistically significant decrease from initial evaluation (x=19.09) to 90-day follow-up (16.95). From 90 day follow-up to 1 year (x=17.98), scores showed a non-significant gain (p<.05). Analysis of individual subject responses showed that only 26.8% (11/41) of subjects reported higher life satisfaction at the 90 day follow-up period. The remainder of the subjects either indicated no change (6/41) or a decrease in life satisfaction (24/41). However, of those 30 subjects reporting no or decreased life satisfaction at 90 day follow-up, 21 indicated higher life satisfaction at one year follow-up. Of the 11 subjects reporting higher life satisfaction at 90 day follow-up, 7 indicated reduced satisfaction at one year follow-up.

	Baseline - mean (SD)	90 day follow-up - mean (SD)	1 year follow-up - mean (SD)
Total CIQ	9.75 (3.75)	13.1 (4.63) A. (p=.000)**	14.56 (3.58) B. (p=.000)** C. (p=.078)
Home Management - CIQ	2.68 (2.04)	4.01 (1.70) A. (p=.000)**	3.95 (1.40) B. (p=.002)** C. (p=.770)
Social Integration - CIQ	5.51 (2.02)	6.39 (2.20) A. (p=.006)**	6.73 (2.19) B. (p=.001)** C. (p=.395)
Productivity - CIQ	1.60 (1.37)	2.80 (1.87) A. (p=.000)**	3.90 (1.91) B. (p=.000)** C. (p=.002)**
Satisfaction with Life - SWLS	19.10 (8.84)	16.95 (6.77) A. (p=.050)*	18.00 (9.45) B. (p=.545) C. (p=.125)

Table I. Mean comparisons among study variables. A = baseline and 90 day reevaluation comparison; B = baseline and one year reevaluation comparison; and C = 90 day reevaluation and one year comparison.

4.3 Relationships among variables

Spearman rank order correlations were used to determine the level of association between community integration and satisfaction with life. The results indicated no such relationship at baseline and follow-up periods with the exception of total integration and social integration where, at one-year follow-up, significant correlations were found with life satisfaction. The relationships (indicated by Spearman's rho) are summarized in table 2.

5. Discussion

The current study evaluated the effectiveness of an intensive, transitional living rehabilitation program with a group of individuals following moderate to severe TBI. The program evaluation was consistent with the International Classification of Functioning, Disability and Health (ICF) (WHO, 2001) through its examination of the interface between the person following TBI and the environment. The notion of societal participation served as a primary dependent variable in the study and was measured using the Community Integration Questionnaire (CIQ), an instrument derived to measure the relative impact of an impaired body system on community integration (Kaplan, 2001). The CIQ was developed with special consideration of the challenges that individuals face during the process of recovery from TBI (Willer, et al., 1993; Dijkers, 1997). Community integration was conceptualized as participation in home, social, vocational, and community activities. In using the CIQ, this study expanded upon the current state of TBI research using this measure by evaluating post-acute rehabilitation outcomes.

The scope of the present study expanded beyond community participation to include a measure of self-reported satisfaction with life. Life satisfaction has been frequently identified as an important indicator of health and hence serves as a critical adjunct to the determination of rehabilitation program outcome (Fuhrer et al., 1992). The construct of life satisfaction was evaluated in study participants using the Satisfaction with Life Scale (SWLS) (Diener et al., 1985). Using both CIQ and SWLS simultaneously allowed separate evaluation of the impact of life skills coaching on community participation and life satisfaction as well as examination of the relationship between community participation and satisfaction with life. Such a relationship has received increased attention among researchers working with individuals with TBI and other disability populations (Heinemann & Whiteneck, 1995; Huebner, et al., 2003).

	SWLS 1	SWLS 2	SWLS 3
CIQ Total - baseline	.138	.042	.139
CIQ Total – 90 day	.100	.029	.139
CIQ Total – 1 year	.380	.303 *	.428 **
CIQ Home - baseline	.154	.079	.236
CIQ Home – 90 day	.040	-.049	.059
CIQ Home – 1 year	.257	.053	.143
CIQ Social - baseline	.079	.097	.164
CIQ Social – 90 day	.064	-.036	.220
CIQ Social – 1 year	.272	.266	.490 **
CIQ Prod. - baseline	.173	-.002	.141
CIQ Prod. – 90 day	.160	.286	-.043
CIQ Prod. – 1 year	.297	.286	.127

*Significant at $p<.05$ ** Significant at $p<.01$

Table II. Correlations among overall CIQ and subscale scores with SWLS scores.

It was hypothesized that the interdisciplinary transitional living program would improve community participation and increase self-reported life satisfaction with a group of moderately to severely brain-injured individuals. In this study, improvement in overall level of community integration showed statistically significant improvement between baseline and ninety day follow-up. These gains were maintained at one year follow-up. The study's findings did not support the hypothesis that such an improvement results in increased self-reported life satisfaction however. Subjects reported a significant decrease in satisfaction at 90 day follow-up before returning to baseline levels of life satisfaction at one year follow-up.

5.1 Community participation

The findings from the study support the effectiveness of community-based rehabilitation in facilitating community integration in terms of home management, social participation, and productive activity. Participants of the study demonstrated significant gains across all areas measured by the Community Integration Questionnaire at 90-day follow-up. Overall, these gains were maintained at 1 year follow-up in home integration and social participation and further significantly improved from 90 day to one year for the CIQ productivity subscale which looks at paid work, volunteer work, or involvement in school. This finding was consistent with that by Willer et al. (1999) who reported a significant improvement in productivity at discharge for persons participating in a post-acute rehabilitation program over a group of matched comparisons.

The possibility that RRS interpersonal learning model can positively influence the attainment of occupational roles with this population warrants some discussion. Individuals with severe TBI have historically been considered "too disabled" (Wehman, et al., 1999, p. 327) to benefit from rehabilitation and as a result have received little support from state vocational rehabilitation programs. In a study by McCordie, et al. (1990), it was reported that of individuals with a length of coma greater than one day, only 5% of those surveyed had returned to full-time work an average of 6.7 years post-injury. Wehman et al. (1999) point out that the emergence of services for persons with severe disabilities in combination with mandates from the Rehabilitation Act Amendments of 1992 show promise in reversing these historical trends for this group of individuals. The life skills training inherent in the RRS model evaluated in this study appears well suited to the return to work process by emphasizing the functions of skill teaching, evaluating worker performance, and advocating for the worker. Each of these steps represents essential aspects of vocational rehabilitation following TBI (Wehman et al., 1999). As described by Jones et al. (1991), life coaching involves not only skill acquisition, but also the application of these skills in everyday environments. Not all studies on post-acute rehabilitation have reported statistically significant increases in productivity however. In the Goranson et al. (2003) study, in which follow-up was conducted at 6-18 months post-discharge, improvement in CIQ productivity score were described as *non-significant* when compared to a group of matched control subjects.

In the present study, home integration scores also significantly improved between baseline and follow-up periods. Home integration, as measured by the CIQ involves performance of normal household activities such as cleaning, meal preparation, and child-care. Such activities represent responsibilities of typical adult roles and are often targeted treatment areas of a TBI rehabilitation program (Huebner et al., 2003). Cognitive deficits commonly associated with TBI contribute to issues in home safety and hence become a treatment plan priority (McNeny, 1999). With market pressures to shorten the length of stay of acute hospitalizations, persons with TBI are leaving acute settings with greater severity of acute deficits.

While the CIQ measures participation in home management activities, scores do not however represent the degree of safety by which such tasks are completed (Seale et al., 2002). In the present study, subjects reporting home integration status may or may not have been performing these activities safely. No data was collected in this study to investigate the qualitative aspects related to the performance of these tasks.

In this study, the level of social integration by subjects over the ninety-day follow-up period showed statistically significance improvement. This finding contrasts with other studies that demonstrated no difference in social integration after post-acute TBI rehabilitation at one-year follow-up (Willer et al. 1999), at 6-18 month follow-up (Goranson et al. ,2003), at 90 day follow up (Wheeler, et al., 2007) ,or least one month post-discharge (Seale et al. 2002). It is possible that the extent focus of the RRS program on group work and community activities facilitated a higher degree of social participation.

As with most other rehabilitation programs, continuation in the RRS transitional living treatment program is based on a number of factors including financial resources, discharge planning, and treatment goal attainment. As a result, study participants were likely at various stages of their individualized programs - some discharged and others relatively early in their involvement in the program. Admission and discharge decisions were the sole responsibility of the program administration and hence could not be controlled or influenced by the researchers.

5.2 Satisfaction with life

Hagen (2003) describes loss of purpose and meaning in one's life as the major long-term consequence of traumatic brain injury. Additionally, social isolation is common because a number of factors including the inability to both understand and respond to another's needs, wants, thoughts, and feelings (Hagen, 2003). He concludes that profound psychosocial disability and social isolation result in decreased life satisfaction and he emphasizes the need for treatment to address this. In the present study, it was hypothesized that a program designed to improve one's skills and abilities related to home and community functioning would also result in an increase in self-reported life satisfaction. Such a relationship was not supported suggesting the need for a greater understanding of the concept of life satisfaction and the factors that influence it following TBI.

Wheeler, et al. (2007) did not find a significant increase in self-reported life satisfaction at 90-day follow-up despite increases in community integration as measured by the CIQ. In the current study, a significant decrease in life satisfaction was reported over this period followed by a return to baseline levels at one year. Such findings may lend insights into the development of self-awareness and the impact of intensive life skills training and group work. It is possible that individuals working on life skill deficits and receiving ongoing feedback within the therapeutic community became increasingly dissatisfied as they became more aware of the amount and extent of their difficulties.

There is some support for this notion in the literature. Prigatano and Schacter (1986) describe awareness, also referred to as insight, as a complex construct involving the information from both external reality and inner experience. Given that awareness of deficits, including the nature of psychosocial and physical problems, influences ones perception of their severity, the relationship between this and life satisfaction requires further exploration. Dirette (2002) explains that attaining awareness following TBI is a slow process that involves comparing performance on functional tasks in a familiar setting with their pre-morbid functional level. If participation in treatment raises awareness of problems previously not perceived as present by the individual, it is reasonable to presume a negative impact on life satisfaction despite functional treatment gain. Struchen, et al. (2011) noted an unexpected increase in depressive symptoms at the conclusion of a three month peer mentoring program. The researchers concluded that this may have been the result of an increased self-awareness of depressive symptoms resulting from the intervention. Peer mentors in the study discussed with their client TBI related issues, such as recovery course and social, family, and vocational changes experienced after injury. While awareness was not measured in the study, the researchers found it conceivable that clients experienced increased awareness through these interactions. Anson and Ponsford (2006) found that those with poorer self-awareness showed an increase in depressive symptoms following participation in a coping skills group intervention. They also hypothesized that increased depression was related to increased awareness of injury related deficits.

In the present study, life satisfaction was viewed as a highly personal and subjective matter and hence would be prone to considerable variation among individuals. These individual differences in all likelihood contributed to the relative absence of relationships between life satisfaction and community participation. Warren et al. (1996) emphasize that rehabilitation researchers must recognize that living with a disability invariably holds different meanings for different individuals. The qualitative nature of such an experience perhaps limited the study's attempt to capture life satisfaction following TBI through quantitative methods.

The current study found a positive relationship between overall community integration and life satisfaction at one year follow-up. These findings suggest that an extended period of rehabilitation may be required to allow clients to adjust to their disability and appreciate the functional progress that they are making. If continued progress is a required for rehabilitation support, then life satisfaction appears to represent an inaccurate indicator of treatment effectiveness in the early stages. In fact, it appears that an initial decrease in life satisfaction may be a necessary component of treatment for those persons whose lack of awareness of deficits is impeding successful community participation.

The positive relationship between social integration and life satisfaction at one year follow-up, after the significant decrease in life satisfaction at 90 day follow-up, supports the notion that many individuals need an extended period of time to develop self-awareness and manage the dissatisfaction that may accompany it. Additionally, this relationship supports the impact of the RRS model on improving both of these historically treatment resistant constructs. Hagen (2003) theorized that a sense of belonging among friends, family, and community is critical to experiencing life satisfaction and that patient needs in this area are not addressed in traditional rehabilitation interventions. Burleigh, et al. (1998) indicates that over time, many persons with TBI lose their pre-injury social network and become socially isolated because they lack the skills to develop new relationships. These authors found a statistically significant correlation between life satisfaction and the social integration subscale of the CIQ with the TBI population. Having a good family life and being married are among those factors found to contribute to life satisfaction in neurological populations (Warren et al., 1996). Sokol, et al. (1999) also reported higher life satisfaction for persons that were married and who perceived that their friendships had not changed for the worse since their injury.

In this study, no relationships were found between CIQ productivity scores and life satisfaction. This contrasts with findings with numerous other studies. According to Csikzentmihaly (1997), the ability to perform an occupation that is meaningful to the individual is of vital importance for life satisfaction. In the Wheeler, et al. study of 18 subjects, individuals with higher levels of productivity (school, work, volunteer activities, and time in community) did report significantly greater satisfaction with life. This finding was consistent with larger scale studies investigating this relationship. Heinemann and Whiteneck (1995) studied the relationship between disability, using the CIQ, and self reported life satisfaction among a sample of 758 individuals with TBI and found that both social integration and productivity were related to satisfaction with life. The positive productivity–life satisfaction relationship following TBI was also reported by Underhill et al. (2003) in a study where persons employed post-injury reported higher life satisfaction over a 36-month follow-up period as well as in other studies (Steadman-Pare et al., 2001; O'Neill et al., 1998).

In the present study, no statistically significant relationships were found between improvements in home integration activities, such as housework and cooking, and self reported life satisfaction. It has been postulated that the impact of improving home integration is not enough to enhance satisfaction with life because individuals desire additional independence in the community (Huebner et al., 2003). For some, these activities may be outside their personal interests or perceived as undesirable (Huebner, et al., 2003). In the Heinemann and Whiteneck (1995) study, home integration was the only one of the CIQ subscales not related to life satisfaction.

6. Conclusions

Findings from the study support the value of the RRS transitional living program to address various aspects of community participation and life satisfaction. The impact of the program on social integration is perhaps most noteworthy given that published research on post-acute treatment programs has demonstrated little effectiveness in social integration following TBI. Brain injury experts point to the challenges of addressing social functioning after TBI. Hagen (2003) suggests a community based treatment approach that involves training and feedback in natural environments to overcome issues such poor social awareness and resultant socially inappropriate behaviors. McNeny (1999) emphasizes social skill retraining that involves group therapy and family involvement and describes the implications of poor social skills. These include troubling families, destroying friendships, and limiting vocational opportunities. The findings of this study suggest that the combination of the therapeutic community, social learning, group therapy, and individual skill building inherent in the RRS model may be an effective approach.

There were a number of limitations in the study which impact its internal and external validity. The absence of control subjects and the use of a relatively small convenience sample limit the confidence by which findings can be generalized to the brain injury population. Additionally, while efforts were made to use sensitive and relevant measures for evaluating community integration and life satisfaction, interpretation of subject performance on the chosen tools revealed their limitations. Such was particularly the case with regards to the CIQ. Despite its popularity, the CIQ may not have had sufficient specificity to capture some aspects of the gains made by subjects. For example, questions addressed participation in areas such as home, community, leisure, work, and school but did not assess whether supervision was required during accomplishment of the tasks or activities. Also, the measure does not differentiate between sheltered and regular work environments, which should be reflected in rehabilitation program outcomes. Similarly, questions on social integration allow performance of social activities within the treatment program to improve scores without necessarily improving performance in the community.

7. References

Anson, K. & Ponsford, J. (2006). Evaluation of a coping skills group following traumatic brain injury. *Brain Injury, 20,* 167-178.

Arrindell, Meeuweesen, Huyse, F. (1991). The Satisfaction with Life Scale: Psychometric properties in a non-psychiatric medical outpatient sample. *Individual Differences, 12,* 117-123.

Asikainen, I., Kaste, M., & Sarna, S. (1998). Predicting late outcome for patients with traumatic brain injury referred to a rehabilitation programme: A study of 508 Finnish patients 5 or more years after injury: *Brain Injury, 12,* 95-107.

Ben-Yishay, Y., Silver, S., Plasetsky, E., & Rattok, J.(1987). Relationship between employability and vocational outcome after intensive holistic cognitive rehabilitation. *Journal of Head Trauma Rehabilitation, 2, 25-48.*

Berg, K. & Latin, R. (2004). *Essentials of Research Methods in Health, Physical Education, Exercise Science, and Recreation.* Philadelphia, PA: Lippincott Williams & Wilkins.

Bogner, J., Corrigan, J., Mysiw, J., Clinchot, D., & Fugate, L. (2001). A comparison of substance abuse and violence in the prediction of long-term rehabilitation outcomes after traumatic brain injury. *Archives of Physical Medicine and Rehabilitation,* 82, 571-577.

Bond, M. (1984). The psychiatry of closed head injuries. In N. Brooks (Ed.), *Closed Head Injury: Psychological, Social, and Family Consequences* (pp.148-178). Oxford: Oxford University Press.

Brooks, N., McKinlay, W., Symington, C., Beattie, A., & Campsie, L.(1987) Return to work within the first seven years of severe head injury. *Brain Injury, 1,* 5-19.

Burleigh, S., Farber, R., & Gillard, M. (1998). Community integration and life satisfaction after traumatic brain injury: Long term findings. *The American Journal of Occupational Therapy, 52,* 45-52.

Canadian Institute for Health Information, (2008). *Inpatient Rehabilitation in Canada, 2006-2007.* Ottawa, Ontario: Author.

Cope, D., Cole, J., Hall, K., & Barkin, H. (1991). Brain injury: analysis of outcome in a postacute rehabilitation system. Part I: general analysis. *Brain Injury, 5,* 111-125.

Corrigan, J., Bogner, J., Mysiw, W., Clinchot, D., & Fugate, L. (2001). Life satisfaction after traumatic brain injury. *Journal of Head Trauma Rehabilitation, 16,* 543-555.

Corrigan, J. & Deming, R. (1995). Psychometric characteristics of the Community Integration Questionnaire: replication and extension. *Journal of Head Trauma Rehabilitation, 10,* 41-53.

Corrigan, J., Smith-Knapp, K., & Granger, C. (1998). Outcomes in the first 5 years after traumatic brain injury. *Archives of Physical Medicine and Rehabilitation, 79,* 298-305.

Csikzentmihaly, M. (1997). *Living Well: The Psychology of Everyday Life.* London, England: Phoenix.

Department of Health and Human Services. (2001). Chapter 6: Disability and secondary conditions. In *Healthy People 2010* (pp. 6-1 - 6-28). Rockville, MD: US Department of Health and Human Services.

Diener, E., Emmons, R., Larsen, J., & Griffin, S. (1985). The Satisfaction with Life Scale. *Journal of Personality Assessment, 49,* 71-75.

Dijkers, M. (1999). Measuring quality of life: methodological issues. *American Journal of Physical Medicine and Rehabilitation, 78,* 286-300.

Dijkers, M. (1997). Measuring the long-term outcomes of traumatic brain injury: a review of the Community Integration Questionnaire. *Journal of Head Trauma Rehabilitation, 12,* 74-91.

Dirette, D. (2002). The development of awareness and the use of compensatory strategies for cognitive deficits. *Brain Injury, 16,* 861-871.

Doig, E., Fleming, J., & Tooth, L. (2001). Patterns of community integration 2-5 years post-discharge from brain injury rehabilitation. *Brain Injury, 15,* 747-762.

Feeney, T. Ylvisaker, M., Rosen, B., & Greene, P. (2001). Community supports for individuals with challenging behavior after brain injury: An analysis of the New York State Behavioral Resource Project. *Journal of Head Trauma Rehabilitation, 16,* 61-75.

Flanagan, J. (1982). Measurement of quality of life: current state of the art. *Archives of Physical Medicine and Rehabilitation, 63,* 56-59.

Fraser, R. & Baarslag-Benson, R. (1994). Crossdisciplinary collaboration in the removal of work barriers after traumatic brain injury. *Topics in Language Disorders, 15,* 55-67.

Fuhrer, M., Rintala, D., Hart, K., Clearman, R., & Young, M. (1992) Relationship of life satisfaction to impairment, disability, and handicap among persons with spinal cord injury living in the community. *Archives of Physical Medicine and Rehabilitation, 73,* 552-557.

Goranson, T., Graves,R., Allison, D., & LaFreniere, R. (2003). Community integration following multidisciplinary rehabilitation for traumatic brain injury. *Brain Injury, 17,* 759-774.

Gordon, W., Hibbard, M., Brown, M., Flanagan, S., & Korves, M. (1999). Community integration and quality of life of individuals with traumatic brain injury. In M. Rosenthal, E. Griffith, J. Kreutzer, & B. Pentland (Eds.), *Rehabilitation of the Adult and Child with Traumatic Brain Injury* (pp.312-325). Philadelphia, PA: FA Davis.

Hagen, C. (2003, December). Traumatic Brain Injury: A Team Approach to Rehabilitation for Children and Adults. Presentation for the Continuing Education Programs of America, Atlanta, GA.

Hallett, J., Zasler, N., Maurer, P., and Cash, S. (1994). Role change after traumatic brain injury in adults. *American Journal of Occupational Therapy, 3,* 241-246.

Hanks, R. Rapport, L., Millis, S., & Deshpande, S. (1999). Measures of executive functioning as predictors of functional ability and social integration in a rehabilitation sample. *Archives of Physical Medicine and Rehabilitation, 80,* 1030-1037.

Harrick, L., Krefting, L., Johnston, J., Carlson, P. & Minnes, P. Stability of functional outcomes following transitional living programme participation: 3 year follow-up. *Brain Injury, 8,* 439-447.

Hayden, M., Moreault, A., LeBlanc, J., & Plenger, P. (2000). Reducing level of handicap in traumatic brain injury: An environmentally based model of treatment. *Journal of Head Trauma Rehabilitation, 15,* 1000-1021.

Heinemann A. & Whiteneck, G. (1995) Relationships among impairment disability handicap and life satisfaction in persons with traumatic brain injury. *Journal of Head Trauma Rehabilitation, 10,* 54-63.

Hoofien, D., Gilboa, A., Vakil, E., & Donovick, P. (2001). Traumatic brain injury (TBI) 10-20 years later: A comprehensive outcome study of psychiatric symptomatology, cognitive abilities, and psychosocial functioning. *Brain Injury, 15,* 189-209.

Huebner, R., Johnson, K., Bennett, & Schneck, C. (2003). Community participation and quality of life outcomes after traumatic brain injury. *The American Journal of Occupational Therapy, 57,* 177-185.

Implement Neurorehabilitation, LLC. (2000). *Implement Neurorehabilitation, LLC: Providing the Tools for Life.* [Brochure]. Huntington, WV: James P. Phifer.

Jean-Bay, E. (2000). The biobehavioral correlates of post-traumatic brain injury depression. *Journal of Neuroscience Nursing, 32,* 169-176.

Johansson, U. & Bernspang, B. (2001). Predicting return to work after brain injury using occupational therapy assessments. *Disability and Rehabilitation, 23,* 474-480.

Johnston, M. & Lewis, F. (1991). Outcomes of community re-entry programmes for brain injury survivors. Part I: Independent living and productive activities. *Brain Injury, 5,* 141-154.

Jones, M., Patrick, P. Evans, R., & Wulff, J. (1991). The life coach model of community re-entry. In B. McMahon & L. Shaw (Eds.), *Work Worth Doing: Advances in Brain Injury Rehabilitation* (pp.279-302). Orlando, FL: Paul M. Deutsch Press, Inc.

Kersel, D., Marsh, N., Havill, J. & Sleigh, J. (2001). Neuropsychological functioning during the first year following severe traumatic brain injury. *Brain Injury, 15*(4), 283-296.

Koskinen, S. (1998). Quality of life 10 years after a very severe traumatic brain injury (TBI): the perspective of the injured and the closest relative. *Brain Injury, 8,* 631-648.

Kowalske, K., Plenger, P., Lusby, B., & Hayden, M. (2000). Vocational reentry following TBI: An enablement model. *Journal of Head Trauma Rehabilitation, 15,* 989-999.

Law, M. & Mills, J. (1998). Client-centered occupational therapy. In M. Law (Ed), *Client centered occupational therapy* (pp.1 -18). Thorofare, NJ: Slack, Inc.

Leahy, B. & Lam, C. (1998). Neuropsychological testing and functional outcome for individuals with traumatic brain injury. *Brain Injury, 12,* 1025-1035.

Levin, H., Grossman, R., Rose, J., & Teasdale, G. (1979). Long-term neuropsychological outcome of closed head injury. *Journal of Neurosurgery, 50,* 412-422.

Lindberg, M. (1995). Quality of life after subarachnoid hemorrhage and its relationship to impairments, disabilities, and depression. *Scandinavian Journal of Occupational Therapy, 2,* 105-112.

Malec, J., Smigielski, J., DePompolo, R., & Thompson, J. (1993). Outcome evaluation and prediction in a comprehensive- integrated post-acute outpatient brain injury rehabilitation programme. *Brain Injury, 7,* 15-29.

McCleary, C., Satz, P., Forney, D., Light, R., Zaucha, K., Asarnow, R. & Namerow, N. (1998). Depression after traumatic brain injury as a function of Glascow outcome score. *Journal of Clinical and Experimental Neuropsychology, 20,* 270-279.

McColl, M. & Bickenbach, J. (1998). Consequences of disability. In M. McColl & J. Bickenbach (Eds.), *Introduction to Disability* (pp.131-133). Philadelphia, PA: WB Saunders.

McColl, M., Carlson, P., Johnston, J., Minnes, K., Shue, K., Davies, D. et al. (1998). The definition of community integration: perspectives of people with brain injuries. *Brain Injury, 12*(1), 15-30.

McColl, M.A., Davies, D., Carlson, P, Johnston, J. & Minnes, P. (2001). The Community Integration Measurement: Development and preliminary validation. *Archives of Physical Medicine and Rehabilitation, 82*, 429-434.

McCordie, W., Barker, S., & Paolo, T. (1990) Return to work after head injury. *Brain Injury, 4*, 57-68.

McKinlay, W. & Watkiss, A. (1999). Cognitive and behavioral effects of brain injury. In M. Rosenthal, E. Griffith, J. Kreutzer & B. Pentland (Eds.), *Rehabilitation of the Adult and Child with Traumatic Brain Injury* (pp.74-86). Philadelphia, PA: FA Davis.

McMahon, B. & Shaw, L. (1991). The outpatient setting: the preferred context for post- acute rehabilitation. In B. McMahon & L. Shaw (Eds.), *Work Worth Doing: Advances in Brain Injury Rehabilitation*, (pp.31-41). Orlando, FL: Paul M. Deutsch Press, Inc.

McNeny, R. (1999). Activities of daily living. In M. Rosenthal, E. Griffith, J. Kreutzer, & B. Pentland (Eds.), *Rehabilitation of the Adult and Child with Traumatic Brain Injury* (pp.242-253). Philadelphia, PA: FA Davis.

Melamed, S., Groswasser, Z., & Stern, M. (1992). Acceptance of disability, work involvement and subjective rehabilitation status of traumatic brain injured (TBI) patients. *Brain Injury, 3*, 233-243.

Morton, M. & Wehman, P. (1995). Psychosocial and emotional sequelae of individuals following traumatic brain injury: a literature review and recommendations. *Brain Injury, 9*, 81-92.

Munro, B. (1997). *Statistical Methods for Health Care Research*. Philadelphia, PA: Lippincott.

National Institutes of Health. (1998). Rehabilitation of persons with traumatic brain injury. *NIH Consensus Statement, 16*, 1 -41.

Neto, F. (1993). The Satisfaction with Life Scale: Psychometric properties with an adolescent sample. *Journal of Youth and Adolescence, 22*, 125-134.

O'Hara, C., & Harrell, M. (1991). The empowerment rehabilitation model: Meeting the unmet needs of survivors, families, and treatment providers. *Cognitive Rehabilitation, 9*, 14-21.

Olver, J., Ponsford, J., & Curan, C. (1996). Outcome following traumatic brain injury: A comparison between 2 and 5 years after injury. *Brain Injury, 10*, 841-848.

O'Neill, J., Hibbard, M., Brown, M., Jaffe, M., Sliwinski, M., Vandergoot, D., & Weiss, M. (1998). The effect of employment on quality of life and community integration after traumatic brain injury. *Journal of Head Trauma Rehabilitation, 13*, 68-79.

Ownsworth, T. & Oei, T. (1998). Depression after traumatic brain injury: conceptualization and treatment considerations. *Brain Injury, 12*, 735-751.

Pavot, W. & Diener, E. (1993). Review of the Satisfaction with Life Scale. *Psychological Assessment, 5*, 164-172.

Pavot, W., Diener, E., Colvin, C., & Sandvik, E. (1991). Further validation of the Satisfaction with Life Scale: Evidence for the cross-method convergence of well-being measures. *Journal of Personality Assessment, 57*, 149-161.

Paniak C, Phillips K, Toller-Lobe G, Durand A, & Nagy J. (1999). Sensitivity of three recent questionnaires to mild traumatic brain injury: Related effects. *Journal of Head Trauma Rehabilitation, 14*, 211-219.

Pavot, W. & Diener, E. (1993). Review of the Satisfaction with Life Scale. *Psychological Assessment, 5,* 164-172.

Pavot, W., Diener, E., Colvin, C., & Sandvik, E. (1991). Further validation of the Satisfaction with Life Scale: Evidence for the cross-method convergence of well-being measures. *Journal of Personality Assessment, 57,* 149-161.

Ponsford, J., Olver, J. & Curran, C. (1996). A profile of outcome: 2 years after traumatic brain injury. *Brain Injury, 10,* 1-10.

Prigatano, G., Fordyce, D., Zeiner, H., Roueche, J., Pepping, M., & Wood, B. (1984). Neuropsychological rehabilitation after closed head injury in young adults. *Journal of Neurosurgical Psychiatry, 4,* 505-513.

Prigatano, G. & Schacter, D. (1986). Introduction. In G. Prigatano & D. Schacter (Eds.), *Awareness of Deficit after Brain Injury: Clinical and Theoretical Issues* (pp. 1-17). Baltimore, MD: Johns Hopkins University Press.

Reilly, M. (1962). Occupational therapy can be one of the greatest ideas of 20th century medicine. *American Journal of Occupational Therapy, 16,* 1-9.

Rice, R., Near, J., & Hunt, R. (1980). The job satisfaction/life satisfaction relationship: A review of empirical research. *Basic and Applied Social Psychology, 7,* 37-64.

Rosenthal, M., Christensen, B. & Ross, T. (1998). Depression following traumatic brain injury. *Archives of Physical Medicine and Rehabilitation, 79,* 90-103.

Rowlands, A. (2001). Ability or disability? Strength-based practice in the area of traumatic brain injury. *Families in Society: The Journal of Contemporary Human Services,* May/June, 273-286.

Sander, A., Fuchs, K., High Jr., Hall, Kreutzer, & Rosenthal. (1999). The Community Integration Questionnaire revisited: An assessment of structural validity. *Archives of Physical Medicine and Rehabilitation, 80,* 1303-1309.

Sander, A., Roebuck, T., Struchen, M., Sherer, & M., High, Jr., W. (2001). Long term maintenance of gains obtained in post -acute rehabilitation by persons with traumatic brain injury. *Journal of Head Trauma Rehabilitation, 16,* 356-373.

Sander A., Seel R., Kreutzer J., Hall K., High W., & Rosenthal M.(1997). Agreement between persons with traumatic brain injury and their relatives regarding psychosocial outcome using the Community Integration Questionnaire. *Archives of Physical Medicine and Rehabilitation, 78,* 353-357.

Seale, G., Caroselli, J., High, W., Becker, C., Neese, L., & Scheibel, R. (2002). Use of the Community Integration Questionnaire (CIQ) to characterize changes in functioning for individuals with traumatic brain injury who participated in a post-acute rehabilitation programme. *Brain Injury, 16,* 955-967.

Seibert, P., Reedy, D., Hash, J., Webb, A., Stridh-Igo, P., Basom, J., & Zimmerman, C. (2002). Brain injury: quality of life's greatest challenge. *Brain Injury, 16,* 837-848.

Shevlin, M., Brunsden, V., & Miles, J. (1998). Satisfaction with Life Scale: Analysis of factorial invariance, mean structures, and reliability. *Personality and Individual Differences, 25,* 911-916.

Sokol, K., Heinemann, A., Bode, R., Shin, J., Van de Veteer, L. (1999). Community participation after TBI: Factors predicting return to work and life satisfaction. Poster Presentation at the 127th Annual Meeting of the American Public Health Association, Chicago, IL.

Steadman-Pare, D., Colantonio, A., Ratcliff, G., Chase, S., & Vernich, L. (2001). Factors associated with perceived quality of life many years after traumatic brain injury. *Journal of Head Trauma Rehabilitation, 16*, 330-342.

Struchen, Davis, Bogaards, Hudler-Hull, Clark, Mazzei, Sander, & Caroselli. (2011). Making connections after brain injury: Development and evaluation of a social peer-mentoring program for persons with traumatic brain injury. *The Journal of Head Trauma Rehabilitation, 26*(1), 4-19.

Thomsen, I. (1987). Late psychosocial outcome in severe blunt trauma. Brain Injury, *1*, 131-143.

Underhill, A., Lobello, S., Stroud, T., Terry, K., Devivo, M., & Fine, P. (2003). Depression and life satisfaction in patients with traumatic brain injury: a longitudinal study. *Brain Injury, 17*, 973-982.

Varney, N. & Menefee, L. (1993). Psychosocial and executive deficits following closed head injury: Implications for orbito -frontal cortex. *Journal of Head Trauma Rehabilitation, 8*, 32-44.

Verbrugge, L. & Jette, A. (1994). The disablement process. *Social Science and Medicine, 38*, 1-14.

Viitanen, M., Fugl-Meyer, A. Bernspang, B., & Fugl-Meyer, A. (1988). Life satisfaction in long-term survivors after stroke. *Scandinavian Journal of Rehabilitation Medicine, 20*, 17-28.

Vitaliano, P., Russo, J., Young, H., Becker, J., & Maiuro, R. (1991). The screen for caregiver burden. *Gerontologist, 31*, 76-83.

Warden, D., Salazar, A., Martin, E., Schwab, K., Coyle, M., & Walter, J. (2000). A home program of rehabilitation for moderately severe traumatic brain injury patients. *Journal of Traumatic Brain Injury, 15*, 1092-1102.

Warren, L., Wrigley, J., Yoels, W., & Fine, P. (1996). Factors associated with life satisfaction among a sample of persons with neurotrama. *Journal of Rehabilitation Research and Development, 33*, 404-408.

Watt, S., Shores, A., & Knoshita, S. (1999). Effects of reducing attentional resources on implicit and explicit memory after severe traumatic brain injury. *Neuropsychology. 13*, 338-349.

Webb, C., Wrigley, M., Yoels, W., and Fine, P. (1995). Explaining quality of life for persons with traumatic brain injuries 2 years after injury. *Archives of Physical Medicine and Rehabilitation, 76*, 1113-1119.

Wehman, P., West, M., Johnson, A., & Cifu, D. (1999). Vocational rehabilitation for individuals with traumatic brain injury. In M. Rosenthal, E. Griffith, J. Kreutzer, & B. Pentland (Eds.), *Rehabilitation of the Adult and Child with Traumatic Brain Injury* (pp.326-341). Philadelphia, PA: FA Davis.

Wheeler, S., Lane, S, & McMahon, B. (2007). Community Participation and Life Satisfaction following Intensive Community Based Rehabilitation using a Life Skills Training Approach. *OTJR: Occupation, Participation and Health,27*(1), 13 -22.

Willer, B., Allen, K., Durnam, M., & Ferry, A. (1990). Problems and coping strategies of mothers, siblings, and young adult males with traumatic brain injury. *Canadian Journal of Rehabilitation, 2*, 167-173.

Willer, B. & Corrigan, J. (1994). A model for community based services: The whatever it takes model. *Brain Injury, 8*, 647 -659.

Willer, B., Ottenbacher, K., & Coad, M. (1994). The Community Integration Questionnaire: A comparative examination. *The American Journal of Physical Medicine and Rehabilitation, 73,* 103-111.

Willer B., Rosenthal M., Kreutzer J., Gordon W., & Rempel R. (1993). Assessment of community integration following rehabilitation for traumatic brain injury. *Journal of Head Trauma Rehabilitation, 8,* 5-87.

World Health Organization. (2001). *International Classification of Functioning, Disability, and Health.* Geneva, Switzerland: WHO.

7

Cognitive Recovery and Rehabilitation After Brain Injury: Mechanisms, Challenges and Support

Jesper Mogensen
The Unit for Cognitive Neuroscience, Department of Psychology
University of Copenhagen
Denmark

1. Introduction

When the brain is injured by vascular incidents (stroke) or mechanical impact leading to traumatic brain injury (TBI), the consequences for the patient are almost inevitably impairments within the motor, sensory, and/or cognitive domains. Such impairments may initially appear more disturbing and devastating to the patient – as well as to her/his loved ones – if the motor abilities are affected. The future of the patients in terms of quality of life, ability to return to independent living and potentially work may, however, depend more crucially on the degree to which the cerebral injury has caused impairments within cognitive domains such as language, attention, learning, memory, and problem solving (e.g. Moore & Stambrook, 1995). In spite of the devastating impact cognitive impairments frequently have on the future life of brain injured patients, there has historically been a disproportional focus of both research and therapeutic efforts on the motor symptoms. While research and therapeutic development within the motor domains are still in need of greater efforts, there is an even more compelling need for such efforts within the area of cognitive consequences of brain injury.

2. Cognitive recovery after brain injury

When injury severs the input or output pathways of the brain (e.g. the optic nerve or the major descending motor pathways) the consequences may be a rather chronic loss of sensory input or the ability to execute motor action, respectively. In such cases the degree of posttraumatic functional recovery may remain limited although processes of an obviously "compensational" nature may allow the patient to achieve at least some degree of "recovery". In case of the complete loss of sensory input within one modality, a degree of intermodal plasticity may allow input via other modalities to substitute somewhat for the lost input (e.g. Bach-y-Rita et al., 1969, 1998; Kaczmarek et al., 1991; Ptito et al., 2005). And spared parts of the motor output pathways may allow the patient to achieve at least some level of mobility (e.g. Levin et al., 2009). Within the cognitive domains, however, a certain level of posttraumatic functional recovery and clinical rehabilitation appears to be more the rule than the exception.

When posttraumatic functional recovery is defined as a more or less complete return to the pretraumatic level of behavioural/cognitive proficiency of task performance and/or conscious representation, such a recovery is documented in numerous studies in both patients and animal models (e.g. Buller & Hardcastle, 2000; Carney et al., 1999; León-Carrión & Machuca-Murga, 2001; Mogensen, 2011a, 2011b, 2011c; Mogensen & Malá, 2009; Mogensen et al., 2004a, 2007; Overgaard & Mogensen, 2011; J. Panksepp & J.B. Panksepp, 2000; Ramachandran & Blakeslee, 1998; Rohling et al., 2009). Mostly, such instances of posttraumatic functional recovery are demonstrated in association with formalized rehabilitative training. There are, however, also instances of what is termed "spontaneous" recovery (e.g. León-Carrión & Machuca-Murga, 2001). A recovery process is normally defined as being "spontaneous" if the subjects - patients or experimental animals - have not been subjected to a specific posttraumatic training procedure, and it is frequently implied that the "spontaneous" recovery is the result of one or another type of experience-independent process. It may, however, be naïve automatically to assume that recovery in the absence of formalized training is necessarily experience-independent. Even in the absence of formalized training, patients and experimental animals alike are constantly exposed to the challenges of daily living. Under almost all circumstances, daily activities such as (more or less successful) coordination of movements, communication (or attempted communication), feeding and other basic activities constitute in themselves informal types of "training". Consequently, it is hard to discriminate between experience-dependent and experience-independent types of recovery processes. There can, however, be no doubt that truly experience-independent processes do occur. One example is recovery associated with disappearance of an injury-associated "penumbra". Briefly described, the penumbra phenomenon is a situation in which injury within one part of the brain causes other brain areas to receive a reduced level of blood supply. Although the reduced blood supply within the penumbra region is sufficient for the survival of the neurons, normal levels of functionality are not possible within the tissue affected by the penumbra. Consequently, the symptoms observed during the presence of the penumbra are a combination of the consequences of the actually lost tissue and the functional impairments within the brain regions affected by the penumbra. Penumbras mostly disappear spontaneously and when that happens, a normal level of functional performance is restored within the affected part of the brain (e.g. Choi et al., 2007).

Both clinically and in animal models the degree to which the functional recovery manages to eliminate the trauma-associated symptoms varies greatly. In some instances, even extensive rehabilitative training can only achieve limited degrees of functional recovery, while in other instances the recovery turn out to be "complete" - when defined as the acquisition of a posttraumatic proficiency equal to that seen in the absence of any brain injury (e.g. Mogensen et al., 2004a). It is important to stress that in animal models such a "complete" functional recovery can be demonstrated even under circumstances ensuring the complete removal of the brain structure in question - and utilizing comparisons to a well-established pretraumatic functional baseline. From a theoretical point of view such a functional recovery - but for the few instances in which it may be ascribed to the disappearance of penumbras or similar phenomena - poses a severe challenge to the concept of "functional localization".

2.1 Functional localization and recovery

Within the neuroscientific literature there is a widespread consensus that a regional specialization exists within the brain. Various structures and substructures are functionally specialized and it appears to make sense to speak about a "localization" of various "functions" (e.g. Coltheart, 2001; Kringelbach & Rolls, 2004; Monakow, 1914; Selnes, 2001). Support for the idea of a functional specialization within the structures of the brain mainly comes from two sources: (1) various types of neuroimaging techniques (e.g. PET and fMRI) reveal rather consistent patterns of regional cerebral activation when subjects are stimulated in particular ways, perform particular tasks, etc., and (2) "lesion experiments" (be it clinical examinations of brain injured patients or controlled experiments in animal models) demonstrate that lesions or regional inactivations within a particular brain structure are associated with specific patterns of symptoms.

Especially the latter source of evidence for a functional localization is directly related to the mentioned contradiction between "functional localization" and posttraumatic "functional recovery". While it seems logical that loss (lesion) of a specialized brain structure leads to a predictable type of impairment (reflecting the posttraumatic absence of that functional contribution) it appears illogical to expect a "recovery" of the lost "function" after lesions of a specialized brain structure - since regrowth of the missing brain region appears not to occur. Nevertheless, localization as well as posttraumatic recovery of functions are highly documented empirical facts (see above and e.g. Mogensen, 2011a, 2011c; Mogensen & Malá, 2009). To resolve this apparent contradiction is not only an important theoretical challenge in order to understand the functional organization and reorganization of the brain. It is also an important issue in the context of developing new clinical methods aiming at improving, supporting and completing the rehabilitative efforts within cognitive domains.

Aphasia may be one of the best-studied clinical conditions when it comes to the attempted mapping of the neural substrate of functional recovery. Aphasias primarily result from injury to the left hemisphere, and ipsilateral contributions to the mediation of reacquired linguistic functions have been documented by for instance Szaflarski et al. (2011), Perani et al. (2003), Specht et al. (2009), and Meinzer et al. (2008). Meinzer et al. (2008) demonstrated treatment-induced reintegration of various perilesional areas. However, the most commonly asked question in the field of posttraumatic reacquisition of language is, whether the contralateral (right) hemisphere contributes significantly to the mediation of posttraumatic recovery? Numerous studies have found the apparent involvement of structures within the right hemisphere in the mediation of posttraumatic recovery of language (e.g. Ansaldo & Arguin, 2003; Ansaldo et al., 2002; Baumgaertner et al., 2005; Perani et al., 2003; Specht et al., 2009; Thomas et al., 1997; Thulborn et al., 1999). There are indications (e.g. Thomas et al., 1997) that the pattern of shift towards right hemisphere mediation of linguistic functions may differ between types of aphasia. Additionally, changes in the direction of right hemisphere mediation of language may be accompanied by internal reorganizations within the left hemisphere (shifts to ipsilateral mediation by uninjured regions). These reorganizations may lead to a more bilateral representation of language - due to the concurrent shift of linguistic mediation within the left hemisphere and to the contralateral, right hemisphere (e.g. Thompson et al., 2010). Mostly, the recovery-associated shifts towards right hemisphere mediation of linguistic functions seem to occur without rehabilitative training specifically aimed at such a shift (instead, rehabilitation has been aimed in a more general way towards recovery of linguistic abilities). However, in some cases aphasic patients have - somewhat successfully - been subjected to training aimed at achieving a higher degree of right hemisphere mediation of linguistic tasks (e.g. Crosson et al., 2009). Crosson et al. (2009) used a manipulation task performed with the patient's left hand to initiate naming trials and thereby obtain an independent right hemisphere activation, which presumably can ease an interhemispheric shift of linguistic task mediation. It may be questioned to what extent the changes in neural activity observed via for instance fMRI in a recovering or recovered aphasic patient are specifically related to the reacquisition of language. Posttraumatic changes in activity within a given structure may be the consequences of any trauma-related process - e.g. "disinhibition" due to lack of input from the injured brain region. Or for that matter any other process, which is not directly related to the recovery of linguistic abilities. Such reservations may be less prominent in certain cases. For instance, Meinzer et al. (2007) studied the recovery of a bilingual aphasic patient. In this case, activation of parts of the superior temporal lobe of the right hemisphere was exclusively associated with the use of the trained language while no such activation was observed associated with the untrained language.

3. Mechanisms of posttraumatic functional recovery

In spite of technical reservations in many individual instances, studies such as these on the posttraumatic functional recovery of linguistic abilities clearly indicate that there is a degree of "shift" of functional mediation to other structures - and presumably cases of "vicariation" (the phenomenon that brain areas with different functions can assume or "take over" the function of an injured brain region (e.g. Finger & Stein, 1982; Slavin et al., 1988)). In philosophy of mind such plastic properties of the brain have been taken as evidence for multiple realization and as an argument in favour of functionalism (e.g. Block & Fodor, 1972). As argued by Overgaard & Mogensen (2011), conclusions regarding multiple realizations require a much deeper and detailed analysis in order to utilize for instance the results of studies mapping posttraumatic task mediation. And, only by addressing more thoroughly the detailed mechanisms of posttraumatic reorganization of the brain can one achieve a thorough understanding of the degree to which functions are "relocalized" (e.g. Mogensen, 2011a, 2011c; Mogensen & Malá, 2009).

A very basic issue in this context is to address the likelihood that the basic circuitry of the brain regions lost to injury is (re)established elsewhere in the brain. This topic is discussed in detail by Mogensen (2011a, 2011c) and although even the adult brain possesses an impressive level of plasticity, it appears unlikely that the posttraumatic processes include such a recreation of lost circuitry. During maturation neurons undergo a number of changes making them less similar to those immature neurons, which originally formed the local circuitry of the brain (e.g. D.F. Chen et al., 1995; Fawcett et al., 1989; Goldberg et al., 2002). There is, however, an ongoing neurogenesis in the adult brain and this neurogenesis is potentiated by injury to the brain (e.g. Arvidsson et al., 2002; J. Chen et al., 2004; Magavi et al., 2000; Nakatomi et al., 2002; Scharff et al., 2000). Such newly formed neurons may - compared to more mature neurons - be better equipped to recreate a particular circuitry. And they may receive support in reaching the relevant brain regions since, upon injury, mature astrocytes are able to transform themselves into radial glial cells similar to those guiding the neural migration during development (Leavitt et al., 1999; Rakic, 1971, 1985). While these observations may create a level of optimism regarding the potential for recreation of lost circuitry, there is one crucial factor, which appears to prevent the adult brain (uninjured or injured) from recreating such networks. From the final stages of the original ontogenic development - and formation of the basic circuitry of the brain - a number of factors associated with glial cells and myelin appear to prevent restructuring and presumably recreation of such a basic circuitry (e.g. Berry, 1982; Schäfer et al., 2008; Schwab

& Thoenen, 1985). An especially important such factor appears to be the astrocyte-produced chondroitin sulphate proteoglycans (CSPGs). The CSPGs play an important role in termination of the developmentally "critical periods" and they are believed to "consolidate" the originally formed circuitry in its "final" form (e.g., Berardi et al., 2004; Del Rio & Soriano, 2007; McGee et al., 2005; Pizzorusso al., 2002; Schäfer et al., 2008). Apparently, the presence of these CSPGs blocks the possibility of an adult recreation of traumatically lost networks (e.g. Del Rio & Soriano, 2007; Schäfer et al., 2008). Consequently, the recreation of the basic circuitry lost to TBI or vascular incidents is unlikely to occur. Which further stresses the need for an improved understanding of the posttraumatic reorganizations and recovery-associated processes of the brain.

While clinical studies (for instance the analyses of ipsi- and contralateral contributions to posttraumatic reacquisition of language - see above) are obviously of significant importance, only well-controlled animal models (e.g. Mogensen, 2011b) can avoid some of the shortcomings of clinical studies (for instance the occurrence of subtotal lesions of brain structures as well as multiple brain regions being simultaneously affected by injury). Such animal models can also allow a degree of experimental manipulation, which is impossible to achieve in human studies. An extensive animal model-based research program (e.g. Mogensen et al., 2002, 2003, 2004a, 2005, 2007) has scrutinized the mechanisms of post-traumatic recovery processes. Utilizing a spectrum of organic and behavioural/cognitive "challenge" methods (e.g. Mogensen, 2011b; Mogensen & Malá, 2009) these studies have provided insights into the neural and cognitive processes mediating the posttraumatic functional recovery of various cognitive processes.

As reviewed by Mogensen (2011a, 2011c) and Mogensen & Malá (2009) a pattern of principles of posttraumatic functional recovery has emerged from the above-mentioned studies and others. Three general principles are especially important and describe the situation after a successful posttraumatic rehabilitation:

1. *Modification of the degree of contribution to task mediation by individual brain structures:*
   Some structures exhibit an increased or decreased level of contribution to task mediation.
2. *Task dependent and dissimilar neural substrates:*
   After a given lesion, the functional recovery of various cognitive tasks is mediated by unique and dissimilar neural substrates.
3. *Application of new cognitive strategies:*
   The fully posttraumatically recovered individuals solve the task by applying new strategies that are dissimilar to those applied pretraumatically.

Supporting the above-mentioned conclusion that posttraumatic recreation of the lost basic circuitry is unlikely, point 2 and 3 of these principles emphasize that the lost information processing (i.e. the destroyed circuitry) appear not to have returned even in case of a situation in which the individual has obtained a full functional recovery. If - within any part of the brain - the rehabilitative training had been accompanied by a recreation of a circuitry similar to that available in the pretraumatic situation, one would expect all cognitive domains affected by the lesion to posttraumatically receive equal contributions to functional recovery from the brain region within which the circuitry had been recreated. Such a situation is contradicted by Principle 2. Principle 3 contradicts the re-establishment of the information processing lost to injury. If posttraumatic processes had re-established the information processing of the injured brain structure, one would expect not only task solutions of a proficiency similar to that seen preoperatively (which is, indeed, seen in some instances), but also that such a task solution would employ similar strategies to those of the pretraumatic situation.

3.1 The REF-model

It has to be concluded that although the brain is posttraumatically capable of a high degree of behaviourally defined functional recovery (even up to the level of a "full" recovery enabling a proficiency similar to that seen prior to injury), the brain does so without recreating the basic circuitry, which has been lost to injury. In order to account for this situation Mogensen (2011a, 2011c) and Mogensen & Malá (2009) have proposed the so-called REF (Reorganization of Elementary Functions) model. While the REF-model has primarily been developed on the basis of research focusing on posttraumatic functional recovery within the cognitive domains, it is believed to account for neural and cognitive processes, which have evolved in order to mediate behavioural and cognitive flexibility (including problem solving) in the intact brain (see Mogensen (2011a, 2011c) for further discussions).
According to the REF-model, three levels of analysis are important to the understanding of the mechanisms of posttraumatic functional recovery (see Table 1). At the lowest of these three levels are the basic information processing modules named Elementary Functions (EFs). Each EF contributes a "modular" type of information processing. The EFs are truly localized. They are at the level of true "functional localization" - in the sense that each EF is mediated by a specific substructure of a brain region. Traditionally defined brain structures (e.g. the hippocampus or the prefrontal cortex) contain the neural substrate of numerous EFs. When a brain structure is lost to injury, all EFs mediated by the subregions within that structure are irreversibly lost. Presently, the functional properties of the individual EFs are poorly characterized. The conceptual distance between the EFs and what is traditionally defined as cognitive or "psychological" functions is significant. When characterization of an EF becomes possible, it is likely that the functional properties of EFs may best be described in mathematical terms rather than in the vocabulary of cognitive psychology. At the top of these three levels are the surface phenomena of behavioural and/or mental manifestations - including cognitive awareness. It is at the level of these surface phenomena that the symptoms upon brain injury are normally characterized (in terms of behavioural and/or cognitive impairments) and it is also at the level of the surface phenomena that post-traumatic functional recovery is normally observed - be it in clinics or in most cases of animal model-based experiments. To bridge the gab between the non-recovering EFs and these surface phenomena, the level of Algorithmic Strategies (ASs) has been inserted.
Each AS consists of numerous interacting EFs. ASs are primarily established as a consequence of experience and learning - although some may be genetically preprogramed. The neural substrate of an AS consists of the neural substrates of all its constituent EFs plus the interconnections between the neural substrates of these EFs. Therefore, while an EF is strictly localized to a particular subregion of a brain structure, most ASs are distributed across many regions of the brain. The information processing of an AS is the mechanism mediating a specific surface phenomenon (e.g. a specific solution of a specific task). Most surface phenomena can be realized via the activity of a multitude of ASs. The task solutions achieved via activation of various ASs may provide outcomes of similar proficiency and unless special analytical techniques are employed, it is at the surface level not possible to discriminate between behavioural phenomena reflecting two related but different ASs. When injury destroys the neural substrate of one or more of the constituent EFs within an

AS, that AS (and as a consequence the surface phenomenon relying on that AS) is lost and posttraumatically this surface phenomenon is impaired.

SURFACE PHENOMENA (Mental/Behavioural manifestation level) • Final products in terms of mental states (potentially conscious) and overt behaviour • Realized by a multitude of individual Algorithmic Strategies (ASs) ALGORITHMIC STRATEGIES (ASs) • Consists of numerous interacting Elementary Functions (EFs) • Mostly a result of experience and learning *Neural substrate:* The substrate of the constituent EFs plus the interconnections between these EFs - that is: most ASs are distributed across many regions of the brain ELEMENTARY FUNCTIONS (EFs) • Truly localized • Perform basic information-processing *Neural substrate:* Substructures/local circuits - within a given brain structure - that is: EFs are fully localized

Table 1. The three levels of analysis of the REF-model - including some of the characteristics of Algorithmic Strategies (ASs) and Elementary Functions (EFs). For further details, see the present text as well as Figs. 1 and 2 in Mogensen & Malá (2009) and Fig. 1 in Mogensen (2011a).

An individual may encounter the demand for a task solution for which there is no established procedure available in at least two different contexts. The situation (and task) may be of a novel nature, thereby presenting the intact individual with a previously unexperienced situation (to which there is no obvious generalization from previous experience). Or the situation may in reality be known from previous experience, but brain injury has robbed the individual of the possibility of utilizing previously established procedures. Whether for one or the other of these reasons - in the terminology of the REF-model - the situation is not a priori associated with activation of a specific AS. In such situations, a process of activation of individual ASs as mediators of behaviour is initiated (see Fig. 1). The quality of the resultant behaviour and/or conscious representation is evaluated and in case of success a future association between that situation and the tested AS is established. In case of failure, an alternative AS is activated and evaluated - thereby continuing a process potentially including the evaluation of numerous pre-existing ASs (for further descriptions see Mogensen (2011a, 2011c) and Mogensen & Malá (2009)). This process bears some resemblance to what was described as the "hypothesis" evaluation of Krechevsky (1932, 1933). The selector/evaluator mechanism controlling the activation and evaluation of ASs resembles (but is not identical to) the "Supervisory Attentional System" (SAS) of Norman & Shallice (1986). If a pre-existing AS is eventually found to successfully give rise to the required surface phenomenon, the situation will in the future be associated with activation of that AS. The neural plasticity involved in this process consists of modified connections within the selector/evaluator mechanism. This plasticity mediates the future association between the situation in question and the selection and activation of successfully utilized AS.

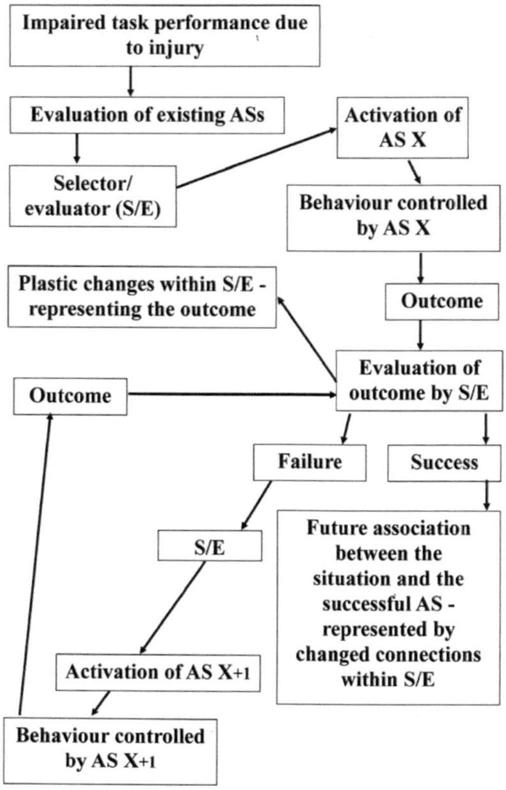

Fig. 1. Flow diagram depicting the sequence of events which according to the REF-model leads to a successful functional recovery after brain injury - provided that a pre-existing AS can achieve a successful task solution. For further details see the present text as well as Figs. 3, 4, and 5 in Mogensen & Malá (2009), Fig. 1 in Mogensen (2011c), and Fig. 2 in Mogensen (2011a).

If the evaluation of existing ASs does not lead to a successful task solution, a novel AS will have to be created and associated with the situation in question. The creation of a novel AS involves a reorganization of the functional interactions between EFs and is the actual "Reorganization of Elementary Functions" (REF) process. This reorganization (see Mogensen, 2011a, 2011c; Mogensen & Malá, 2009) includes a type of process resembling the backpropagation algorithm (e.g. Rumelhart & McClelland, 1986; Werbos, 1994). A schematic and simplified representation of this process is illustrated in Fig. 2 (and in Fig. 5 in Mogensen & Malá, 2009). Utilizing such a backpropagation-resembling process, a set of EFs - which previously did not constitute an interacting entity - is functionally united to form a novel AS. Most likely, backpropagation mechanisms constantly modify the connectivity between EFs. The outcome of an attempted task solution (whether successful or not) results (in parallel to the feedback to the selector/evaluator mechanism regarding the degree of success of the attempted task solution) also in a backpropagation process modifying the connectivity (and consequently functional interaction) between individual EFs. This is illustrated in Panel B of Fig. 2 while Panel A and C, respectively, illustrates the (highly simplified) functional interactions (and connectivity between neural substrates) of individual EFs. While many of the interconnections between EFs remain unchanged between Panel A and C, a number of changes have occurred. The most striking may be that EF 22 and EF 47 - which originally (Panel A) did not participate in AS X and AS X+1, respectively - are now integrated into the network of these two ASs. Furthermore, EF 53 - which originally (Panel A) was part of AS X+2 - no longer (Panel C) participates in the information processing of AS X+2. Examples of other changes are a strengthening of the connectivity and functional interaction between EF 2 and EF 16 as well as a weakening of the connectivity and functional interaction between EF 39 and EF 16. As is illustrated in Panel D of Fig. 2, the backpropagation mediated plastic changes - and thereby reorganization of functional relationships between EFs - can result in the creation of a network, which in itself constitutes the basis for a novel AS - in this case AS X+3.

It is important to notice that what is modified as a result of this backpropagation-mechanism is the connectivity between EFs rather than any aspect of the internal circuitry of the EFs. According to the REF-model, the circuitry of individual EFs as well as their information processing remains unchanged by these processes. They do, however, perform that information processing in a novel context and on information of novel sources. Within the domains of sensory and perceptual analysis examples of a somewhat related process can be found. In individuals in whom one of the hands has been amputated, the region of somatosensory cortex, which used to represent the now missing hand, does not remain "vacant". Instead, the neighbouring somatosensory regions (representing the arm and face, respectively) encroaches on the "vacant" area in such a way that the original hand area is eventually fully taken over by inputs from arm and face, respectively (e.g. Karl et al., 2001; Weiss et al., 2000; Yang et al., 1994). Also, training restricted to part of the body may be associated with relative shifts within the somatosensory representations (e.g. Elbert et al., 1995; Merzenich & Jenkins, 1993; Münte et al., 2002; Xerri et al., 1996). Somewhat similar processes are found within the auditory system where the tonotopic representations at various levels may be reorganized as a result of both partial loss of input (e.g. due to restricted cochlear lesions) and learning experiences in intact individuals (e.g. Irvine, 2007; Recanzone et al., 1993; D. Robertson & Irvine, 1989; Scheich, 1991; Thai-Van et al., 2007). In all of these instances neural "modules", which originally performed their information processing (and contribution to sensory and perceptual processes) on information from one part of the body or aspect of the tonotopic spectrum, respectively, received a modified input but most likely continued to perform identical or rather similar information processing on information from another part of the body or tonotopic spectrum, respectively (for further discussion: see Mogensen, 2011a, 2011c; Overgaard & Mogensen, 2011). At least some cases of intermodal plasticity (e.g. Bach-y-Rita et al., 1969, 1998; Kaczmarek et al., 1991; Ptito et al., 2005) may provide somewhat related examples. For instance, in "early blind" individuals Ptito et al. (2005) found a spatial orientation discrimination performed on somatosensory information to be partly mediated by a cortical region, that in sighted individuals is associated with the performance of visual tasks in which the spatial orientation of figures are to be determined. As discussed further by Mogensen (2011a, 2011c), the cortical region in question may have contributed the same type of information processing in sighted and blind individuals, respectively, but receiving the relevant inputs from visual and somatosensory inputs, respectively.

As mentioned above, the processes described by the REF-model are likely to have evolved in the context of problem solving, and behavioural as well as conscious flexibility in the intact individual (Mogensen, 2011a, 2011c). They, however, automatically also become the

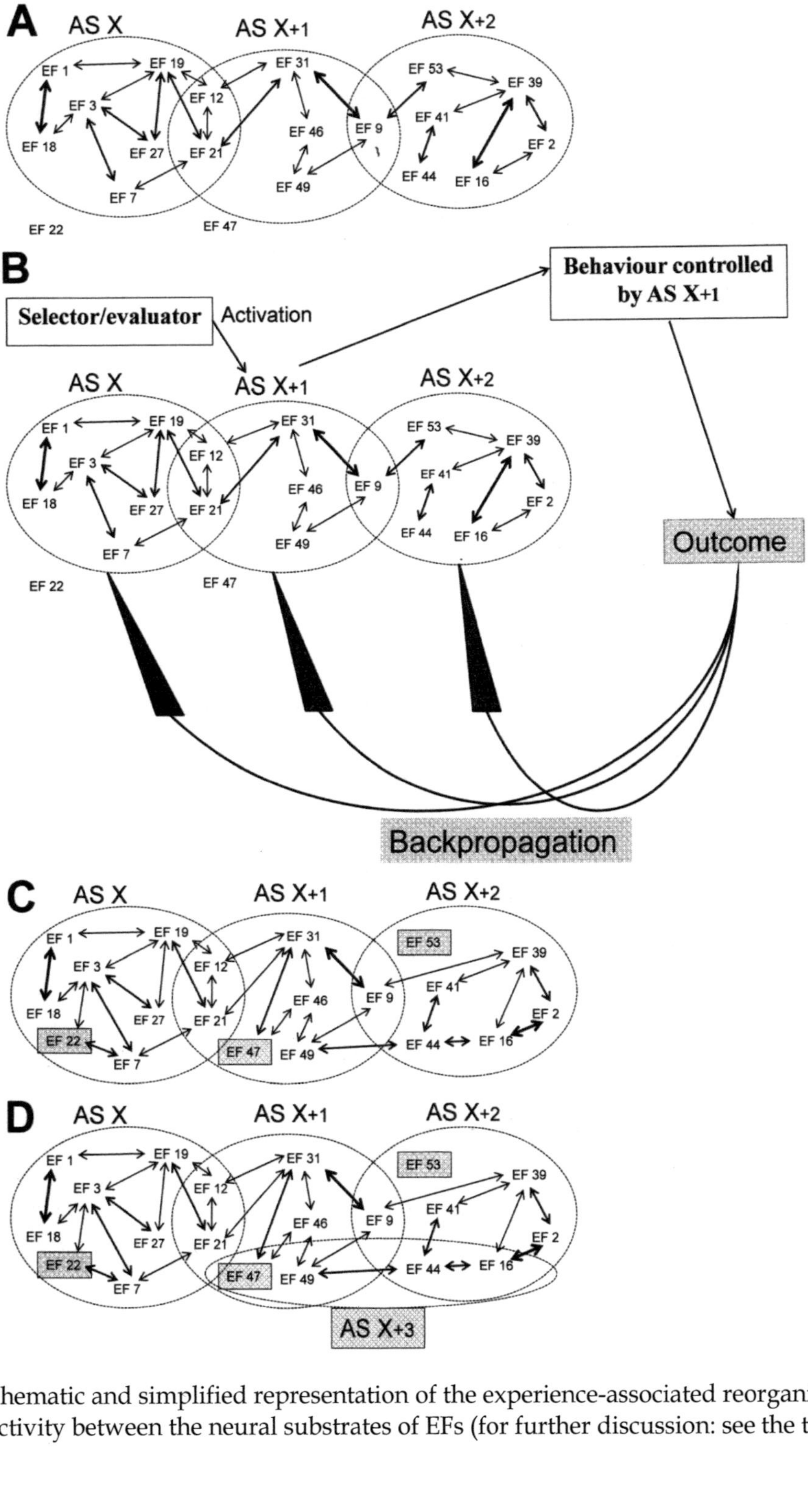

Fig. 2. Schematic and simplified representation of the experience-associated reorganizations of connectivity between the neural substrates of EFs (for further discussion: see the text).

mechanisms of posttraumatic functional recovery when brain injury robs the individual of the EFs, ASs, and thereby mechanisms, which pretraumatically allowed a particular task to be solved. What was pretraumatically associated with an efficient task solution (activation of an appropriate AS in the terminology of the REF-model) is posttraumatically equivalent to a "novel problem solving situation" and thereby calls for the above-described mechanisms of search for an adequate AS and potentially the creation of a novel AS.

Posttraumatically, the behaviourally defined "complete functional recovery" is in the context of the REF-model to be seen as a situation in which the posttraumatic task solution is accomplished via an AS, that allows behavioural manifestation which cannot - but for a detailed (and most often not performed) behavioural/cognitive analysis - be distinguished from the behaviour occurring pretraumatically. The apparent contradiction between "functional localization" and "functional recovery" is, according to the REF-model, the result of a "confusion of levels" regarding the term "function". The term "function" is used in two different contexts. What is truly localized is the information processing of the individual EFs - an information processing which is permanently lost when the neural substrate of those EFs are destroyed by injury. On the other hand, the "functional recovery" is observed and defined according to the surface phenomena, which can posttraumatically be achieved at a more or less similar proficiency to that seen pretraumatically via the activation of alternative ASs (which do not depend on the EFs lost to injury) (for further discussion: see Mogensen, 2011a, 2011c; Mogensen & Malá, 2009).

4. Implications of the REF-model for posttraumatic rehabilitative training

One of the implications of the REF-model is that the neuroplastic changes, which are essential to the mediation of posttraumatic cognitive recovery, are "instructed" by two types of feedback regarding the outcome of the processes in which the behavioural manifestations of a particular AS meet the current environment: the feedback to the selector/evaluator mechanism (e.g. Fig. 1) and the backpropagation mechanism instructing the reorganization of the connectivity between EFs (Fig. 2) (see further discussions in Mogensen, 2011a, 2011c; Mogensen & Malá, 2009). As stressed by Mogensen (2011a) it can be argued, that it is at the level of the surface phenomena that the primary causation of plastic changes is to be found. When the functional manifestations at the surface level interact with a specific environment, the feedback and backpropagation mechanisms lead to a "downward causation" according to which AS-selection and potentially creation of a novel AS is achieved. This is a situation with important implications for clinical practise in terms of rehabilitative training.

The outcome of the specific interaction between the individual and the current environment is the source of both the plastic modifications within the selector/evaluator mechanism and the modified connectivity between individual EFs. Consequently, the future nature as well as selection of ASs related to a particular task depends crucially on the situation in which the training leading to posttraumatic functional recovery has occurred. One may, in other words, expect a potentially worrying degree of situational dependence of the outcome of the rehabilitative training. As discussed elsewhere (e.g. Mogensen, 2011a, 2011c; Mogensen & Malá, 2009; Wilms & Mogensen, 2011) a rehabilitative training program may lead to highly proficient task solutions in the particular task and training setting administered in the clinical context - while unfortunately having little or no generalization to the everyday life situation of the patient. Therefore, patients might appear fully "recovered" when subjected to formal testing in a hospital or other clinical setting while subsequently demonstrating severe recidual problems in non-institutionalized contexts (e.g. Mogensen, 2011a; Wilms & Mogensen, 2011).

An important implication of this situation is that as far as possible rehabilitative training should be conducted under circumstances optimizing generalization to the everyday environment of the patient. Ideally, training within clinical institutions should be organized in manners resembling the everyday challenges of the patient's home and potentially workplace. Furthermore, training should be continued as seemlessly as possible into the daily environment to which the patient eventually returns after leaving the hospital and/or other institutions. Utilization of advanced technology is a growing and important field within neurorehabilitation. The use of such technologies may contribute towards realizing the ideal of "life-like" training situations in the institution and the possibility of continuing rehabilitative training in an "out-of-institution" setting. The development of virtual reality settings and utilization of these in rehabilitative training holds the promise of much more life-like training situations in the institution. Utilization of various hand-held micro-computers and similar devises may allow a relatively formalized but highly flexible "training" to continue into the daily life of the patient. An example of the latter may be the success of the "NeuroPage" project (e.g. Wilson et al., 1997) in which hand-held devises support and ease the daily life of amnestic patients - while also producing apparent training effects, which makes the NeuroPage not only a "cognitive prosthesis" but makes it part of an actual rehabilitative training process (e.g. Wilson et al., 2001).

The utilization of computers and other types of advanced technology in the rehabilitative training of brain injured patients obviously holds significant promise - not the least regarding possibilities of creating a more "ecologically valid" cognitive training by "bringing reality into the institution" (e.g. via utilization of virtual reality settings) and "bringing training into the real world" (e.g. by utilizing devices like the above-mentioned NeuroPage and even more advanced hand-held devices) (for further discussions, see for instance Wilms & Mogensen, 2011). In parallel to the important potentials to provide a more "ecologically valid" training situation, the use of advanced technologies also promise a number of other already realized and not the least potential benefits. Rehabilitative training may, for instance, become more intensive by supplementing the (time and financially highly demanding) face-to-face therapeutic sessions with a therapist with training sessions in which the patient exclusively interacts with technological devises (e.g. Katz, 2009; Rizzo et al., 2004; Tsirlin et al., 2009). Also, utilization of computer systems based on artificial intelligence (e.g. Wilms, 2011) can allow advanced technology-based training systems to adapt in highly flexible and dynamic manners to many aspects of the progress of the patient. The pattern of progressions in task performance during cognitive recovery after brain injury is often highly dissimilar between patients and therefore requires a dynamic and adjustable approach in order to provide the optimal training parameters (e.g. I.H. Robertson & Murre, 1999). Another way in which the effects of training may be measured and utilized in the guidance of the progression of training is by inclusion of the novel - but promising - area of brain-computer interactions (e.g., Coyle et al., 2003). Such techniques may allow the training situation - including the demands and feedback to the patient - to be steered by direct measurements of neural activity (e.g. Coyle et al., 2003; Daly & Wolpaw, 2008; Sitaram et al., 2009). Obviously, in order to obtain the optimal utilization of such brain-computer interactions, one needs a thorough (and presently only partly existing) knowledge of the neural processes mediating the desired functional rehabilitative process.

When utilizing advanced technologies in the context of cognitive neurorehabilitation one needs, however, to exert a high degree of caution (as well as extensive subsequent testing of methods) when translating more traditional types of training to for instance a computer-based setting. As is stressed by Wilm & Mogensen (2011), naïve "translations" from for example a "paper and pencil" version of a test or training procedure to a computer-based version may create unexpected discrepances between the two versions. While this situation poses a significant challenge to the clinical utilization of advanced technologies, it also provides a "window" through which cognitive neuroscience may gain an improved understanding of some of the cognitive mechanisms mediated by the intact and injured brain. Such an example can be seen in the results of Wilms & Malá (2010). In patients suffering hemispatial neglect (e.g. Rossetti et al., 1998) the so-called Prism Adaptation Therapy (PAT) (e.g. Frassinetti et al., 2002; Rossetti et al., 1998) may be used successfully. In PAT, the patients are trained in a task requiring them to point (without being able to follow their arm visually during the pointing movement) to targets defined by the therapist. While doing so, the patient is wearing prism goggles, which diverts the visual field ten degrees to the right (the patients are exhibiting a hemispatiel neglect of the left hemispace). In the traditional version of PAT, the feedback provided to the patient is the sight of the pointing finger at the moment when the pointing movement has been terminated. In most cases, the patient gradually adapts to the perceptual shift and eventually shows an after-effect in the form of a relative shift of the pointing movement. This shift even persists after the removal of the goggles. In other words, the procedure constitutes an at least partial therapeutic intervention regarding the neglect of the left hemispace. An essential element of the procedure is the feedback regarding the precision of the pointing movements during the training period (e.g. Frassinetti et al., 2002; Sarri et al., 2008; Serino et al., 2006, 2007). Wilms & Malá (2010) included in their study this traditional version of the PAT-procedure and compared it directly to a procedure in which the patients pointed to a touch-sensitive computer screen and feedback was provided graphically (in the form of an X) on the screen rather than via the direct sight of the pointing finger. Surprisingly, in both patients and uninjured subjects the outcome from the two procedures differed significantly - the version in which an icon on the computer screen provided the feedback resulted in significantly less after-effects than the traditional version. While being unexpected, these results emphasize - as is stressed by the REF-model - that the exact setting of the training procedure as well as the nature of the feedback provided to the patient are crucial factors for the outcome of neurorehabilitative training (e.g. Wilms & Mogensen, 2011). Furthermore, the results are potentially reflecting some of the same processes as those emphasized by a model published by Milner & Goodale (1995, 2008) - a model stressing the likelihood that visual feedback may be processed along different channels depending on the circumstances of its presentation.

Amongst the important factors shaping the outcome of rehabilitative cognitive training after brain injury are not only the therapeutic setting (e.g. institutionalised/daily life environment) and the details of the type of feedback provided to the patient. Equally important components spring from the pretraumatic experience and cognitive profile of the patient. As is obvious from the REF-model, the spectrum of ASs available during posttraumatic functional recovery is crucial to the efficacy of training. This effect is not limited to cases where activation of a pre-existing AS may achieve successful task solution (as indicated in Fig. 1). Even if no spared AS, in itself, is able to mediate a successful task solution, the interconnectivity between the neural substrates of EFs - viewed at the cognitive level: the pre-existing interactions between individual EFs - are crucial "building blocks" in the process of shaping new and successful ASs (as shown in Fig. 2). On such a basis one can expect the speed, efficacy and for that matter eventual outcome of rehabilitative training to be highly dependent on the pretraumatic cognitive status of the patient. If the brain injured individual posttraumatically still possesses varied and proficient ASs within a number of cognitive domains related to the area in which the symptoms are seen, one will - all other factors equal - expect a more proficient and potentially quicker recovery process.

But not only the efficacy of rehabilitative training but also the cognitive nature of the outcome achieved via such training may depend crucially upon pretraumatic cognitive factors (i.e. the nature of available ASs). An example of this may be seen in a series of fascinating observations regarding training-induced increases in utilization as well as subjective awareness of originally not consciously perceived stimuli in the metacontrast masking experimental setup (e.g. Schwiedrzik et al., 2009). The context of these experiments is that both clinical and experimental data point to the fact that brain injured individuals exhibiting "blindsight" can improve their task performance with training. For instance, improved performance in a forced choice procedure can be seen in both monkeys suffering bilateral ablation of the primary visual cortex (V1) (Dineen & Keating, 1981; Humphrey, 1974) and in patients demonstrating blindsight (e.g. Bridgeman & Staggs, 1982; Chokron et al., 2008; Henriksson et al., 2007; Raninen et al., 2007; Stoerig, 2006; Zihl, 1980; Zihl & Werth, 1984). Often, such improvements are not accompanied by any change in subjective awareness of the stimulus - in general, patients exhibit blindsight by behavioural demonstrations of a "perceptual processing" of the stimulus without showing any conscious awareness of the stimulus. However, there is now a growing body of evidence demonstrating that perceptual training can also increase the reported perceptual awareness of stimuli in blindsight patients (e.g. Sahraie et al., 2006). Also, studies in intact subjects exposed to subliminal presentation of visual stimuli (mostly utilizing the above-mentioned metacontrast masking in a "stimulus onset asynchrony" paradigm) have demonstrated that even in individuals without injury to the brain, training can increase the degree of perceptual awareness of a stimulus originally unavailable to consciousness (e.g. Albrecht et al., 2010; Schwiedrzik et al., 2009). In the context of such metacontrast masking experiments (e.g. Schwiedrzik et al., 2009) it appears that individual differences between normal subjects reflect dissimilar solution strategies (i.e. selection of dissimilar ASs) (Albrecht et al., 2010). When individuals displaying such dissimilarities at the outset of training are subjected to identical training procedures, it turns out that the solution strategies become even more dissimilar during the period of training - demonstrating a potentiation rather than an elimination of these strategy differences (Albrecht et al., 2010). Results such as these emphasize that subjecting individuals with pre-existing differences in the available ASs as well as the potential differences in "biases" of the selector/evaluator mechanisms to identical rehabilitative training may not necessarily shape the cognitive processes in question in one particular direction. Rather, it may produce different outcomes depending on the pretraumatic condition of the patients.

Especially in the context of Alzheimer's dementia - but also with references to traumatic and vascular acquired brain injury - a somewhat related discussion deals with the issues of "brain reserve" (e.g. Scheibel et al., 2009) and "cognitive reserve" (e.g. Fuentes et al., 2010; Kesler et al., 2010; Ropacki & Elias, 2003; Stern, 2002). Both of these concepts refer to situations in which the pretraumatic condition influences the degree to which patients posttraumatically (or, for instance, during degenerative neural processes such as those seen in Alzheimer's dementia) are able to "compensate" for the neural and cognitive loss sustained due to injury and/or degeneration. While "brain reserve" primarily emphasizes structural aspects of the brain (e.g. density of synaptic contacts), the emphasis in "cognitive reserve" is on the availability of cognitive processes and strategies. In the context of the REF-model, "brain reserve" should be seen as an analysis of the degree of connectivity between the neural substrates of individual EFs, while "cognitive reserve" in general refers to more or less the same - but analysed at the cognitive level of the ASs. There may in "brain reserve" be a tendency to (over-)stress the quantitative aspects of synaptic connectivity, while according to both the idea of "cognitive reserve" and the REF-model it must be emphasized that what may be most important to the posttraumatic performance and potential of the patient is rather the quality (shape) of the patterns of synaptic connections (as opposed to the potentially less informative raw count of synaptic connections). A somewhat related phenomenon may be found within the research area dealing with the potentially "cognitively enhancing" effects of an upbringing in an "enriched" (varied and stimulating) environment (e.g. Rosenzweig, 1971). Much of the initial research within this area (e.g. Bennett et al., 1964, 1969; Renner & Rosenzweig, 1987; Rosenzweig et al., 1961) primarily focused on biochemical and anatomical effects on the brain - directly or indirectly assuming such changes to manifest themselves in cognitively "enhancing" consequences. It has, however, turned out that such environments may not always be "cognitively enhancing" in a more global sense. Rather, the consequences may be a changed tendency to select particular solution strategies (ASs in the terminology of the REF-model) (e.g. Mogensen, 1991). In other words: to fully understand the potential consequences of the prehistory of an experimental animal or a patient, one needs to address not only the quantitative but also the qualitative aspects of modified connectivity of the brain.

5. Supporting the posttraumatic rehabilitative process

As described above, according to the REF-model some of the essential aspects of the mechanisms mediating posttraumatic cognitive rehabilitation are the reorganization (and to an extent recruitment) of preserved networks more or less distal from the site of trauma as well as plastic modifications of the neural connectivity between such networks. Consequently, it is likely that the posttraumatic rehabilitative processes can be supported by interventions which are able to (1) promote the optimal survival of originally undamaged networks (i.e. the integrity of originally unaffected EFs), and (2) create the optimal conditions for plastic reorganizations of the connectivity between such networks.

A prerequisite for the optimal functioning - including plastic abilities - and ultimately the survival of neurons is an adequate supply of neurotrophic factors (including the neurotrophin Brain Derived Neurotrophic Factor (BDNF)) (e.g. Kafitz et al., 1999; Levi-Moltalcini, 1982, Lewin & Barde, 1996). BDNF is produced by glial cells as well as neurons and the supply to a neuron - in the form of synaptic take-up followed by retrograde axonal transport - is mostly achieved as part of the synaptic interaction within an efficient functional network (e.g. Hamburger, 1934, 1975; Hollyday & Hamburger, 1976; Levi-Montalcini, 1982; Levi-Montalcini & Levi, 1942). When the brain is injured, the primary injury (mechanical impact or immediate and local consequences of a vascular incident) is followed by further degeneration within more distal parts of the brain - known as secondary and tertiary degeneration. One of the many (e.g. B.K. Siesjo & P. Siesjo, 1996) mechanisms of this secondary and tertiary degeneration is that neurons within these parts of the brain have lost the possibility to interact (and receive for instance BDNF as part of that interaction) with neurons lost to the primary injury (e.g. Sofroniew et al., 1993). Therefore, it may be assumed that interventions which can boost the production (transcription) - and thereby availability - of BDNF (as well as other neurotrophic factors) may have the potential to support the posttraumatic rehabilitative process by both preserving as much as possible of the originally uninjured parts of the brain and by optimizing the neuroplastic potentials of these preserved brain regions.

The hormone erythropoietin (EPO) has long been recognized as crucial to the production of erythrocytes (and utilized clinically in this capacity). More recently, however, it has been demonstrated that there is a separate production of EPO and EPO-receptors in the brain (e.g. Baciu et al., 2000; Hasselblatt et al., 2006; Silva et al., 2006). In the central nervous system, EPO has a broad range of effects (e.g. Mammis et al., 2009) - including stimulation of the production of BDNF (e.g. Viviani et al., 2005; F. Zhang et al., 2006). EPO significantly increases BDNF-production when administered 6 or 24 hours after a traumatic brain injury (Mahmood et al., 2007).

By now, numerous techniques have demonstrated the neuroprotective abilities of EPO (e.g. Grasso et al., 2007; Mammis et al., 2009; Y. Zhang et al., 2009). The close association between EPO and blood-related processes originally provoked a primary research focus around the use of EPO in vascular brain injury (e.g. Alafaci et al., 2000; Brines et al., 2000; Buemi et al., 2000; Calapai et al., 2000; Grasso, 2001; Siren et al., 2001; Springborg et al., 2002). Subsequently, however, it turned out that EPO possesses a strong therapeutic potential even in TBI - including the ability to reduce posttraumatic cognitive impairments and support the cognitive rehabilitative processes (e.g. Lu et al., 2005; Malá et al., 2005, 2007; Mogensen et al., 2004b, 2008a, 2008b; Wang et al., 2006). The degree to which such therapeutic effects are mediated via stimulation of BDNF remains unknown, but it is obvious that further research is needed in order to clarify some of the intricacies of the therapeutic use of EPO. For instance, it appears that EPO administered at the moment of TBI may have a more pronounced ability to support posttraumatic cognitive recovery, if the rehabilitative training is initiated relatively soon after injury as opposed to later (Malá et al., 2005, 2007). Also, the relationship between EPO and BDNF is not restricted to the EPO-provoked stimulation of BDNF-production (e.g. Viviani et al., 2005; F. Zhang et al., 2006) - another aspect of the relationship is that BDNF induces EPO-expression - demonstrated at the levels of both the mRNA and protein (Wu et al., 2010).

The production of BDNF may also be enhanced by physical activity in the form of exercise (e.g. Griesbach et al., 2004a, 2004b, 2009; Moltini et al., 2004; Vaynman et al., 2003; M. Gajhede, E. Wogensen, G. Wörtwein & J. Mogensen, in preparation). And although much needs to be explored within this area, a growing number of publications from recent years (e.g. Arida et al., 2009; Devine & Zafonte, 2009; Griesbach et al., 2004a, 2004b, 2009; Hayes et al., 2008; Luo et al., 2007; Malá et al., 2008; Seo et al., 2010) have demonstrated that various types of physical activation and exercise are able to promote the posttraumatic functional recovery and rehabilitation after various types of brain injury. At least in certain instances, it has been shown that the exercise-induced improvements of cognitive abilities after brain injury depend upon stimulation of the production of BDNF (Griesbach et al., 2009). In animal models, exercise and other types of physical activation are studied under conditions of both "voluntary" and "forced" exercise - where the "forced" variants typically are associated with at least a certain level of stress and consequently increased production of the "stress-hormone" corticosterone

(CORT). Increased serum concentrations of CORT has been found to reduce the production of BDNF (e.g.. Adlard & Cotman, 2004; Duman et al., 1997). On this background, it is not surprising that Luo et al. (2007) have demonstrated that while voluntary exercise acts therapeutically in brain injured individuals, the stressful and forced variant has no such effects. But even in this context, a highly promising avenue in the support of posttraumatic rehabilitation after brain injury is in clear need of additional research. In contrast to the results of Luo et al. (2007), Hayes et al. (2008) and Malá et al. (2008) have independently documented significant therapeutic effects of forced and stress-associated types of physical activation. Furthermore, the stress-associated method originally published by Malá et al. (2008) has been found to be associated with both an increase in the serum concentration of CORT and (surprisingly) an increased concentration of BDNF in the hippocampus and the prefrontal cortex (M. Gajhede, E. Wogensen, G. Wörtwein & J. Mogensen, in preparation). Clearly, the optimal utilization of several of these highly promising ways of supporting the posttraumatic rehabilitative processes can only be fully utilized (not to mention understood) in the light of future research.

6. Conclusion

The neuroplasticity mediated cognitive rehabilitative processes upon brain injury are frequently divided into two phases: initially a relearling of compromized and/or lost "functions" followed by later compensational processes which support the behavioural abilities without re-establishing what has been lost to injury (e.g. Stein & Hoffman, 2003). According to the REF-model, such a distinction is likely to be somewhat artificial and potentially misleading regarding the possibility of major re-establishment of lost functions - at least if "function" is considered at the level of the EFs. As mentioned above and discussed extensively elsewhere (Mogensen, 2011a), re-establishment of the lost neural substrate of EFs is unlikely to occur. However, as noted by Mogensen & Malá (2009), subtotal lesions of various structures (or more likely substructures) of the brain may allow a degree of "re-establishment" of the original substrate of task mediation via mechanisms such as those suggested by I.H. Robertson & Murre (1999). If such a process leads to re-establishment of the substrate of EFs originally lost to trauma, an actual "relearning" may indeed take place. But in general, a distinction between "relearning" and "compensation" will (according to the REF-model) in most if not all cases reflect the degree to which the surface level phenomena can easily be distinguished from those seen pretraumatically - while both "relearning" and "compensation" in reality reflect the REF-processes.

At the theoretical level, the REF-model has provided a framework within which the concepts of localization of function and functional recovery can co-exist. But it has also provided a structure within which connectionist networks (e.g. McClelland et al., 1986; McLeod et al., 1998; Rumelhart & McClelland, 1986) can co-exist with "modularity" (e.g. Fodor, 2000; Pinker, 1999). The functionally very specialized EFs place the REF-model within the framework of what is called "Massive Modularity" (e.g. Barrett & Kurzban, 2006) and it consequently embraces the idea of "rules of computation" associated with such modularity-based models. Since, however, at the level of the ASs the REF-model must be considered connectionist and distributed - and the ASs are established and modified according to backpropagation mechanisms - the basis for an AS is more or less a connectionist network of interconnected EFs. Via this combination, the REF-model can accommodate both the modularity-based predictability of for instance lesion effects and the connectionist flexibility and potential for dynamic reorganizations, which allow behavioural and cognitive flexibility in the intact individual as well as the posttraumatic cognitive rehabilitation of the brain injured patient.

As stressed above, the way the REF-model conceptualizes the mechanisms of posttraumatic cognitive recovery points to a number of important issues to consider clinically:

It is important to provide supportive therapeutic interventions which can limit secundary and tertiary neurodegeneration as well as create the optimal conditions for the plasticity required for the reorganization of connectivity between the neural substrates of EFs (as well as within the selector/evaluator mechanisms). As mentioned, this may be done utilizing pharmacological interventions and/or exercise. And there is little doubt that future research will provide additional ways of accomplishing this - potentially by combining for instance environmental enrichment and various types of training (e.g. Hicks et al., 2007).

And perhaps the most important aspect in at least a short term clinical perspective is the ways in which the REF-model puts focus on the fact that rehabilitative training is situationally dependent - and not the least the dependence on the specific types of feedback provided during training. In order to achieve a cognitive rehabilitative training that can generalize to the everyday situation of the patient - and thereby provide the types of ecologically valid "recovery" which remains the goal of all such efforts - significant efforts and progress must be invested in optimizing training methods. Including the creation of training which can bridge the therapeutic situation in an institution and the subsequent life of the recovering brain injured patient.

In order to achieve all of these goals, progress within technology, medical practise as well as research at the conceptual and empirical levels is required. And an adequate synthesis between the results from all of these (and many other) areas must be achieved. The REF-model is a theoretical framework within which some of these steps may be achieved. However, in its present form it is but a first sketch. Further improvements and refinements of the REF-model as well as our understanding of cognitive rehabilitation after brain injury will grow from the continued research as well as the daily marriage between clinical and research efforts.

7. Acknowledgements

The present study was supported by a grant from the Danish Research Council.

8. References

Adlard, P.A. & Cotman, C.W. (2004). Voluntary exercise protects against stress-induced decreases in brain-derived neurotrophic factor protein expression. *Neuroscience,* Vol.124, pp. 985-992.

Alafaci, C., Salpietro, F., Grasso, G., Sfacteria, A., Passalacqua, M., Morabito, A., Tripodo, E., Calapai, G., Buemi, M. & Tomasello, F. (2000). Effect of recombinant human erythropoietin on cerebral ischemia following experimental subarachnoid hemorrhage. *European Journal of Pharmacology,* Vol.406, pp. 219-225.

Albrecht, T., Klapötke, S. & Mattler, U. (2010). Individual differences in metacontrast masking are enhanced by perceptual learning. *Consciousness and Cognition*, Vol.19, pp. 656-666.

Ansaldo, A.I. & Arguin, M. (2003). The recovery from aphasia depends on both the left and right hemispheres: three longitudinal case studies on the dynamics of language function after aphasia. *Brain and Language,* Vol.87, pp. 177-178.

Ansaldo, A.I., Arguin, M. & Lecours, A.R. (2002). The contribution of the right cerebral hemisphere to the recovery from aphasia: a single longitudinal case study. *Brain and Language,* Vol.82, pp. 206-222.

Arida, R.M., Scorza, F.A., Scorza, C.A. & Cavalheiro, E.A. (2009). Is physical activity beneficial for recovery in temporal lobe epilepsy? Evidences from animal studies. *Neuroscience and Biobehavioral Reviews,* Vol.33, pp. 422-431.

Arvidsson, A., Collin, T., Kirik, D., Kokaia, Z. & Lindvall, O. (2002). Neuronal replacement from endogenous precursors in the adult brain after stroke. *Nature Medicine,* Vol.8, pp. 963-970.

Bach-y-Rita, P., Collins, C.C., Saunders, F.A., White, B. & Scadden, L. (1969). Vision substitution by tactile image projection. *Nature,* Vol.221, pp. 963-964.

Bach-y-Rita, P., Kaczmarek, K.A., Tyler, M.E. & Garcia-Lara, J. (1998). Form perception with a 49-point electrotactile stimulus array on the tongue: a technical note. *Journal of Rehabilitation Research and Development,* Vol.35, pp. 1-7.

Baciu, I., Oprisiu, C., Derevenco, P., Vasile, V., Muresan, A., Hriscu, M. & Chris, I. (2000). The brain and other sites of erythropoietin production. *Romanian Journal of Physiology,* Vol.37, pp. 3-14.

Barrett, H.C. & Kurzban, R. (2006). Modularity in cognition: framing the debate. *Psychological Review,* Vol.113, pp. 628-647.

Baumgaertner, A., Schraknepper, V. & Saur, D. (2005). Differential recovery of aphasia and apraxia of speech in an adolescent after infarction of the left frontal lobe: longitudinal behavioral and fMRI data. *Brain and Language,* Vol.95, pp. 211-212.

Bennett, E.L., Diamond, M.L., Krech, D. & Rosenzweig, M.R. (1964). Chemical and anatomical plasticity of brain. *Science,* Vol.146, pp. 610-619.

Bennett, E.L., Rosenzweig, M.R. & Diamond, M.C. (1969). Rat brain: effects of environmental enrichment on wet and dry weights. *Science,* Vol.163, pp. 825-826.

Berardi, N., Pizzorusso, T. & Maffei, L. (2004). Extracellular matrix and visual cortical plasticity: freeing the synapse. *Neuron,* Vol.44, pp. 905-908.

Berry, M. (1982). Post-injury myelin-breakdown products inhibit axonal growth: an hypothesis to explain the failure of axonal regeneration in the mammalian central nervous system. *Bibliotheca Anatomica,* Vol.23, pp. 1-11.

Block, N. & Fodor, J. (1972). What psychological states are not. *Philosophical Review,* Vol.81, pp. 159-181.

Bridgeman, B. & Staggs, D. (1982). Plasticity in human blindsight. *Vision Research,* Vol.22, pp. 1199-1203.

Brines, M.L., Ghezzi, P., Keenan, S., Agnello, D., de Lanerolle, N.C., Cerami, C., Itri, L.M. & Cerami, A. (2000). Erythropoietin crosses the blood-brain barrier to protect against experimental brain injury. *Proceedings of the National Academy of Sciences, USA,* Vol.97, pp. 10526-10531.

Buemi, M., Grasso, G., Corica, F., Calapai, G., Salpietro, F.M., Casuscelli, T., Sfacteria, A., Aloisi, C., Alafaci, C., Sturiale, A., Frisina, N. & Tomasello, F. (2000). In vivo evidence that erythropoietin has a neuroprotective effect during subarachnoid hemorrhage. *European Journal of Pharmacology,* Vol.392, pp. 31-34.

Buller, D.J. & Hardcastle, V.G. (2000). Evolutionary psychology, meet developmental neurobiology: against promiscuous modularity. *Brain and Mind,* Vol.1, pp. 307-325.

Calapai, G., Marciano, M.C., Corica, F., Allegra, A., Parisi, A., Frisina, N., Caputi, A.P. & Buemi, M. (2000). Erythropoietin protects against brain ischemic injury by inhibition of nitric oxide formation. *European Journal of Pharmacology,* Vol.401, pp. 349-356.

Carney, N., Chesnut, R.M., Maynard, H., Mann, N.C., Patterson, P. & Helfand, M. (1999). Effect of cognitive rehabilitation on outcomes for persons with traumatic brain injury: a systematic review. *Journal of Head Trauma Rehabilitation,* Vol.14, pp. 277-307.

Chen, D.F., Jhaveri, S. & Schneider, G.E. (1995). Intrinsic changes in developing retinal neurons result in regenerative failure of their axons. *Proceedings of the National Academy of Sciences, USA,* Vol.92, pp. 7287-7291.

Chen, J., Magavi, S.S. & Macklis, J.D. (2004). Neurogenesis of corticospinal motor neurons extending spinal projections in adult mice. *Proceedings of the National Academy of Sciences, USA,* Vol.101, pp. 16357-16362.

Choi, J.Y., Lee, K.H., Na, D.L., Byun, H.S., Lee, S.J., Kim, H., Kwon, M., Lee, K-H. & Kim, B-T. (2007). Subcortical aphasia after striatocapsular infarction: quantitative analysis of brain perfusion SPECT using statistical parametric mapping and a statistical probabilistic anatomic map. *Journal of Nuclear Medicine,* Vol.48, pp. 194-200.

Chokron, S., Perez, C., Obadia, M., Gaudry, I., Laloum, L. & Gout, O. (2008). From blindsight to sight: cognitive rehabilitation of visual field defects. *Restorative Neurology and Neuroscience,* Vol.26, pp. 305-320.

Coltheart, M. (2001). Assumptions and methods in cognitive neuropsychology. In: *The Handbook of Cognitive Neuropsychology,* B. Rapp, (Ed.), pp. 3-21, Psychology Press, Philadelphia PA.

Coyle, S., Ward, T. & Markhan, C. (2003). Brain-computer interfaces: a review. *Inter-disciplinary Science Reviews,* Vol.28, pp. 112-118.

Crosson, B., Moore, A.B., McGregor, K.M., Chang, Y-L., Benjamin, M., Gopinath, K., Sherod, M.E., Wierenga, C.E., Peck, K.K., Briggs, R.W., Rothi, L.J.G. & White, K.D. (2009). Regional changes in word-production laterality after a naming treatment designed to produce a rightward shift in frontal activity. *Brain and Language,* Vol.111, pp. 73-85.

Daly, J.J. & Wolpaw, J.R. (2008). Brain-computer interfaces in neurological rehabilitation. *The Lancet Neurology,* Vol.7, pp. 1032-1043.

Del Rio, J.A. & Soriano, E. (2007). Overcoming chondroitin sulphate proteoglycan inhibition of axon growth in the injured brain: lessons from chondroitinase ABC. *Current Pharmacological Design,* Vol.13, pp. 2485-2492.

Devine, J.M. & Zafonte, R.D. (2009). Physical exercise and cognitive recovery in acquired brain injury: a review of the literature. *Physical Medicine and Rehabilitation,* Vol.1, pp. 560-575.

Dineen, J. & Keating, E.G. (1981). The primate visual system after bilateral removal of striate cortex. Survival of complex pattern vision. *Experimental Brain Research,* Vol.41, pp. 338-345.

Duman, R.S., Heninger, G.R. & Nestler, E.J. (1997). A molecular and cellular theory of depression. *Archives of General Psychiatry,* Vol.54, pp. 597-606.

Elbert, T., Pantev, C., Weinbruch, C., Rockstroh, B. & Taub, E. (1995). Increased cortical representation of the fingers of the left hand in string players. *Science,* Vol.270, pp. 305-307.

Fawcett, J.W., Housden, E., Smith-Thomas, L. & Meyer, R.L. (1989). The growth of axons in three-dimensional astrocyte cultures. *Developmental Biology,* Vol.135, pp. 449-458.

Finger, S. & Stein, D.G. (1982). Vicariation theory and radical reorganization of function. In: *Brain Damage and Recovery: Research and Clinical Perspectives,* S. Finger & D.G. Stein, (Eds.), pp. 287-302, Academic Press, New York.

Fodor, J. (2000). *The Mind Doesn't Work That Way: The Scope and Limits of Computational Psychology.* MIT Press, Cambridge, MA.

Frassinetti, F., Angeli, V., Meneghello, F., Avanzi, S. & Ladavas, E. (2002). Long-lasting amelioration of visuospatial neglect by prism adaptation. *Brain,* Vol.125, pp. 608-623.

Fuentes, A., McKay, C. & Hay, C. (2010). Cognitive reserve in paediatric traumatic brain injury: relationship with neuropsychological outcome. *Brain Injury,* Vol.24, pp. 995-1002.

Goldberg, J.L., Klassen, M.P., Hua, Y. & Barres, B.A. (2002). Amacrine-signaled loss of intrinsic axon growth ability by retinal ganglion cells. *Science,* Vol.296, pp. 1860-1864.

Grasso, G. (2001). Neuroprotective effect of recombinant human erythropoietin in experimental subarachnoid hemorrhage. *Journal of Neurosurgical Sciences,* Vol.45, pp. 7-14.

Grasso, G., Sfacteria, A., Meli, F., Fodale, V., Buemi, M. & Iacopino, D.G. (2007). Neuroprotection by erythropoietin administration after experimental traumatic brain injury. *Brain Research,* Vol.1182, pp. 99-105.

Griesbach, G.S., Gomez-Pinilla, F. & Hovda, D.A. (2004a). The upregulation of plasticity-related proteins following TBI is disrupted with acute voluntary exercise. *Brain Research,* Vol.1016, pp. 154-162.

Griesbach, G.S., Hovda, D.A., Molteni, R., Wu, A., Gomez-Pinilla, F. (2004b). Voluntary exercise following traumatic brain injury: brain-derived neurotrophic factor upregulation and recovery of function. *Neuroscience,* Vol.125, pp. 129-139.

Griesbach, G.S., Hovda, D.A. & Gomez-Pinilla, F. (2009). Exercise-induced improvement in cognitive performance after traumatic brain injury in rats is dependent on BDNF activation. *Brain Research,* Vol.1288, pp. 105-115.

Hamburger, V. (1934). The effects of wing bug extirpation in chick embryos on the development of the central nervous system. *Journal of Experimental Zoology,* Vol.68, pp. 449-494.

Hamburger, V. (1975). Cell death in the development of the lateral motor column of the chick embryol. *Journal of Comparative Neurology,* Vol.160, pp. 535-546.

Hasselblatt, M., Ehrenreich, H. & Siren, A. (2006). The brain erythropoietin system and its potential for therapeutic exploitation in brain disease. *Journal of Neurosurgical Anesthesiology,* Vol.18, pp. 132-138.

Hayes, K., Sprague, S., Guo, M., Davis, W., Friedman, A., Kumar, A., Jimenez, D.F. & Ding, Y. (2008). Forcecd, not voluntary, exercise effectively induces neuroprotection in stroke. *Acta Neuropathologica,* Vol.115, pp. 289-296.

Henriksson, L., Raninen, A., Näsänen, R., Hyvärinen, L. & Vanni, S. (2007). Training-induced cortical representation of a hemianopic hemifield. *Journal of Neurology, Neurosurgery, and Psychiatry,* Vol.78, pp. 74-81.

Hicks, A.U., Hewlett, K., Windle, V., Chernenko, G., Ploughman, M., Jolkkonen, J., Weiss, S. & Corbett, D. (2007). Enriched environment enhances transplanted subventricular zone stem cell migration and functional recovery after stroke. *Neuroscience,* Vol.146, pp. 31-40.

Hollyday, M. & Hamburger, V. (1976). Reduction of the naturally occurring motor neuron loss by enlargement of the periphery. *Journal of Comparative Neurology,* Vol.170, pp. 311-320.

Humphrey, N.K. (1974). Vision in a monkey without striate cortex: a case study. *Perception,* Vol.3, pp. 241-255.

Irvine, D.R.F. (2007). Auditory cortical plasticity: does it provide evidence for cognitive processing in the auditory cortex? *Hearing Research,* Vol.229, pp. 158-170.

Kaczmarek, K.A., Webster, J.G., Bach-y-Rita, P. & Tompkins, W.J. (1991). Electrotactile and vibrotactile displays for sensory substitutionsystems. *Biomedical Engineering,* Vol.38, pp. 1-16.

Kafitz, K.W., Rose, C.R., Thoenen, H. & Konnerth, A. (1999). Neurotrophin-evoked rapid excitation through TrkB receptors. *Nature,* Vol.401, pp. 918-921.

Karl, A., Birbaumer, N., Lutzenberger, W., Cohen, L.G. & Flor, H. (2001). Reorganization of motor and somatosensory cortex in upper extremity amputees with phantom limb pain. *Journal of Neuroscience,* Vol.15, pp. 3609-3618.

Katz, R.C. (2009). Application of computers to the treatment of US veterans with aphasia. *Aphasiology,* Vol.23, pp. 1116-1126.

Kesler, S.R., Adams, H.F., Blasey, C.M. & Bigler, E.D. (2010). Premorbid intellectual functioning, education, and brain size in traumatic brain injury: an investigation of the cognitive reserve hypothesis. *Applied Neuropsychology,* Vol.10, pp. 153-162.

Krechevsky, I. (1932). "Hypotheses" in rats. *Psychological Reviews,* Vol.39, pp. 516-532.

Krechevsky, I. (1933). Hereditary nature of "hypotheses". *Journal of Comparative Psychology,* Vol.16, pp. 99-116.

Kringelbach, M.L. & Rolls, E.T. (2004). The functional neuroanatomy of the human orbitofrontal cortex: evidence from neuroimaging and neuropsychology. *Progress in Neurobiology*, Vol.7, pp. 341-372.

Leavitt, B.R., Hernit-Grant, C.S. & Macklis, J.D. (1999). Mature astrocytes transform into transitional radial glia within adult mouse neocortex that supports directed migration of transplanted immature neurons. *Experimental Neurology*, Vol.157, pp. 43-57.

León-Carrión, J. & Machuca-Murga, F. (2001). Spontaneous recovery of cognitive functions after severe brain injury: when are neurocognitive sequelae established? *Revista Española de Neuropsicologia*, Vol.3, pp. 58-67.

Levi-Montalcini, R. (1982). Developmental neurobiology and the natural history of nerve growth factor. *Annual Review of Neuroscience*, Vol.5, pp. 341-362.

Levi-Montalcini, R. & Levi, G. (1942). Les conséquences de la destruction d'un territoire d'innervation périphérique sur le développement des centres nerveux correspondants dans l'embryon de poulet. *Archives of Biology*, Vol.53, pp. 537-545.

Levin, M.F., Kleim, J.A. & Wolf, S.L. (2009). What do motor "recovery" and "compensation" mean in patients following stroke? *Neurorehabilitation and Neural Repair*, Vol.23, pp. 313-319.

Lewin, G.R. & Barde, Y.A. (1996). Physiology of the neurotrophins. *Annual Review of Neuroscience*, Vol.19, pp. 289-317.

Lu, D., Mahmood, A., Qu, C., Goussev, A., Schallert, T. & Chopp, M. (2005). Erythropoietin enhances neurogenesis and restores spatial memory in rats after traumatic brain injury. *Journal of Neurotrauma*, Vol.22, pp. 1011-1017.

Luo, C.X., Jiang, J., Zhou, Q.G., Zhu, X.J., Wang, W., Zhang, Z.J., Han, X. & Zhu, D.Y. (2007). Voluntary exercise-induced neurogenesis in the postischemic dentate gyrus is associated with spatial memory recovery from stroke. *Journal of Neuroscience Research*, Vol.85, pp. 1637-1646.

Magavi, S.S., Leavitt, B.R. & Macklis, J.D. (2000). Induction of neurogenesis in the neocortex of adult mice. *Nature*, Vol.405, pp. 951-955.

Mahmood, A., Lu, D., Qu, C., Goussev, A., Zhang, Z.G., Lu, C. & Chopp, M. (2007). Treatment of traumatic brain injury in rats with erythropoietin and carbamylated erythropoietin. *Journal of Neurosurgery*, Vol.107, pp. 392-397.

Malá, H., Alsina, C.G., Madsen, K.S., la Cour Sibbesen, E., Stick, H. & Mogensen, J. (2005). Erythropoietin improves place learning in an 8-arm radial maze in fimbria-fornix transected rats. *Neural Plasticity*, Vol.12, pp. 329-340.

Malá, H., Castro, M.R., Jørgensen, K.D. & Mogensen, J. (2007). Effects of erythropoietin on posttraumatic place learning in fimbria-fornix transected rats after a 30-day postoperative pause. *Journal of Neurotrauma*, Vol.24, pp. 1647-1657.

Malá, H., Castro, M.R., Knippel, J., Køhler, P.J., Lassen, P. & Mogensen, J. (2008). Therapeutic effects of a restraint procedure on posttraumatic place learning in fimbria-fornix transected rats. *Brain Research*, Vol.1217, pp. 221-231.

Mammis, A., McIntosh, T.K. & Maniker, A.H. (2009). Erythropoietin as a neuroprotective agent in traumatic brain injury. Review. *Surgical Neurology*, Vol..71, pp. 527-531.

McClelland, J.L., Rumelhart, D.E. & The PDP Research Group (1986). *Parallel Distributed Processing: Vol. 2. Psychological and Biological Models.* MIT Press, Cambridge, MA.

McGee, A.W., Yang, Y., Fischer, Q.S., Daw, N.W. & Strittmatter, S.M. (2005). Experience-driven plasticity of visual cortex limited by myelin and Nogo receptor. *Science,* Vol.309, pp. 2222-2226.

McLeod, P., Plunkett, K. & Rolls, E.T.. (1998). *Introduction to Connectionist Modelling of Cognitive Processes.* Oxford University Press, Oxford.

Meinzer, M., Obleser, J., Flaisch, T., Eulitz, C. & Rockstroh, B. (2007). Recovery from aphasia as a function of language therapy in an early bilingual patient demonstrated by fMRI. *Neuropsychologia,* Vol.45, pp. 1247-1256.

Meinzer, M., Flaisch, T., Breitenstein, C., Wienbruch, C., Elbert, T. & Rockstroh, B. (2008). Functional re-recruitment of dysfunctional brain areas predicts language recovery in chronic aphasia. *NeuroImage,* Vol.39, pp. 2038-2046.

Merzenich, M.M. & Jenkins, W.M. (1993). Reorganization of cortical representations of the hand following alterations of skin inputs induced by nerve injury, skin island transfers, and experience. *Journal of Hand Therapy,* Vol.6, pp. 89-104.

Milner, A.D. & Goodale, M.A. (1995). *The Visual Brain in Action.* Oxford University Press, Oxford.

Milner, A.D. & Goodale, M.A. (2008). Two visual systems re-viewed. *Neuropsychologia,* Vol.46, pp.774-785.

Mogensen, J. (1991). Influences of the rearing conditions on functional properties of the rat's prefrontal system. *Behavioural Brain Research,* Vol.42, pp. 135-142.

Mogensen, J. (2011a). Almost unlimited potentials of a limited neural plasticity: levels of plasticity in development and reorganization of the injured brain. *Journal of Consciousness Studies,* Vol.18: pp. 13-45.

Mogensen, J. (2011b). Animal models in neuroscience, In: *Handbook of Laboratory Animal Science, Third Edition, Volume II. Animal Models.* J. Hau & S.J. Schapiro, (Eds.), pp. 47-73, CRC Press LLC, Boca Raton, FL.

Mogensen, J. (2011c). Reorganization in the injured brain: implications for studies of the neural substrate of cognition. *Frontiers in Psychology,* Vol.2:7, pp. 1-10.

Mogensen, J. & Malá, H. (2009). Post-traumatic functional recovery and reorganization in animal models. A theoretical and methodological challenge. *Scandinavian Journal of Psychology,* Vol.50, pp. 561-573.

Mogensen, J., Christensen, L.H., Johansson, A., Wörtwein, G., Bang, L.E. & Holm, S. (2002). Place learning in scopolamine treated rats: the roles of distal cues and catecholaminergic mediation. *Neurobiology of Learning and Memory,* Vol.78, pp. 139-166.

Mogensen, J., Wörtwein, G., Plenge, P. & Mellerup, E.T. (2003). Serotonin, locomotion, exploration, and place recall in the rat. *Pharmacology, Biochemistry, and Behavior,* Vol.75, pp. 381-395.

Mogensen, J., Lauritsen, K.T., Elvertorp, S., Hasman, A., Moustgaard, A. & Wörtwein, G. (2004a). Place learning and object recognition by rats subjected to transection of the fimbria-fornix and/or ablation of the prefrontal cortex. *Brain Research Bulletin*, Vol.63, pp. 217-236.

Mogensen, J., Miskowiak, K., Sørensen, T.A., Lind, C.T., Olsen, N.V., Springborg, J.B. & Malá, H. (2004b). Erythropoietin improves place learning in fimbria-fornix transected rats and modifies the search pattern of normal rats. *Pharmacology, Biochemistry, and Behavior*, Vol.77, pp. 381-390.

Mogensen, J., Moustgaard, A., Khan, U., Wörtwein, G. & Nielsen, K.S. (2005). Egocentric spatial orientation in a water maze by rats subjected to transection of the fimbria-fornix and/or ablation of the prefrontal cortex. *Brain Research Bulletin*, Vol.65, pp. 41-58.

Mogensen, J., Hjortkjær, J., Ibervang, K.L., Stedal, K. & Malá, H. (2007). Prefrontal cortex and hippocampus in posttraumatic functional recovery: spatial delayed alternation by rats subjected to transection of the fimbria-fornix and/or ablation of the prefrontal cortex. *Brain Research Bulletin*, Vol.73, pp. 86-95.

Mogensen, J., Boyd, M.H., Nielsen, M.D., Kristensen, R.S. & Malá, H. (2008a). Erythropoietin improves spatial delayed alternation in a T-maze in rats subjected to ablation of the prefrontal cortex. *Brain Research Bulletin*, Vol.77, pp. 1-7.

Mogensen, J., Jensen, C., Kingod, S.C., Hansen, A., Larsen, J.A.R. & Malá, H. (2008b). Erythropoietin improves spatial delayed alternation in a T-maze in fimbria-fornix transected rats. *Behavioural Brain Research*, Vol.186, pp. 215-221.

Molteni, R., Wu, A., Vaynman, S., Ying, Z., Bernard, R.J. & Gomez-Pinella, F. (2004). Exercise reverses the harmful effects of consumption of a high-fat diet on synaptic and behavioral plasticity associated to the action of brain-derived neurotrophic factor. *Neuroscience*, Vol.123, pp. 429-440.

Monakow, C.V. (1914). *Die Lokalisation im Grosshirn und der Abbau der Funktion durch Kortikale Herde*, Bergmann, Wiesbaden.

Moore, A.D. & Stambrook, M. (1995). Cognitive moderators of outcome following traumatic brain injury: a conceptual model and implications for rehabilitation. *Brain Injury*, Vol.9, pp. 109-130.

Münte, T.F., Altenmüller, E. & Jäncke, L. (2002). The musician's brain as a model of neuroplasticity. *Nature Reviews. Neuroscience*, Vol.3, pp. 473-478.

Nakatomi, H., Kuriu, T., Okabe, S., Yamamoto, S-C., Hatano, O., Kawahara, N., Tamura, A., Kirino, T. & Nakafuku, M. (2002). Regeneration of hippocampal pyramidal neurons after ischemic brain injury by recruitment of endogenous neural progenitors. *Cell*, Vol.110, pp. 429-441.

Norman, D.A. & Shallice, T. (1986). Attention to action: Willed and automatic control of behavior. In: *Consciousness and Self-Regulation (Vol. 4)*, R.J. Davidson, G.E. Schwartz & D. Shapiro, (Eds.), pp. 1-18, Plenum Press, New York.

Overgaard, M. & Mogensen, J. (2011). A framework for the study of multiple realizations: the importance of levels of analysis. *Frontiers in Psychology*, Vol.2:79, pp. 1-10.

Panksepp, J. & Panksepp, J.B. (2000). The seven sins of evolutionary psychology. *Evolution and Cognition*, Vol.6, pp. 108-131.

Perani, D., Cappa, S.F., Tettamanti, M., Rosa, M., Scifo, P., Miozzo, A., Basso, A. & Fazio, F. (2003). A fMRI study of word retrieval in aphasia. *Brain and Language*, Vol.85, pp. 357-368.

Pinker, S. (1999). *How the Mind Works*. Penguin Books, London.

Pizzorusso, T., Medini, P., Berardi, N., Chierzi, S., Fawcett, J.W. & Maffei, L. (2002). Reactivation of ocular dominance plasticity in the adult visual cortex. *Science,* Vol.298, pp. 1248-1251.

Ptito, M., Moesgaard, S.M., Gjedde, A. & Kupers, R. (2005). Cross-modal plasticity revealed by electrotactile stimulation of the tongue in the congenitally blind. *Brain,* Vol.128, pp. 606-614.

Rakic, P. (1971). Guidance of neurons migrating to the fetal monkey neocortex. *Brain Research,* Vol.33, pp. 471-476.

Rakic, P. (1985). Mechanisms of neuronal migration in developing cerebellar cortex. In: *Molecular Basis of Neural Development,* G.M. Edelman, W.M. Cowan & E. Gull, (Eds.), pp. 139-160, Wiley, New York.

Ramachandran, V.S. & Blakeslee, S. (1998). *Phantoms in the Brain: Probing the Mysteries of the Human Mind.* William Morrow, New York.

Raninen, A., Vanni, S., Hyvärinen, L. & Näsänen, R. (2007). Temporal sensitivity in a hemianopic visual field can be improved by long-term training using flicker stimulation. *Journal of Neurology, Neurosurgery, and Psychiatry,* Vol.78, pp. 66-73.

Recanzone, G.H., Schreiner, C.E. & Merzenich, M.M. (1993). Plasticity in the frequency representation of primary auditory cortex following discrimination training in adult owl monkeys. *Journal of Neuroscience,* Vol.13, pp. 87-103.

Renner, M.J. & Rosenzweig, M.R. (1987). *Enriched and Impoverished Environments: Effects on Brain and Behavior.* Springer, New York.

Rizzo, A.A., Schultheis, M., Kerns, K.A. & Mateer, C. (2004). Analysis of assets for virtual reality applications in neuropsychology. *Neuropsychological Rehabilitation,* Vol.14, pp. 207-239.

Robertson, D. & Irvine, D.R.F. (1989). Plasticity of frequency organization in auditory cortex of guinea pigs with partial unilateral deafness. *Journal of Comparative Neurology,* Vol.282, pp. 456-471.

Robertson, I.H. & Murre, J.M.J. (1999). Rehabilitation of brain damage: brain plasticity and principles of guided recovery. *Psychological Bulletin,* Vol.125, pp. 544-575.

Rohling, M.L., Faust, M.E., Beverly, B. & Demakis, G. (2009). Effectiveness of cognitive rehabilitation following acquired brain injury: a meta-analytic re-examination of Cicerone et al.'s (2000, 2005) systematic reviews. *Neuropsychology,* Vol.23, pp. 20-39.

Ropacki, M.T. & Elias, J.W. (2003). Preliminary examination of cognitive reserve theory in closed head injury. *Archives of Clinical Neuropsychology,* Vol.18; pp. 643-654.

Rossetti, Y., Rode, G., Pisella, L., Farne, A., Li, L., Boisson, D. & Perenin, M-T. (1998). Prism adaptation to a rightward optical deviation rehabilitates left hemispatial neglect. *Nature,* Vol.395, pp. 166-169.

Rosenzweig, M.R. (1971). Effects of environment of development of brain and behavior. In: *The Biopsychology of Development,* E. Tobach, L.R. Aronson & E. Shaw, (Eds.), pp. 303-342, Academic Press, New York.

Rosenzweig, M.R., Krech, D. & Bennett, E.L. (1961). Heredity, environment, brain biochemistry, and learning. In: *Current Trends in Psychological Theory,* pp. 87-110. University of Pittsburg Press, Pittsburgh, PA.

Rumelhart, D. & McClelland, J. (1986). *Parallel Distributed Processing*. MIT Press, Cambridge, MA.

Sahraie, A., Trevethan, C.T., MacLeod, M.J., Murray, A.D., Olson, J.A. & Weiskrantz, L. (2006). Increased sensitivity after repeated stimulation of residual spatial channels in blindsight. *Proceedings of the National Academy of Sciences, USA,* Vol.103, pp. 14971-14976.

Sarri, M., Greenwood, R., Kalra, L., Papps, B., Husain, M. & Driver, J. (2008). Prism adaptation aftereffects in stroke patients with spatial neglect: pathological effects on subjective straight ahead but not visual open-loop pointing. *Neuropsychologia,* Vol.46, pp. 1069-1080.

Schäfer, R., Dehn, D., Burbach, G.J. & Deller, T. (2008). Differential regulation of chondroitin sulfate proteoglycan mRNAs in the denervated rat fascia dentata after unilateral entorhinal cortex lesion. *Neuroscience Letters,* Vol.439, pp. 61-69.

Scharff, C., Kirn, J.R., Grossman, M., Macklis, J.D. & Nottebohm, G. (2000). Targeted neuronal death affects neuronal replacement and vocal behavior in adult songbirds. *Neuron,* Vol.25, pp. 481-492.

Scheibel, R.S., Newsome, M.R., Troyanskaya, M., Steinberg, J.L., Goldstein, F.C., Mao, H. & Levin, H.S. (2009). Effects of severity of traumatic brain injury and brain reserve on cognitive-control related brain activation. *Journal of Neurotrauma,* Vol.26, pp. 1447-1461.

Scheich, H. (1991). Auditory cortex: comparative aspects of maps and plasticity. *Current Opinion in Neurobiology,* Vol.1, pp. 236-247.

Schwab, M.E. & Thoenen, H. (1985). Dissociated neurons regenerate into sciatic but not optic nerve explants in culture irrespective of neurotrophic factors. *Journal of Neuroscience,* Vol.5, pp. 2415-2423.

Schwiedrzik, C.M., Singer, W. & Melloni, L. (2009). Sensitivity and perceptual awareness increase with practice in metacontrast masking. *Journal of Vision,* Vol.9, pp. 1-18.

Selnes, O.A. (2001). A historical overview of contributions from the study of deficits. In: *The Handbook of Cognitive Neuropsychology,* B. Rapp, (Ed.), pp. 23-41, Psychology Press, Philadelphia PA.

Seo, T-B., Kim, B-K., Ko, I-G., Kim, D-H., Shin, M-S., Kim, C-J., Yoon, J-H. & Kim, H. (2010). Effect of treadmill exercise on Purkinje cell loss and astrocytic reaction in the cerebellum after traumatic brain injury. *Neuroscience Letters,* Vol.481, pp. 178-182.

Serino, A., Angeli, V., Frassinetti, F. & Ladavas, E. (2006). Mechanisms underlying neglect recovery after prism adaptation. *Neuropsychologia,* Vol.44, pp, 1068-1078.

Serino, A., Bonifazi, S., Pierfederici, L. & Ladavas, E. (2007). Neglect treatment by prism adaptation: what recovers and for how long. *Neuropsychological Rehabilitation,* Vol.17, pp. 657-687.

Siesjo, B.K. & Siesjo, P. (1996). Mechanisms of secondary brain injury. *European Journal of Anaesthesiology,* Vol.13, pp. 247-268.

Silva, M., Grillot, D., Benito, A., Richard, C., Nunez, G. & Fernandez-Luna, J.L. (2006). Erythropoietin can promote erythroid progenitor survival by repressing apoptosis through Bcl-XL and Bcl-2. *Blood,* Vol.88, pp. 1576-1582.

Siren, A.L., Fratelli, M., Brines, M., Goemans, C., Casagrande, S., Lewczuk, P., Keenan, S., Gleiter, C., Pasquali, C., Capobianco, A., Mennini, T., Heumann, R., Cerami, A.,

Ehrenreich, H. & Ghezzi, P. (2001). Erythropoietin prevents neuronal apoptosis after cerebral ischemia and metabolic stress. *Proceedings of the National Academy of Sciences, USA,* Vol.98, pp. 4044-4049.

Sitaram, R., Caria, A. & Birbaumer, N. (2009). Hemodynamic brain-computer interfaces for communication and rehabilitation. *Neural Networks,* Vol.22, pp. 1320-1328.

Slavin, M.D., Laurence, S. & Stein, D.G. (1988). Another look at vicariation. In: *Brain Injury and Recovery: Theoretical and Controversial Issues,* S. Finger, T.E. LeVere, C.R. Almli, & D.G. Stein, (Eds.), pp. 165-178, Plenum Press, New York.

Sofroniew, M.V., Cooper, J.D., Svendsen, C.N., Crossman, P., Ip, N.Y., Lindsay, R.M., Zafra, F. & Lindholm, D. (1993). Atrophy but not death of adult septal cholinergic neurons after ablation of target capacity to produce mRNAs for NGF, BDNF, and NT3. *Journal of Neuroscience,* Vol.13, pp. 5263-5276.

Specht, K., Zahn, R., Willmes, K., Weis, S., Holtel, C., Krause, B.J., Herzog, H. & Huber, W. (2009). Joint independent component analysis of structural and functional images reveals complex patterns of functional reorganisation in stroke aphasia. *NeuroImage,* Vol.47, pp. 2057-2063.

Springborg, J.B., Ma, X.D., Rochat, P., Knudsen, G.M., Amtorp, O., Paulson, O.B., Juhler, M. & Olsen, N.V. (2002). A single subcutaneous bolus of erythropoietin normalizes cerebral blood flow autoregulation after subarachnoid haemorrhage in rats. *British Journal of Pharmacology,* Vol.135, pp. 823-829.

Stein, D.G. & Hoffman, S.W. (2003). Concepts of CNS plasticity in the context of brain damage and repair. *Journal of Head Trauma Rehabilitation,* Vol.18, pp. 317-341.

Stern, Y. (2002). What is cognitive reserve? Theory and research application of the reserve concept. *Journal of the International Neuropsychological Society,* Vol.8, pp. 448-460.

Stoerig, P. (2006). Blindsight, conscious vision, and the role of primary visual cortex. *Progress in Brain Research,* Vol.155, pp. 217-234.

Szaflarski, J.P., Eaton, K., Ball, A.L., Banks, C., Vannest, J., Allendorfer, J.B., Page, S. & Holland, S.K. (2011). Poststroke aphasia recovery assessed with functional magnetic resonance imaging and a picture identification task. *Journal of Stroke and Cerebrovascular Diseases,* Vol.20, pp. 336-345.

Thai-Van, H., Micheyl, C., Norena, A., Veuillet, E., Gabriel, D. & Collet, L. (2007). Enhanced frequency discrimination in hearing-impaired individuals: a review of perceptual correlates of central neural plasticity induced by cochlear damage. *Hearing Research,* Vol.233, pp. 14-22.

Thomas, C., Altenmüller, E., Marckmann, G., Kahrs, J. & Dichgans, J. (1997). Language processing in aphasia: changes in lateralization patterns during recovery reflect cerebral plasticity in adults. *Electroencephalography and Clinical Neurophysiology,* Vol.102, pp. 86-97.

Thompson, C.K., den Ouden, D-B., Bonakdarpour, B., Garibaldi, K. & Parrish, T.B. (2010). Neural plasticity and treatment-induced recovery of sentence processing in agrammatism. *Neuropsychologia,*Vol.48, pp. 3211-3227.

Thulborn, K.R., Carpenter, P.A. & Just, M.A. (1999). Plasticity of language-related brain function during recovery from stroke. *Stroke,* Vol.30, pp. 749-754.

Tsirlin, I., Dupierrix, E., Chokron, S., Coquillart, S. & Ohlmann, T. (2009). Uses of virtual reality for diagnosis, rehabilitation and study of unilateral spatial neglect: review and analysis. *CyberPsychology and Behavior,* Vol.12, pp. 175-181.

Vaynman, S., Ying, Z. & Gomez-Pinilla, F. (2003). Interplay between brain-derived neurotrophic factor and signal transduction modulators in the regulation of the effects of exercise on synaptic-plasticity. *Neuroscience,* Vol.122, pp. 647-657.

Viviani, B., Bartesaghi, S., Corsini, E., Villa, P., Ghezzi, P., Garau, A., Galli, C.L. & Marinovich, M. (2005). Erythropoietin protects primary hippocampal neurons increasing the expression of brain-derived neurotrophic factor. *Journal of Neurochemistry,* Vol.93, pp. 412-421.

Wang, K.W., Larner, S.F., Robinson, G. & Hayes, R.L. (2006). Neuroprotection targets after traumatic brain injury. *Current Opinion in Neurology,* Vol.19, pp. 514-519.

Weiss, T., Miltner, W.H.R., Huonker, R., Friedel, R., Schmidt, I. & Taub, E. (2000). Rapid functional plasticity of the somatosensory cortex after finger amputation. *Experimental Brain Research,* Vol.134, pp. 199-203.

Werbos, P.J. (1994). *The Roots of Backpropagation: From Ordered Derivatives to Neural Networks and Political Forecasting*. John Wiley & Sons, New York.

Wilms, I. (2011). Using artificial intelligence to control and adapt level of difficulty in computer based, cognitive therapy - an explorative study. *Journal of Cybertherapy and Rehabilitation,* in press.

Wilms, I. & Malá, H. (2010). Indirect versus direct feedback in computer-based Prism Adaptation Therapy. *Neuropsychological Rehabilitation* i*First,* pp. 1-24.

Wilms, I. & Mogensen, J. (2011). Dissimilar outcomes of apparently similar procedures as a challenge to clinical neurorehabilitation and basic research - when the same is not the same. *NeuroRehabilitation,* Vol.29, in press.

Wilson, B.A., Evans, J.J., Emslie, H. & Malinek, V. (1997). Evaluation of NeuroPage: a new memory aid. *Journal of Neurology, Neurosurgery, and Psychiatry,* Vol.63, pp. 113-115.

Wilson, B.A., Emslie, H.C., Quirk, K. & Evans, J.J. (2001). Reducing everyday memory and planning problems by means of a paging system: a randomised control crossover study. *Journal of Neurology, Neurosurgery, and Psychiatry,* Vol.70, pp. 477-482.

Wu, C-L., Chen, S-D., Yin, J-H., Hwang, C-S. & Yang, D-I. (2010). Erythropoietin and sonic hedgehog mediate the neuroprotective effects of brain-derived neurotrophic factor against mitochondrial inhibition. *Neurobiology of Disease,* Vol.40, pp. 146-154.

Xerri, C., Coq, J., Merzenich, M. & Jenkins, W. (1996). Experience-induced plasticity of cutaneous maps in the primary somatosensory cortex of adult monkeys and rats. *Journal of Physiology,* Vol.90, pp. 277-287.

Yang, T.T., Gallen, C.C., Ramachandran, V.S., Cobb, S., Schwartz, B.J. & Bloom, F.E. (1994). Noninvasive detection of cerebral plasticity in adult human somatosensory cortex. *Neuroreport,* Vol.5, pp. 701-704.

Zhang, F., Signore, A.P., Zhou, Z., Wang, S., Cao, G. & Chen, J. (2006). Erythropoietin protects CA1 neurons against global cerebral ischemia in rat: potential signalling mechanisms. *Journal of Neuroscience Research,* Vol.83: pp. 1241-1251.

Zhang, Y., Xiong, Y., Mahmood, A., Meng, Y., Qu, C., Schallert, T. & Chopp, M. (2009). Therapeutic effects of erythropoietin on histological and functional outcomes following traumatic brain injury in rats are independent of hematocrit. *Brain Research,* Vol.1294, pp. 153-164.

Zihl, J. (1980). "Blindsight": improvement of visually guided eye movements by systematic practice in patients with cerebral blindness. *Neuropsychologia,* Vol.18, pp. 71-77.

Zihl, J. & Werth, R. (1984). Contributions to the study of "blindsight" – II. The role of specific practice for saccadic localization in patients with postgeniculate visual field defects. *Neuropsychologia*, Vol.22, pp. 13-22.

8

Communicative Impairment After Traumatic Brain Injury: Evidence and Pathways to Recovery

Francesca M. Bosco[1,2] and Romina Angeleri[1]
[1]*Center for Cognitive Science and Department of Psychology, University of Turin*
[2]*Neuroscience Institute of Turin*
Italy

1. Introduction

Traumatic brain injury (TBI) patients show a series of communicative difficulties, loading on all the dimensions that characterize satisfying communicative interactions. This chapter has three aims: first, it reviews the current literature on this topic in order to provide a complete picture of the communicative impairment in TBI patients; second, it examines the relationship between cognitive functions - i.e. executive functions and theory of mind - and pragmatic deficits resulting as a consequence of traumatic brain injury; third, it reviews the current literature on treatment planning in rehabilitation therapy and provides suggestions for the clinical practice.

2. Communicative deficit in TBI

The literature has shown that traumatic brain injury, (TBI), results in a range of communicative deficits that cannot be adequately explained in terms of linguistic impairment. Patients affected by TBI do not display classical aphasic symptoms: their syntactical and lexical abilities are often normal and their performance on standardized aphasia batteries is good (McDonald, 1993). However, communicative ability involves going beyond the comprehension and production of correct lexical and syntactical aspects: patients have substantial difficulty managing interactions in their everyday life, since for example they may have confused verbal behavior, inaccurate and confabulated speech (Hartley & Jensen, 1992). The discourse of TBI patients may be long-winded, poorly organized and tangential (Glosser, 1993), while some patients may have a lower than normal level of linguistic productivity, resulting in an inability to communicate their basic needs (Hartley & Levin, 1990).
From a pragmatic viewpoint, TBI patients encounter difficulties at various levels of comprehension: they cannot go beyond the literal meaning of utterances since they are not able to understand what is implied, as in the case of comprehension of sarcastic utterances (McDonald & Pearce, 1996), humor (Braun et al., 1989; Docking et al., 2000) or commercial messages which require inferential processes in order to be understood (Pearce et al., 1998). TBI patients are also impaired on the production side, to varying degrees of severity: for

example, they may have difficulty producing correct requests (McDonald & Van Sommers, 1993) or giving the interlocutor sufficiently detailed information (McDonald, 1993; for a complete review of pragmatic disorders in adults with language impairment see Cummings, 2007).

Dardier and coll. (2011) recently conducted a detailed analysis of pragmatic aspects of language use by TBI individuals, examining both comprehension - i.e., direct requests, indirect requests, and hints - and production ability - i.e., conversation during an interview situation-. The authors showed that the pragmatic skills of persons with TBI vary across tasks: patients demonstrated weakness (in topic maintenance) but also strengths (in turn-taking, comprehension of requests and hints). The authors also argued that the specific deficits observed in patients were not systematically linked to executive function performance, even if lesion unilaterality (right or left) seems help to preserve patients' pragmatic performance.

It is not only the linguistic modality that may be impaired after traumatic brain damage, but also the extralinguistic modality, that is the ability to communicate through gestures (Bara et al., 2001), and the paralinguistic modality, that is the ability to mark one's own communicative acts appropriately using cues such as tone, prosody and rhythm. For example Rousseaux and coll. (2010) evaluated the verbal and non-verbal aspect of communication in TBI patients during a dyadic interaction and found that in the chronic phase patients showed marked difficulties in speech outflow and pragmatic language - i.e. responding to open questions, presenting new information and introducing new themes, organizing discourse and adapting to interlocutor language. As far as non-verbal communication is concerned, patients were impaired in understanding and producing gestures, in affective expressivity, in feedback management and pragmatics (i.e., prosody, orienting gaze, using regulatory mimogestuality and turn-taking).

Focusing on paralinguistic communication, some authors (e.g., Ylvisaker et al., 1987) have suggested that the inability to recognize emotions expressed by other people, both through their voice and through their facial expression, may even be the causal factor for the antisocial behavior and poor social relationships of TBI patients. After traumatic brain injury it is difficult to understand prosodic aspects of speech (Joanette & Brownell, 1990), especially in cases in which prosodic elements would help in disambiguating utterances (Marquardt et al., 2001). Furthermore, the social difficulties experienced after traumatic brain injury spread to the management of social interactions, with the inability to resume and carry on normal personal relationships.

Angeleri and coll. (2008) provided a comprehensive picture of communicative performance in TBI patients, encompassing both comprehension and production of a series of pragmatic tasks, such as for example direct and indirect speech acts, irony and deceit. They analyzed a great variety of expressive modalities, including linguistic, extralinguistic, and paralinguistic communication, conversational exchange management and the ability to evaluate the appropriateness of a communicative act with respect to a given social context. The authors showed that in the linguistic and extralinguistic modalities TBI patients performed worse than controls in both comprehension and production of each investigated phenomenon, i.e. direct and indirect, ironic and deceitful communication acts. However, while impaired in comparison with normal controls, some pragmatic tasks have been found to be better preserved than others. In particular, direct and indirect speech acts are better preserved than deceit, which is in turn better preserved than irony, the most difficult task to manage. Furthermore TBI patients showed a pronounced impairment in comprehending and producing paralinguistic aspects, remaining attached to the expressed semantic content and neglecting the emotional meaning expressed through other modalities, such as, for example, prosody. However TBI patients are still competent in understanding communication acts adequate to the context (i.e., formal vs. informal) in which they are uttered, but they have difficulty in grasping subtler conversational violations of Grice's (1989) cooperation principle (i.e., the speaker is ambiguous or confused). Lastly, TBI patients achieve good conversational performance when the interaction is principally directed by another person through simple and superficial topics, although they have a pronounced tendency to persevere on the same topic during the dialogue. All their results considered, Angeleri and coll. (2008) concluded that the TBI patients they studied had a communicative deficit but preserved abilities in some areas. Furthermore, the authors point out that even when communication is damaged some pragmatic abilities are less damaged than others, such as for example direct and indirect speech acts with respect to deceit, and deceit with respect to the comprehension and production of irony.

Some authors have suggested that the communicative inappropriateness of TBI patients represents the most impressive obstacle to patients' social reintegration, due to impairments in social communication (Dahlberg et al., 2006; Turkstra et al., 2001). All these aspects are central to communication because of their role in setting and maintaining social relationships; it appears to be extremely important to assess this in patients affected by TBI since changes in social ability after brain injury represent one of the most destabilizing and invalidating sides of the condition (McDonald et al., 2004).

3. Cognitive functioning in communication

In recent years, there has been increasing interest in the cognitive aspects underlying pragmatic impairment (e.g., Perkins, 2000). In particular, some authors have suggested that cognitive abilities, such as executive functions and theory of mind, play a central role in the pragmatic performance of brain-damaged subjects (Happé et al., 1999; Martin & McDonald, 2003). TBI patients often suffer damage in the frontal lobe, the brain area involved in executive functioning - the construct used to describe goal-directed behavior - and some authors have explained the pragmatic deficit displayed by these individuals as being caused mainly by executive function impairment (McDonald & Pearce, 1998).

Theory of Mind (ToM) is the ability to ascribe mental states to oneself and to other people and to use such knowledge to interpret one's own as well as other people's behavior. Some authors highlight the role of ToM in human communication (Happé & Loth, 2002; Tirassa et al., 2006) and argue that a developed and intact capacity to mindread is necessary to comprehend a partner's communicative intention (Frith, 1992).

The relation between Theory of Mind and communicative ability is particularly apparent in individuals on the autism spectrum whose communicative and social difficulties have been noticed in several studies (e.g., Frith, 1989; Tager-Flusberg, 2006). Several authors (e.g., Baron-Cohen et al., 1985) have proposed that difficulty in social adjustment and communicative impairments typically demonstrated by autistic children were caused by a specific ToM deficit.

Only a few studies have specifically investigated ToM impairment in TBI patients (Channon & Crawford, 2010). In a focused study Bibby and McDonald (2005) tested patients with TBI on mentalistic (ToM) tasks and non-mentalistic (inferential) tasks. Their results revealed that subjects with TBI performed more poorly than controls on all tasks (mentalistic and non-mentalistic). However a more detailed analysis revealed that inference-making ability and working memory significantly predict the subject's performance on second-order stories and non-verbal ToM tasks but these factors were not significant predictors of subjects' performance on first-order ToM tasks. The authors concluded that further studies are necessary to determine whether a specific ToM deficit can be observed in relation to other tasks that demand a comparable non-mentalizing process. The authors also suggested that a number of factors, in addition to ToM deficit, may influence TBI patients' social performance, including inferential ability, language comprehension, understanding of humor and working memory. The authors concluded that rehabilitative programs should also consider these factors, in addition to ToM. However, to the best of our knowledge, no specific rehabilitative processes focusing on ToM, or on ToM plus such factors, have been created and used in TBI patients' rehabilitative treatment.

4. Cognitive rehabilitation

Generally speaking, cognitive rehabilitation refers to a wide range of methods aimed at remediating or compensating for decreased cognitive abilities. However, in recent decades, it has been emphasized that treatment should focus on the *individual* rather than on cognitive functioning per se; this means that the influence of specific contextual variables on rehabilitation plans, the emotional and social aspects associated with brain injury, and their interactions with cognitive function should be clarified for each patient, in order to precisely assess the patient's particular needs. The goal of treatment is thus a functional change able to bring about meaningful changes in the patient's everyday life, including improved autonomy and satisfactory social relationships.

As researchers have shown (e.g., Chen et al., 2010, Kolb & Gibb, 1999), the brain is a plastic organ capable of considerable reorganization that can be considered the basis for functional recovery; the way in which dendritic growth, structured stimulation, and recovery of lost function are related has been well demonstrated, and this is the starting point for the utility of cognitive treatment.

Rehabilitation programs for individuals with brain injury commonly focus on attention, memory, and executive function. We will now briefly review those cognitive functions that have the greatest impact on communicative abilities, i.e. executive function and theory of mind ability.

For individuals with acquired brain injury, damage to the frontal lobe and its connections throughout the central nervous system could drive impairment in executive functioning, i.e., a cluster of deficits including planning, problem solving, initiating, and regulating behavior (Kramer & Quitania, 2007; Stuss, 2007).

A clinical model of executive functions has been proposed by Mateer (1999). This model conceives the following different domains of executive functions with wide clinical impact: 1. *Initiation and drive (starting behavior)*, 2. *Response inhibition (stopping behavior)*, 3. *Task persistence (maintaining behavior)*, 4. *Organization (organizing actions and thoughts)*, 5. *Generative thinking (creativity, fluency, cognitive flexibility)*, and 6. *Awareness (monitoring and modifying one's own behavior)*. These categories capture the wide range of cognitive and behavioral impairments that may occur when executive functions are damaged; it is important to note that these six categories, as part of the same brain network, are linked, related, and interdependent. Once the cognitive impairment has been carefully assessed, a variety of clinical approaches may be used to address executive function rehabilitation. The choice of clinical approach is dependent upon specific variables that clinicians must consider when planning patient management. For instance, it is important to consider the time after onset, the severity of the executive dysfunction, the co-occurrence of other cognitive problems, the social support available, and the patient's level of awareness. Developing a specific and flexible treatment plan is essential in order to lead to cognitive improvement, and establish the necessary therapeutic alliance.

One of the most common rehabilitative approaches refers to *teaching task-specific routines*, which must be relevant to a specific setting (e.g., dressing, writing letters, traveling on a bus, playing solitaire and so on). After training, the patient should also be able to initiate and maintain the behavioral sequence in her/his daily life (Sohlberg & Raskin, 1996). This kind of routine is designed to produce automatic responses for specific procedures; in contrast, the therapeutic approach called *training the selection and execution of cognitive plans* aims to improve patients' ability to reinforce specific areas of executive functioning, also extending the results to related tasks. This approach considers several critical components (e.g., goal selection, planning/sequencing, initiation and so on) and suggests specific exercises to improve performance in those areas: examples are planning repeated activities in role-play situations, practicing specific tasks also in naturalistic contexts (e.g., getting a bus schedule), and completing activities according to time constraints.

A different rehabilitative approach is *teaching to use metacognitive routines*. In this case, patients have to modulate their own behavior by talking to themselves using self-instructional techniques (Alderman et al., 1995; Fish et al., 2008; Levine et al., 2000). This approach leads patients to regulate their behavior and autonomously complete goal directed activities. In line with these aims, Von Cramon and Matthes-von Cramon (1994) proposed *problem-solving therapy* groups, a treatment based on the idea of substituting the patient's impulsive behavior with a verbally-mediated, systematic analysis of the goal and the means by which it may be achieved. The problem-solving intervention focuses on the development of self-regulation strategies as the basis for maintaining an effective problem orientation (Rath et al., 2003).

Cognitive rehabilitation has also been used to successfully remediate the social perception deficit, i.e. deficit in emotion perception, commonly experienced by TBI patients (Bornhofen & Mcdonald, 2008). The treatment program consists of tasks involving the recognition of specific patterns of changes in facial expressions, voice tone and body posture during the expression of different kinds of emotions. These tasks consist in interpreting conventional emotional contexts (i.e., knowledge regarding emotions typically expressed in scenarios such as birthday parties, funerals, and so on), judging static (i.e., photograph) and dynamic (i.e., video or role-play) emotion cues and making social inferences on the basis of emotional demeanor and situational cues (i.e., regarding whether a speaker is sarcastic or lying, rehearsed via therapist modeling, video sequences and role play).

5. Communicative rehabilitation

People express their communicative ability via different expressive means, for instance, using linguistic, gestural and paralinguistic modalities. However, the majority of studies in the literature have focused primarily on remediation of the linguistic modality.

The major limit of interventions exclusively focused on language is that after the therapy patients are often impaired in solving communicative difficulties in everyday life situations. The pragmatic approach has been developed to overcome this limitation (for a review see Carlomagno et al., 2000). The pragmatic view has shifted the focus of therapeutic practice from the patient's linguistic ability to the effective use of language in a given context and was first used with aphasic patients. Functional pragmatic therapies also focus on a patient's residual communicative abilities, such as for instance gestural and prosodic skills in aphasic patients, and look for alternative and compensatory communicative strategies with respect to the defective ones. Aten, Caligiuri and Holland (1982) were the first to develop a successful formal pragmatic therapy program, the *Functional Communication Treatment*, in which aphasic patients were confronted with simulated everyday life situations and trained in the use of non-verbal communicative strategies. Holland (1991) further expanded this treatment by introducing *Conversational Coaching* therapy. The aim of this method, based on the use of short monologues, is to train patients to control the quality of the monologue depending on the degree of familiarity with the listener - from relatives to unknown persons - and the informativeness of the script - from known information to improbable events. A further example of the use of the functional pragmatic approach, backed by experimental evidence, is *Promoting Aphasics Communicative Effectiveness* (Davis & Wilcox, 1985). The treatment requires that therapist and patient sit facing one another across a table on which are a set of printed stimulus cards. In turn, each participant takes a card and, without showing it, he tries to describe it to the other person. The therapeutic basis of this treatment is that it involves a progressive exercise within the setting of natural conversation, supported by a therapist eliciting compensatory strategies and providing useful feedback, which improves the patient's linguistic and communicative performance.

Within the pragmatic approach, an important setting for practicing pragmatic therapies is the group (Marshall, 1999). Group communication treatments focus on initiating conversation and conveying a message, understanding the communication disorder, being aware of personal goals and progress and having confidence in being able to communicate in personally relevant situations (Elman & Bernstein-Ellis, 1999).

Ehrlich and Sipes (1985) described a model of group intervention specifically for TBI patients based on the functional pragmatic approach. The treatment consisted of four modules focused on improving non-verbal communication, appropriate communication in context, message repair and message cohesiveness. The therapist role-played and videotaped both appropriate and inappropriate examples of target behavior. The videos were examined and reviewed by the group under the supervision of the therapist, who pointed out the inappropriate behavior and suggested possible appropriate alternatives. After treatment patients showed improvements in the reformulation of inappropriate messages, sentence cohesion and in the introduction and development of conversational topics.

TBI patients have been found to have, in particular, social communication problems (Dahlberg et al., 2006). Social communication interventions include therapies such as group discussion, forming communication goals, modeling, role-playing, feedback, self-monitoring, behavioral rehearsal and social reinforcement (Struchen, 2005). For example, Bellon and Rees (2006) examined the role of social context on language and communication skills among TBI patients, demonstrating the notable benefits of carefully structured supportive social networks. The key component of their rehabilitation intervention was the presence of a mentor, who prompted the patients and gave them cues and models of positive behavior; this kind of social support stimulated patients' positive self-image, positive self-talk and inter-personal language. Ylvisaker (2006) presented an intervention for TBI patients based on self-coaching which was aimed at improving planned, goal-oriented and successful behavior.

Lastly, further rehabilitative treatments focus on training the partners who communicate with patients affected by TBI (Togher et al., 2004); the goal of such interventions is to improve the quality of conversational interactions, enhance the listener's ability to comprehend and promote the patient's communicative attempts. The listener's attitude can in fact shape the patient's language, communicative behavior and motivation, reducing the social isolation typically resulting as an outcome of brain injury.

6. Conclusions

Traumatic brain injury, (TBI), patients show a series of communicative difficulties, however such difficulties may vary across the communicative tasks and the expressive modalities investigated, showing large individual differences with specific areas of weakness and strength. One of the first steps in designing an effective rehabilitation program is thus to define an in-depth and articulate assessment of the deficit/preserved ability of a specific patient taking into consideration different pragmatic phenomena and expressive modalities. Empirical studies also suggest that cognitive abilities, such as executive functions and theory of mind, may have a role in the communicative performance of brain-damaged subjects, however only a few studies have systematically investigated the role played in TBI by ToM and executive function impairment and such relationship is not sufficiently explained. Further studies are thus necessary to clarify this relationship and to support the possibility of including specific cognitive training in treatment aimed at improving communicative ability in TBI patients.

Several communicative rehabilitation treatment programs already exist and the effectiveness of functional pragmatic therapy after TBI is supported by empirical data. However, given the limited number of studies in the literature and the small samples considered, further confirmation is necessary.

7. Acknowledgments

This research was supported by the University of Turin (Ricerca scientifica finanziata dall'Università di Torino, fondi ex-60% 2007)

8. References

Alderman, N., Fry, R. K. & Youngson, H. A. (1995). Improvement in self-monitoring skills, reduction of behavior disturbance and the dysexecutive syndrome: Comparison of response cost and a new programme of self monitoring training. *Neuropsychological Rehabilitation,* Vol. 5, No.3, (December, 2008), pp. 193-221, ISNN 0960-2011

Angeleri, R., Bosco, F. M., Zettin, M., Sacco, K., Colle, L. & Bara, B. G. (2008). Communicative impairment in traumatic brain injury: A complete pragmatic assessment. *Brain and Language,* Vol. 107, No.3, (Decembre 2008), pp. 229-245, ISNN 0093-934X

Aten, J. L., Caligiuri, M. P., & Holland, A. L. (1982). L., Caligiuri, M. P., & Holland, A. L. (1982). The efficacy of functional communication therapy for chronic aphasic patients. *Journal of Speech and Hearing Disorders,* Vol. 47, No. 1, (April 1982), pp. 93-96, ISSN 0022-4677.

Bara, B. G., Cutica, I., & Tirassa, M. (2001). Neuropragmatics: Extralinguistic communication after closed head injury. *Brain and Language,* Vol. 77, No. 1, (April 2001), pp. 72-94, ISSN 0093-934X.

Baron-Cohen, S., Leslie, A. & Frith, U. (1985). Does the autistic child have a Theory of Mind? *Cognition,* Vol. 21, No. 1, (April 1985), pp. 37-46, ISSN 0010-0277.

Bellon, M., & Rees, R. (2006). The effect of context on communication: a study of the language and communication skills of adults with acquired brain injury. *Brain Injury*, Vol. 20, No. 10, (January 2006), pp. 1069-1078, ISSN 0269-9052.

Bibby, H., & McDonald, S. (2005). Theory of mind after traumatic brain injury. *Neuropsychologia*, Vol. 43, No. 1, (April 2005), pp. 99-114, ISSN 0028-3932.

Bornhofen, C., & Mcdonald, S. (2008). Treating deficits in emotion perception following traumatic brain injury. *Neuropsychologial Rehabilitation*, (December 2008), Vol. 18, No. 1, pp. (22-44), ISSN 0960-2011.

Braun, C. M. J., Lissier, F., Baribeau, J. M. C., & Ethier, M. (1989). Does severe traumatic closed head injury impair sense of humor? Brain Injury, Vol. 3, No. 4, (Octobe-December 1989), pp. (345-354), ISNN 0269-9052

Carlomagno, S., Blasi, V., Labruna, L., & Santoro, A. (2000). The role of communication models in assessment and therapy of language disorders in aphasic adults', *Neuropsychological Rehabilitation*, Vol. 10, No. 3, (April 2000), pp. (337–363), ISSN 0960-2011

Cummings, L. (2007). Pragmatics and adult language disorders: past achievements and future directions. *Seminars in Speech & Language*. Vol. 28, No. 2. (May 2007), pp. 96-110, ISNN 0734-0478

Chen, B. A., Epstein, J., & Stern, E. (2010). Neural plasticity after acquired brain injury: Evidence from functional neuroimaging. *PM&R*, Vol. 2, No. (12 Supp. 2), (December 2010), pp. S306-S312, ISNN 1934-1482

Crawford, S., & Channon, S. (2010). Mentalising and social problem-solving after brain injury. *Neuropsychological Rehabilitation*, Vol. 20, No. 5, (May 2010), pp. (739-759), ISSN 0960-2011.

Dahlberg, C., Hawley, L., Morey, C., Newman, J., Cusick, C. P., & Harrison-Felix, C. (2006). Social communication skills in persons with post-acute traumatic brain injury: Three perspectives. *Brain Injury*, Vol. 20, No. 4, (April 2006), pp. 425-435, ISNN 0269-9052

Dardier, V., Bernicot, J., Delanoë, A., Vanberten, M., Fayada, C, Chevignard, M., Delaye, C., Laurent-Vannier, A & Dubois B. (2011). Severe traumatic brain injury, frontal lesions, and social aspects of language use: A study of French-speaking adults. *Journal of Communication Disorders*, Vol. 44, No. 3, (June 2011) pp. (359-378), ISNN 0021-9924.

Davis, G., & Wilcox, M. (1985). *Adult Aphasia Rehabilitation: Applied Pragmatics*, NFER-Nelson, ISBN 0-933914-07-4, Windsor.

Docking, K., Murdoch, B. E., & Jordan, F. M. (2000). Interpretation and comprehension of linguistic humor by adolescents with head injury: A group analysis. *Brain Injury*, Vol. 14, No. 1, (January 2000), pp. 89-108, ISNN 0269-9052

Ehrlich, J.S., & Sipes, A.L (1985). Group treatment of communication skills for head trauma patients', *Cognitive Rehabilitation*, Vol. 3, No. 1 (January-February 1985), pp. 32-37, ISNN 1062-2969.

Elman, R. J., & Bernstein-Ellis, E. (1999). The efficacy of group communication treatment in adults with chronic aphasia, *Journal of Speech, Language and Hearing Research*, Vol. 42, No. 2, (April 1999), pp. 411-419, ISNN 1092-4388.

Fish, J., Manly, T., & Wilson, B. A. (2008). Long-term compensatory treatment of organizational deficits in patients with bilateral frontal lobe damage. *Journal of the International Neuropsychological Society*, Vol. 14, No.1 (January 2008), pp. 154-163, 1355-6177

Frith, C. D.. (1992). *The cognitive neuropsychology of schizophrenia*, Hove, UK and Hillsdale, ISBN 0-86377-224-2, NJ: Erlbaum

Frith, U. (1989). Autism and "theory of mind.", In *Diagnosis and treatment of autism*, Gillberg Christopher [Ed], pp. (33-52), ix, 450, Plenum Press, ISBN 0-306-43481-4, New York, NY, US.

Glosser, G. (1993). Discourse production patterns in neurologically impaired and aged populations. In H. H. Brownell & Y. Joannette (Eds.), Narrative discourse in neurologically impaired and normal aging adults, pp. 191–211. Singular Publisher Group, ISBN 1565930835, 9781565930834, San Diego

Grice, H.P. (1989). *Studies in the ways of words*, Harvard University Press, ISBN 0-674-85271-0, Cambridge.

Happé, F. G. E., Brownell, H., & Winner, E. (1999). Acquired theory of mind impairments following stroke. *Cognition*, No. 70, (April 1999), pp. 211-240, ISSN 0010-0277.

Happé, F., & Loth, E. (2002). Theory of mind and tracking speaker's intentions. *Mind and Language*, No. 17, (December 2002), pp. 24-36, ISSN 0268-1064.

Hartley, L. L., & Levin, H. S. (1990). Linguistic deficits after closed head injury: A current appraisal. Aphasiology, 4, 353–370, ISSN 0268-7038

Hartley, L. L., & Jensen, P. J. (1992). Three discourse profiles of closed-head-injury speakers: Theoretical and clinical implications. Brain Injury, Vol. 6, No. 3, (May 1992), pp. 271-282, ISSN 0269-9052.

Holland, A. L. (1991). Pragmatic aspects of intervention in aphasia. *Journal of Neurolinguistics,* Vol. 6, No. 2, (December 1991) pp. 197-211, ISSN 0911-6044.

Joannette, Y., & Brownell, C.A. (Eds.) (1990). *Discourse ability and brain damage: Theoretical and empirical perspectives.* Springer-Verlag, ISBN 0387970444, New York

Kolb, B., & Gibb, R. (1999). Neuroplasticity and revovery of function after brain injury. In D. T. Stuss, G. Winocur, &I. H. Robertson (Eds.), Cognitive Neurorehabilitation, pp. 9–25. Cambridge University Press, ISBN 0521581028, Cambridge, United Kingdom

Kramer, J.H. & Quitania, L. (2007). Beside frontal lobe testing, In: *The human frontal lobes: Functions and disorders, 2nd edition*, B.L. Miller & J.L. Cummings, (Eds.), pp. 279–291, The Guilford Press, ISBN 1593853297, New York

Levine, B., Robertson, I.H., Clare, L., Carter, G., Hong, J., Wilson, B.A., Duncan, J., & Stuss, D.T. (2000). Rehabilitation of executive functioning: An experimental-clinical validation of goal management training. *Journal of the International Neuropsychological Society*, Vol.6, No.3, (March 2000), pp. 299-312, ISSN 1355-6177

Marquardt, T.P., Rios-Brown, M., Richburg, T., Seibert, L.K., & Cannito, M.P. (2001). Comprehension and expression of affective sentences in traumatic brain injury. *Aphasiology*, Vol.15, No.10-11, (May 2000), pp. 1091-1101, ISSN 1464-5041

Marshall, R. (1999). *Introduction to Group Treatment for Aphasia: Design and Management*, Butterworth-Heinemann, ISBN 0750670134, Woburn, Massachussetts

Martin, I. & McDonald, S. (2003). Weak coherence, no theory of mind, or executive dysfunction? Solving the puzzle of pragmatic language disorders. *Brain and Language*, Vol.85, No.3, (June 2003), pp. 451-466, ISSN 0093934X

Mateer, C.A. (1999). The rehabilitation of executive disorders, In: *Cognitive neurorehabilitation* D.T. Stuss, G. Winocur, & I.H. Robertson, (Eds.), pp. 314-332, Cambridge University Press, ISBN 0521691850, Cambridge, United Kingdom

McDonald, S. (1993). Viewing the brain sideways? Right hemisphere versus anterior models of non-aphasic language disorders. *Aphasiology*, Vol.7, No.6, (May-June 1993), pp. 535-549, ISSN 0268-7038

McDonald, S., Flanagan, S., Martin, I., & Saunders, C. (2004). The ecological validity of TASIT: A test of social perception. *Neuropsychological Rehabilitation*, Vol.14, No.3, (July 2004), pp. 285-302, ISSN 0960-2011

McDonald, S., & Pearce, S. (1996). Clinical insight into pragmatic theory: Frontal lobe deficits and sarcasm. *Brain and Language*, Vol.61, No.1, (April 1996), pp. 81-104, ISSN 0093-934X

McDonald, S. & Van Sommers, P. (1993). Pragmatic language skills after closed head injury: Ability to negotiate requests. *Cognitive Neuropsychology*, Vol.10, No.4, (August 1993), pp. 297-315, ISSN 0264-3294

Pearce, S., McDonald, S., & Coltheart, M. (1998). Interpreting ambiguous advertisements: The effect of frontal lobe damage. *Brain and Cognition*, Vol.38, No.2, (November 1998), pp. 150-164, ISSN 0278-2626

Perkins, M.R. (2000). The scope of pragmatic disability: A cognitive approach, In: *Pragmatics and clinical applications*, N. Müller (Ed.), pp. 7-28, John Benjamins Pub Co, ISBN 9027243387, Amsterdam

Rath, J.F., Simon, D., Lagenbahn, D.M., Sherr, R.L., & Diller, L. (2003). Group treatment of problem-solving deficits in outpatients with traumatic brain injury: A randomized outcome study. *Neuropsychological Rehabilitation*, Vol.13, No.4, (September 2003), pp. 461-488, ISSN 0960-2011

Russeaux, M., Vérigneaux, C., & Kozlowski, O. (2010). An analysis of communication in conversation after severe traumatic brain injury. *European Journal of Neurology*, Vol.17, No.7, (July 2010), pp. 922-929, ISSN 1468-1331

Sohlberg, M.M., & Raskin, S. (1996). Principles of generalization applied to attention and memory interventions. *Journal of Head Trauma Rehabilitation*, Vol.11, No.2, (April 1996), pp. 65-78, ISSN 0885-9701

Struchen, M. (2005). Social communication intervention, In: *Rehabilitation for Traumatic Brain Injury*, W.M. High, A.M. Sander, M. Struchen, & K.A. Hart (Eds.), pp. 88-117, Oxford University Press, ISBN 0195173554, Oxford, New York

Stuss, D.T. (2007). New approaches to prefrontal lobe testing, In: *The human frontal lobes: Functions and disorders, 2nd edition* B. L. Miller, & J. L. Cummings (Eds.), pp. 292–305, The Guilford Press, ISBN 1593853297, New York

Tager-Flusberg, H. (2006). Defining language phenotypes in autism. *Clinical Neuroscience Research*, Vol.6, No.3, (October 2006), pp. 219–224, ISSN 1566-2772

Tirassa, M., Bosco, F.M., & Colle, L. (2006). Sharedness and privateness in human early social life, *Cognitive Systems Research*, Vol.7, No.2-3, (June 2006), pp. 128-139, ISSN 1389-0417

Togher, L., McDonald, S., Code, C., & Grant, S. (2004). Training communication partners of people with traumatic brain injury: A randomized controlled trial. *Aphasiology*, Vol.18, No.4, (April 2004), pp. 313-335, ISSN 0268-7038

Turkstra, L., McDonald, S., & DePompei, R. (2001). Social information processing in adolescents: Data from normally developing adolescents and preliminary data from their peers with traumatic brain injury. *Journal of Head and Trauma Rehabilitation*, Vol.16, No.5, (October 2001), pp. 469-483, ISSN 0885-9701

von Cramon, D.Y., & Matthes-von Cramon, G. (1994). Back to work with a chronic dysexecutive syndrome. *Neuropsychological Rehabilitation*, Vol.4, No.4, (December 1994), pp. 399-417, ISSN 0960-2011

Ylvisaker, M. (2006). Self-coaching: a context-sensitive, person-centred approach to social communication after traumatic brain injury. *Brain Impairment*, Vol.7, No.3, (December 2006), pp. 246-258, ISSN 1443-9646

Ylvisaker, M., Szekeres, S., Henry, K., Sullivan, D., & Wheeler, P. (1987). Topics in cognitive rehabilitation therapy, In: *Community re-entry for head injured adults*, M. Ylvisaker & E. Gobble (Eds.), pp. 137-220, Little, Brown Book Group, ISBN 0316968803, United Kingdom

9

Traumatic Brain Injury: Consequences and Family Needs

Edilene Curvelo Hora et al.*
Associate professor, Nursing Department and Graduate Center of Medicine Federal University of Sergipe Brazil

1. Introduction

Traumatic Brain Injury (TBI) is one of the most common injuries resulting from external causes and constitutes a global public health problem of great significance. TBI is mainly caused by traffic accidents, violence and falls, with a strong impact on the population's morbidity and mortality.

TBI is a complex injury caused by a cascade of changes in the brain and throughout the body. Its consequences, especially neuropsychiatric ones, do not appear immediately, a characteristic of a silent epidemic (Hampton, 2011).

It is considered to be a chronic disease process, according to the World Health Organization, presenting one or more of the following characteristics: permanent, caused by non-reversible pathological alterations, requires special treatment to rehabilitate the patient, or a long period of observation, supervision and care (Masel & DeWitt, 2010).

It affects people of all ages, with a higher incidence among those who are 15 to 24 years old and 75 years old or older. It occurs twice as frequently in men as in women, half of all cases are associated with alcohol and can result in physical, cognitive, and psychosocial disability. Due to the large number of cases with disabilities, prevention is of great importance (National Institutes Health [NIH], 1999).

There is a worldwide concern to promote widespread awareness, warning people of all classes and ages about how serious a problem TBI is becoming. Good education, knowledge of risk factors and prevention reduces the incidence of trauma and its consequences.

Regina Márcia Cardoso de Sousa[1], Maria do Carmo de Oliveira Ribeiro[2], Mariangela da Silva Nunes[3], Rita de Cássia Vieira Araújo[4], Ana Carla Ferreira Silva dos Santos[5], Carla Kalline Alves Cartaxo[6] and Liane Viana Santana[7]
[1]*Medical Surgical Department and Graduate Center of Nursing, University of São Paulo*
[2]*Nursing Department and doctoral student, the Graduate Center of Medicine, Federal University of Sergipe,*
[3]*Graduate Center of Medicine, Federal University of Sergipe*
[4]*Medical Surgical Nursing Department, University of São Paulo, Brazil*[5]*Student, Nursing Department, Federal University of Sergipe*
[6]*Graduate Center of Medicine, Federal University of Sergipe*
[7]*Speech and language therapy Center and Master's student at the Graduate Center of Medicine, Federal University of Sergipe*
Brazil

Each year, more than one million people are affected by TBI in the United States. Of these 52,000 die and 800,000 have permanent disabilities at a cost exceeding US$ 40 billion (Torpy, 2003). A study conducted with 8,927 patients in 46 countries found that one-quarter died within six months after the occurrence of TBI (Silva et al., 2009).

Estimates of the prevalence of TBI in United States soldiers who were serving in the wars in Afghanistan and Iraq between 2001 and March 2011 revealed more than 200 thousand cases (AAAS, 2011).

Reports of emergency cases due to external causes in Brazilian cities, between 2006 and 2007, show there is a predominance of mixed race males, teenagers and young adults with low educational levels. Pedestrians and passengers were the majority of victims among children and adults, while the driver is prevalent among adolescents and adults. Among children, bicycle accidents predominated. The motorcycle was the main vehicle involved in accidents among adolescents and adults. Among the elderly, automobiles were the most common means of transport (Brasil, 2009).

For many years, the literature about TBI has remained focused on victims of trauma, however, in recent decades, studies have also sought to portray the impact of TBI and the need to support the family system that also suffers the consequences of trauma (NIH, 1999; Serio et al., 1997).

Due to the importance of this issue, we decided to describe TBI considerations and discuss the consequences and needs of the family who experiences TBI in order to encourage further studies in the field with a consequent improvement in quality of care.

2. Traumatic Brain Injury (TBI)

2.1 Concept

TBI is defined as any anatomic lesion or functional impairment alone or in combination with the following elements in the head: scalp, cranial bones, meninges, brain or cranial nerves produced by a force of external action (Mariani & Paranhos, 2009).

2.2 Classification

TBI is classified according to its intensity, as severe, moderate and mild, and measured by various parameters such as duration of unconsciousness, the time of post-traumatic amnesia and the scores obtained in the initial Glasgow Coma Scale (Souza, 2003).

TBI can be caused by the penetration of a projectile or other sharp instrument through the skull or from blunt trauma due to an impact of the head on a hard surface or by the displacement of the brain within the skull, which is present in the mechanism of acceleration and deceleration trauma (Sousa, 2006).

Injuries resulting from these types of trauma can be categorized as primary and secondary. The primary type occurs at the time of the event and is related to the mechanism of injury and is classified according to the nature of the injury, either as diffuse (concussion and diffuse axonal injury) or localized (abrasion, contusion, laceration, skull fractures and hematoma). Secondary injuries follow primary ones. In this case, there is decreased cerebral blood flow and metabolic changes that result in ischemia, caused by hypoxia, hypercarbia, hypotension and intracranial hypertension (Sousa, 2006).

2.3 Severity

The indices of trauma severity aid the classification of pre- and intra-hospital risk, predict consequences of trauma, provide support for the provision of resources, allow comparison among therapeutic methods, improve the quality of care, aid in the development of programs for accident prevention and for the development of safety equipment, facilitate communication concerning the nature and severity of trauma, and help estimate the costs of care (Sousa, 2009).

Severity indices can be based on anatomical data, which consider the site of injury on the body, the injury type and extent in order to calculate the trauma score, such as the Abbreviated Injury Scale (AIS) and the Injury Severity Score (ISS). Severity of physiological trauma indices can be used as well. These evaluate organic response, measured mainly by means of vital signs and level of consciousness, such as the Glasgow Coma Scale and Revised Trauma Score (RTS) and mixed, which use combined measures, such as the Trauma and Injury Severity Score (TRISS) (Sousa, 2009). A study conducted with 18,002 patients indicates the AIS is a good predictor of the severity of multiple trauma injuries (Grote et al., 2011).

Change of consciousness measured by the Glasgow Coma Scale, a widely accepted instrument, assesses the level of consciousness through eye opening, best verbal response and best motor response, with scores ranging from 3 to 15. A score up to 8 has been viewed as an important indicator of severe TBI, between 9 and 12 indicates moderate trauma, and a score equal to or greater than 13, indicates mild trauma (Sousa, 2006).

The duration of posttraumatic amnesia, which includes the period after TBI in which the victim cannot remember events, is another parameter used to establish the severity of TBI. Memory changes are common after TBI, particularly in temporal lobe lesions, frontal, bilateral hippocampal lesions and diffuse axonal injury. Orientation levels such as time, place and person are assessed through the Galveston Orientation and Amnesia Test (Sousa, 2006).

2.4 Consequences

As previously described, a primary lesion corresponds to direct trauma in the brain associated with vascular lesions, whereas a secondary injury refers to ongoing pathophysiological processes that are triggered by primary injuries and extends for hours, days or weeks. Hypotension, hypoxia, edema and intracranial hypertension (ICH) are common examples of secondary lesions considered to be "enemies" of the brain (Hora& Aguiar, 2010; National Association of Emergency Medical Technicians [NAEMT], 2007).

ICH is the most common intracranial lesion that is secondary in the first week of patient care in hospitalized patients with severe TBI and hemorrhagic stroke (Hora & Aguiar, 2010).

Intracranial Pressure (ICP) is defined as pressure inside the skull caused by brain tissue (80%), cerebrospinal fluid (10%) and blood volume (10%). The increase in ICP (Intracranial Hypertension) occurs when the pressure in the skull reaches 20 mmHg or more, resulting from serious conditions, among which TBI stands out (Hora & Aguiar, 2010).

Cerebral edema is the most common cause of increasing ICP occurrences and refers to the abnormal accumulation of fluid in the interstitial or intracellular spaces. Elevations in ICP are serious because of declining Cerebral Perfusion Pressure (CPP) and Cerebral Blood Flow (CBF), which consequently leads to focal or local ischemia with lesion blood brain barrier, acidosis, vasodilatation and inflammation (Figure 1). Ischemia is a catastrophic event, because neurons do not tolerate hypoxia and the brain requires 50 to 55 ml of blood for every 100g of brain tissue to maintain a normal metabolic state (Arbour, 2004; Diccini & Koizumi).

The initial ischemia leads to anaerobic metabolism, which is an inefficient way to power the cell, resulting in lactic acidosis. This commonly occurs after a TBI and about 60% of the victims who die due to this injury have evidence of ischemia at necropsy (Sousa, 2006).

It is also understood as a syndrome with initial signs and symptoms of headache, vomiting and visual disorders, whose appearance depends on the severity of factors and its etiology, speed of development, location of lesion(s) and degree of intracranial compliance. The treatment for ICH (ICP monitoring, decompressive craniectomy, liquor drainage, osmotic therapy, hyperventilation, barbiturates, among others) is to maintain an adequate perfusion pressure (Hora& Aguiar, 2010).

One of the biggest challenges experienced by the health team is to prevent a secondary brain injury that can be more devastating than the original injury (primary). Controlling damage caused by these lesions is the main focus of care provided to severe patients with brain compromise (Jantzen, 2007; Josephson, 2004).

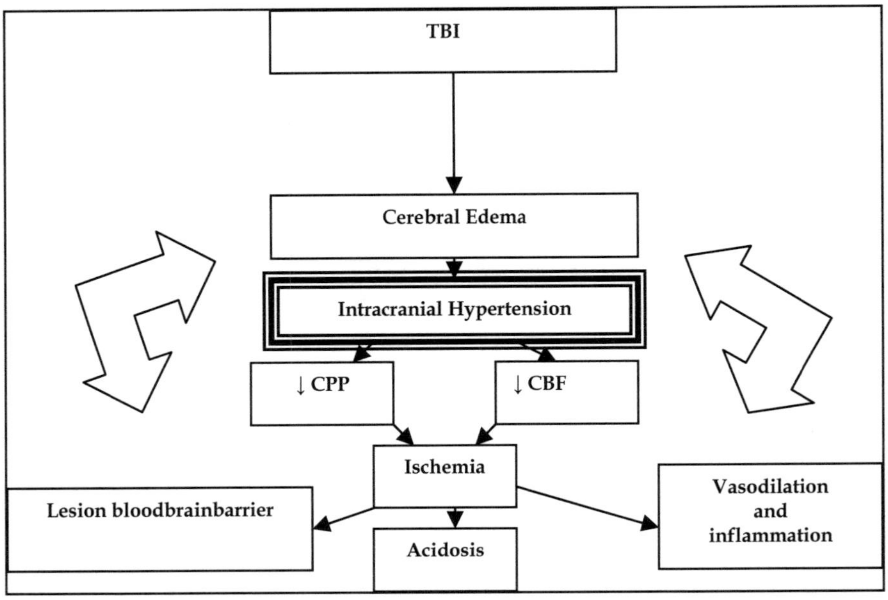

Fig. 1. Schematic representation of TBI during Intracranial Hypertension, 2011.

TBI consequences go beyond the acute phase and may persist for many years. The period up to six months post trauma is when more intense recovery occurs, however, it may take up to one year or more after the trauma. In addition to functional capacity, resuming productivity is an important parameter for analyzing the consequences of TBI (Sousa & Koizumi, 1998; Sousa, 2006).

The use of alcohol and drugs increases the risk of TBI and impairs the recovery of an individual who suffers a trauma, in addition to increasing the risk of relapse and dependence (Bjork & Grant, 2009).

Patients who survive TBI may present impairments and disabilities that can be temporary or permanent, affecting the individual's ability to perform tasks.

The physical and psychological sequelae of TBI patients are dramatic. The neuropsychiatric alterations after a traumatic event are many and diverse and generally include the categories of mood, cognition and behavior disorders, leading many patients to resort to psychiatric evaluation (Nieto et al., 2003).

There are occurrences of neurological disorders after TBI (epilepsy, headaches and sleep disorders), as well as neurodegenerative diseases (decline in cognitive function, Alzheimer's, Parkinson's disease), neuroendocrine disorders (post trauma hypopituitarism), psychiatric disorders (mood disorders, anxiety, depression, compulsive obsessive disorders). There are non-neurological diseases, as well (sexual dysfunction, urinary and bowel incontinence, musculoskeletal dysfunction) and possibly metabolic dysfunction, among other occurrences, that can last for months or years (Masel & DeWitt, 2010).

Post concussion syndrome (PCS) is usually a sequela of TBI and includes headache, dizziness, fatigue, neurocognitive impairment and mood and behavior alterations. Headaches are a key symptom and the most common of PCSs, beginning within seven days after a trauma; it is classified as chronic when it persists for more than three months (Láinez & Pesquera, 2011).

Chronic pain is a common complication of TBI and contributes to morbidity and poor recovery after injury. It is independent of psychological disorders and frequent among mild TBI patients (Nampiaparampil, 2008).

Other consequences were also described in a consensus on the rehabilitation of people with TBI: visual and language impairment, nutritional and gastrointestinal disorders, as well as memory, attention and concentration disorders, aggressiveness, agitation, impulsiveness, social disinhibition, personality change, suicide risk, divorce, and unemployment, among others (NIH, 1999).

Gould et al. (2011) found a significant association between psychiatric disorders after 12 months of TBI and unemployment, pain, poor quality of life and the use of ineffective coping strategies.

A meta-analysis showed an increased risk of schizophrenia following TBI of about 60%, with a larger effect in those people with a genetic predisposition to psychosis (Molloy et al., 2011).

Many studies have focused on severe TBI; however, people with moderate and mild TBI also experience sequelae (Kreutzer et al., 1992). Although this is considered the simplest form of TBI, it can be disabling and its effects are minimized with a certain frequency or discredited by the population. Usually patients are discharged from an emergency department without any guidance concerning cognitive changes that affect how a person acts and thinks, such as forgetfulness, poor attention span and concentration, fatigue, sensitivity to light or sound, changed taste and smell (Maia et al., 1993).

A comparative study conducted in an emergency department at one week and at three months after people suffered a trauma revealed that the group of patients with mild TBI complained about memory and concentration in daily activities (Ponsford et al., 2011). The absence of an imaging abnormality (computed tomography or magnetic resonance) is not equivalent to the absence of an abnormality (Bigler, 2001).

The consequences can also remain in the long term, such as shown by a study conducted 12 months to 21 years after mild TBI. The studied patients complained of significant disorders in sleep patterns (Schreiber et al., 2008) as well as severe and persistent neurobehavioral problems following mild TBI (Hartlage et al., 2001).

McDowell (1995) described a protocol with 18 initial choices to deal with the consequences of mild TBI in a non-traditional way, using homeopathic medicines properly licensed by the U.S. Food and Drug Administration.

A study conducted between 1986 and 2008 with 32,133 elderly Dutch patients revealed a marked increase in hospitalization of these elderly individuals due to TBI caused by falls, particularly in the oldest ones; most were diagnosed with a concussion or contusion injury (57.3%) (Hartholt et al., 2011).

American soldiers who are serving in Iraq and Afghanistan have suffered severe head trauma and persistent physical, emotional and behavioral problems, requiring efforts to develop better ways to diagnose and treat the consequences of such injuries. Mild TBI has been the most common in this context, probably caused by explosions that affect the connections of the brain at the level of capillaries with consequent widespread contusion and tissue damage; as such, it is not evident in structural imagery (Hampton, 2011).

There is a high prevalence of soldiers with posttraumatic stress disorder. Many of the patients with TBI develop depression or other mood disorders that limit their social contact with consequent increased loneliness (Hampton, 2011).

People with TBI become more socially isolated, with few friends, and an increasingly denser and smaller social network (Zasler & Kreutzer, 1990).

According to Sluzki (1997) this isolation is caused mainly by the individual's restricted mobility: when one stops working or attending school, church, community activities, among others, this reduces the opportunity to make social contacts. The author also reports that sometimes the disease can generate new networks, as well, such as those corresponding to social services and health care.

Zasler & Kreutzer (1990) studied sexuality after TBI and observed that most cases of sexual difficulties are attributed to emotional and psychological problems, which are characteristic of people with TBI, who typically have difficulty maintaining emotional stability.

A Canadian study carried out with 104 women, five to 12 years after moderate to severe TBI showed that 46% of them experienced amenorrhea with duration of up to 60 months; 68% experienced irregular cycles and reported difficulties in the postpartum. These results indicate there is a need to provide women's health care after injuries (Colantonio et al., 2010).

According to epidemiological assumptions, Souza (2003) states that patients with TBI can be considered within the parameters of people at "risk of damage" and "lower quality of life"; there are changes in all aspects of life for many years (Hawthorne et al., 2008).

Considering the complexity of trauma as a public health problem worldwide, a group of researchers reached a consensus concerning the categories to be used in research addressing TBI in order to improve comparisons among studies, facilitate meta-analysis of data obtained from patients, standardize data essential for systematic reviews, and advance in patient care. The categories identified were designated as: participant / subject characteristics, participant and family history, injury / disease related events, assessments and examinations, treatments / interventions, protocol experience, adverse events and safety data and outcome, and function (Maas et al., 2011).

The preceding discussion indicates that the importance of deepening knowledge concerning TBI is mainly related to the magnitude of its consequences and the need for planning appropriate care. Mello Jorge & Koizumi (2004) suggest investments not only in relation to aspects of primary and secondary prevention, but also tertiary prevention focused on long-term care, rehabilitation and reintegration to minimize the effects of trauma and reduce hospitalizations.

3. Family

3.1 Organization and concept

Changes observed in contemporary society related to economy, work organization, revolution in human reproduction, changes of values, liberalization of habits and customs, all resulted in radical changes in the organization of families (Mioto, 2004).

Among these changes are the downsizing of families, that is, families used to be large with many children and currently, given the scarcity or absence of family resources, families have fewer children or no children at all (Duarte, 2001).

Another change is related to a variety of family arrangements, the nuclear family with a heterosexual couple united by marriage raising biological children, is increasingly less relevant, both in statistical and legal terms, which reveals itself as something more complex than previously thought (Fonseca, 2004).

The result of such changes is the weakening of family ties, making families more vulnerable to life events such as deaths, disease, unemployment, and self-management in everyday life (Mioto, 2004).

Walsh (2005) uses the term "vulnerable families" to designate those who are overwhelmed and unsupported, facing many challenges and unmet needs. He adds that even in the face of all the problems families experience in today's world, one should not view families as "dysfunctional families" but as “families struggling with many problems”, often beyond their control. Most of the time, the problems are not caused by them.

Due to the diversity of structures and forms of organization of families, the complexity of the institution becomes evident. As stated by Althoff (1999), the concept of family is dynamic in time and space, depending on the structure and functions of each society, and therefore, it is difficult to find a universal definition.

Angelo (1997) states that in order to clarify the focus of attention of someone when speaking of family, one is required to present a definition of it, because it is precisely the definition of family that will determine the questions about this family and instruments used to achieve the defined dimensions. For the author, such a definition somewhat directs the perspective and intention of working with families.

Angelo & Bousso (2001) conceptualize family as a system or a unit whose members may or may not necessarily be related or live together, be with or without children, not necessarily having a single parent. What shall exist is, therefore, a commitment and bond among its members. For Wright & Leahey (2002) " a family is who its members say they are".

The boundaries of the meaningful system of an individual are not limited to the nuclear or extended family but include the full range of interpersonal bonds of an individual. In particular, this consists of his/her personal social network, which includes family, friends, work relationships, study, community embeddedness and social practices (Sluzki, 1997).

Angelo (1999) points out three challenges that must be overcome to facilitate approaching and working with families. The first is "teaching to think about family" that is, being sensitized to it, which involves understanding and appreciating the complexity of family life. The second is "to encourage advanced practice with families" which is to create strategies and institutional mechanisms to promote sensitization of professionals and provide them tools to deal with families. The last is "to help one to build knowledge concerning family" based on doubts, uncertainties, and willingness of people to overcome their own limits to find the truth.

3.2 Consequences of TBI for the family

In the family, the impact of TBI is felt in many consequences, among which are stress and sadness (Tyerman & Booth, 2001; Watanabe et al., 2000), changes in family roles (Serna & Sousa, 2006; Tyerman &Booth , 2001), guilt and anger (Sander & Kreutzer, 1999), difficulties

in sexual and marital relationships (Tyerman & Booth, 2001), depression (Serna & Sousa, 2005), psychiatric disorders (Livingston et al., 1985), anxiety (Marsh et al. 1998a; Marsh et al., 1998b), psychosomatic disorders (Kreutzer et al., 1992), and reduced quality of life (Kolakowski-Hayner et al., 2001).
One third of caregivers of patients who were one to two years post injury were at risk for depression, anxiety, or other forms of psychological distress. Those who care for survivors who are more disabled, unemployed or otherwise uninvolved in productive activity, or have problems with alcohol abuse, are at greatest risk (Kreutzer et al., 2009).
The use of tranquilizers, sleeping medications and alcohol to copy with trauma was also reported (Kreutzer et al., 1992).
These studies indicate that these negative consequences are mainly caused by behavioral, psychosocial and cognitive changes presented by patients with TBI, and those associated with physical impairment, such as visual and motor deficits (Frosh et al., 1997; Marsh et al. 1998a). Hora & Sousa (2005) reported that the behavioral changes of patients that mostly affected the family were explosive temper, aggressiveness, depression, irritability, anxiety, dependency and forgetfulness.
Rolland (2001) argues that different types of disability imply differences in specific adjustments required by the family. The association of cognitive and motor deficits of a patient requires a greater redistribution of family roles than in the case of motor deficit only.
Spouses are more affected than parents by the disease. Common sense suggests that parents should better adjust because they often have a partner to share the care burden (Kreutzer et al., 1992).
Each family member has a different perception of how their lives have been affected and how they will be affected by the patient's trauma. Different perceptions, personalities and coping styles contribute to emotional differences within the family (Sander & Kreutzer, 1999).
Social isolation affecting a patient also affects family members. Sluzki (1997) asserts that there is a positive correlation between a person's social network and health. A chronic illness deteriorates the quality of an individual's social interaction and reduces the size of one's network (the number of people) in the long term and the ability to access it. This negative effect has a negative impact on the individual's health and/or intimate group (especially the family), which in turn increases the shrinkage of the individual's network and so on.
The family with a person with TBI is in crisis, because this event totally changes one's circumstances, ambitions and life in a considerable way (Freeman, 1997). The crisis triggered by a TBI provides families the opportunity to move toward greater cohesion or toward deterioration of its functioning; the quality of education received during such a period is one of the most important factors for its resolution (Gordon, 1989).
There is no doubt that TBI affects not only the person who suffered the trauma, but the family system as well (Cole et al., 2009; Hora & Sousa, 2005; Watanabe et al., 2000). Patients are not the only victims; their families suffer as much, if not more, and can also be considered victims of trauma (Dufor et al., 1992; Fowler, 1997) or occult victims of trauma.

3.3 Family needs

Families experience a lot of needs in the initial period of crisis after a TBI, which may go unnoticed or not be recognized by health professionals. However, because the effects of TBI are often long-term ones, it is important to assess these needs after the initial crisis period, that is, in the long-term (Dufor et al.,1992; Kolakowski-Hayner et al., 200).

Many studies have only focused on short-term needs after the trauma, but little is known about the post acute phase. Considering the duration of sequelae of TBI, however, addressing the needs years after the trauma is a substantial challenge (Sander & Kreutzer, 1999).

After an extensive search in the literature seeking instruments that measure the needs of families, the Family Needs Questionnaire (FNQ) was chosen in the nursing field to be a reliable and valid instrument to be used in the American culture and which present the specific needs of families of people with TBI. This instrument was translated and adapted for the Brazilian Portuguese language and culture (Hora & Sousa, 2009).

The cross-cultural adaptation is a process that comprises five steps or stages, in which an evaluation of semantic, idiomatic, cultural and conceptual equivalences is performed between the original and translated version in order to achieve content validity for the instrument (Hora & Sousa, 2009).

The FNQ was developed in Virginia, United States by Kreutzer and Marwitz (1989) in an effort to standardize the measures of TBI. The instrument lists various psychosocial and educational needs visible in the acute and post-acute phase of TBI. Clinically, the responses obtained from family members can be used for assessment and intervention. The FNQ, therefore, has the potential to improve understanding of family members (Kreutzer et al., 1994).

Thus the FNQ identifies the need for, importance and degree of care, aids in the development of individualized educational programs tailored to the needs established by family members, as well as group support programs. Priorities can also be established to meet these needs, in addition to serving as an index for the effectiveness of the intervention. Its administration in series can help to identify temporal changes of needs (Kreutzer et al., 1994).

The need for information is prominent in the short and long terms (Kolakowski-Hayner et al., 2001; Serio et al. 1997). According to Kleinpell & Powers (1992) such a need can be considered a universal need, due to the high frequency it is found in many studies.

The information needs of families of people with TBI was the subject of a study conducted by Junquera et al. (1997) who emphasize the importance of providing information concerning the consequences of TBI several years after a trauma, highlighting behavioral and emotional disorders, aiming to better cope with these problems, since these were the most noticed by the family. The study also reveals that the understanding of the effects of TBI improves family health and facilitates more adaptive behaviors.

The Brazilian study performed with family members of people with TBI and which used the FNQ also indicated the need for information as the most important. It also observed that most needs were not met; the least addressed need was related to resources for the patient and family (Serna, 2005).

It important to keep in mind that information should not be merely transmitted to family members in a didactic manner, but, reflexively, exploring its significant responses (Man, 1999).

Information is therefore an important mechanism to prevent family crises and should be consistent and realistic (Kreutzer et al., 1994). A well-informed family member is able to provide a more appropriate therapeutic environment for the patient (Eisner & Kreutzer, 1989).

Investigations addressing the identification of family needs correspond to an effort to improve the adaptation of its members to the new condition of having a survivor with TBI (Kolakowski-Hayner et al., 2001).

3.4 Intervention with families

According to Wilkinson (1999) little has been written about the best way to provide such support, which is corroborated by Tyerman & Booth (2001) when they assert that family members often face changes in patients after TBI with little support, especially when there are long-term cognitive and personality changes.

The description of a study carried out in the United Kingdom showed that support for families after TBI starts with an assessment of the family to understand the impact caused by the TBI and, subsequently, conducting educational workshops, family support and individual counseling by a specialist in marital problems, while time for rehabilitation is variable for each family member (Tyerman & Booth, 2001).

The study developed by Acorn (1995) in Canada showed that the identification of family needs precedes the development of a support program. The results revealed the importance of support groups to meet their educational and psychological needs of families.

Regarding the importance of providing support to the family, according to Pelletier & Alfano (2000), when families received greater support, depression diminished.

Family members need to have a safe place to express their feelings and reactions in the face of behaviors they observe and experience, while it is also important that the professionals involved have the ability to listen, offering realistic and individualized advice (Wilkinson, 1999).

According to Silva (2003) resilience represents one of the possible avenues for professionals to work primarily with health, shifting the emphasis from the dimension of the negativity of the disease to the potentialities of the family, because some people are able not only to overcome problems, but also be strengthened by their experiences.

The view of Walsh (2005) is similar. The author describes that addressing family resilience is based on the conviction that even the most distressed families want to be healthy and have the potential for change and growth.

Resilience is a theoretical approach drawn from a concept used in physics and engineering, representing the ability of a system to overcome disorder imposed by an external and unchanged phenomenon. Applied to human life it represents the ability to withstand harsh and persistent conditions, that is, the ability of people, groups or communities not only to withstand adversity, but also to use them in their process of personal development and social growth (Antunes, 2003).

The author adds that all organisms are endowed with some degree of resilience, which can be changed through education; it is possible to instill reliability, security and organizational schemes even in seemingly apathetic people. Thus, it is believed that the family members caring for a person with TBI may be examples of resilient people.

The evaluation of the results of interventions is also of great importance in order to develop a deeper understanding of their effectiveness (Acorn, 1993). This same view is described by Wright & Leahey (2002) when they assert the need to determine the responses of family members to the proposed interventions.

4. Conclusion

Families usually have little or no guidance in how to understand the complex difficulties of TBI. It is believed, therefore, that family support is a valuable intervention to meet the needs of families.

Patients with TBI may feel "lost" after being discharged from the hospital due to a lack of outpatient treatment or rehabilitation, particularly a lack of guidance concerning how to overcome the consequences of trauma.

Trauma must be regarded as a disease rather than an accident or mischance because most deaths and injuries are preventable. Therefore, prevention is the key; it is necessary to educate people to develop awareness of risk behaviors, and especially of individual responsibility and respect for others.

5. References

AAAS. (2011). Healing the Brain, Healing the Mind. *Science*. Vol. 333, pp. 514-517

Acorn, S. (1993). Head- injured survivors: caregivers and support groups. *J Advanc Nurs*. Vol. 18, pp. 39-45

Acorn, S. (1995). Assisting families of head-injured survivors throught a family support programme. *J Advanc Nurs* . Vol. 21, pp. 872-877

Althoff, C.R. (1999). Pesquisando a família: a experiência da enfermagem na UFSC. *Fam Saúde Desenv* Vol. 1 , N ½, pp. 49-56, ISBN 85-7291-126-X

Angelo M, Bousso RS (2001). Fundamentos da Assistência à Família em Saúde. In: *Manual de Enfermagem*, Brasil. Ministério da Saúde (Org) p. 14-7. Ministério da Saúde,

Angelo, M. (1997). *Com a família em tempos difíceis*. [Livre Docência]. São Paulo (SP): Escola de Enfermagem da USP

Angelo, M. (1999). Abrir-se para a família: superando desafios. *Fam Saúde Desenv* . Vol. 1 , N ½, pp. 7-14.

Antunes, C. (2003).*Resiliência: a construção de uma nova pedagogia para uma escola pública de qualidade*. 101 p. Petrópolis

Arbour R. (2004). Intracranial Hypertension : monitoring and nursing assessment. *Crit Care Nurse*. Vol. 24, N 5, pp. 19-32

Bigler, E.D. (2001). The Lesion(s) in Traumatic Brain Injury: Implications for Clinical Neuropsychology. *Archives of Clinical Neuropsychology*, Vol. 16, pp. 95-131

Bjork, J.M.& Grant, S. (2009). Does Traumatic Brain Injury Increase Risk for Substance Abuse? *Journal of Neurotrauma*. Vol. 26, pp. 1077-1082

Brasil, Ministério da Saúde. (2009). *Viva: vigilância de violência e acidentes, 2006 e 2007*, pp. 147-148, Ministério da Saúde, ISBN 978-85-334-1618-5, Brasília

Colantonio, A.; Mar, W.; Escobar, M.; Yoshida, K.; Velikonja, D.; Rizoli, S.; Cusimano, M. & Cullen, N. (2010). Women's Health Outcomes After Traumatic Brain Injury. *Journal of Women's Health*. Vol. 19, N 6, pp. 1109-1116

Cole, W.R.; Paulos, S.K.; Cole, C.A.S.& Tankard, C. (2009). A Review of Family Intervention Guidelines for Pediatric Acquired Brain Injuries. *Dev Disabil Res Rev*. Vol. 15, pp. 159-166

Diccini, S; Koizumi, MS; Resque AP (2006). Hipertensão intracraniana-bases teóricas para o cuidado, In: *Enfermagem em neurociência: fundamentos para a prática clínica*, Koizumi, MS; Diccini MS, (Ed), pp.113-133, Atheneu, ISBN 85-7379-840-8, São Paulo

Duarte YAO (2001). *Família: Rede de suporte ou fator estressor, a ótica de idosos e cuidadores familiares*. [tese]. São Paulo (SP): Escola de Enfermagem da USP

Dufor, LT; Aiken, LC; Gueldner, S. (1992). Traumatic brain injury: a family experience. *J Neurosc Nurs* Vol. 24 , N 6, pp. 317-323.

Eisner, J; Kreutzer, J.S. (1989). A Family information system for education following traumatic Brain Injury.*Brain Inj*. Vol. 3, N1, 79-90

Fonseca, C.(2004). Olhares antropológicos sobre a família contemporânea. In: *Pesquisando a família, olhares contemporâneos*, Althof, C.R; Elsen, I; : Papa-Livro , Nitschke, R.G. ISBN 85-7291-126-X Florianopolis

Fowler, S.B. (1997). Neurotrauma family Interventions. *J Trauma Nurs*. Vol. 4, N. 3, pp. 68-74.

Freeman, E.A. (1997). Community-based rehabilitation of the person with a severe brain injury. *Brain Inj*. Vol. 11, N 2, pp. 143-153

Frosch, S; Gruber, A; Jones, C; Myers, S; Noel, E; Westerlund. A. (1997). The long term effect of traumatic brain injury on the roles of caregivers. *Brain Inj*. Vol 11, N12, pp. 891-906.

Gervasio, A.H; Kreutzer, J.S. (1997). Kinship and family members' psychological distress after traumatic brain injury: a large sample study. *J Head Rehabil*. Vol 12, N 3,pp. 14-26

Gordon, V.L. (1989). Recovery from a head injury: a family process. *Pediatric Nursing*. Vol 15, N 2, pp. 131-133

Gould, K.R.; Ponsford, J.L.; Johnston,L. & Schonberger. (2011). Predictive and Associated Factores of Psychiatric Disorders After Traumatic Brain Injury: A prospective Study. *Journal of Neurotrauma*. Vol. 28, pp. 1155-1163

Grote, S.; Bocker, W.; Mutschler, W.; Bouillon,B. & Lefering, R. (2011). Diagnostic Value of the Glasgow Coma Scale for Traumatic Brain Injury in 18,002 Patients With Severe Multiple Injuries. *Journal of Neurotrauma*. Vol. 28, pp. 527-534

Hampton, T. (2011). Traumatic Brain Injury a Growing Problem Among Serving in Today's Wars. *JAMA*. Vol. 306, N 5, pp. 477-479

Hartholt, K.A.; Van Lieshout, E.M.M.; Polinder, S.; Panneman, J.M.; Van der Carmmen, T.J.M.& Patka, P. (2011). *Journal of Neurotrauma*. Vol. 28, pp. 739-744

Hartlage, L.C; Durant-Wilson, D. & Patch, P.C. (2001). Persistent Neurobehavioral Problems Following Mild Traumatic Brain Injury. *Archives of Clinical Neuropsychology*, Vol. 16, pp. 561-570

Hawthorne, G.; Gruen, R. & Kaye, A.H. (2008). Traumatic Brain Injury and Long-Term Quality of Life: Findings from an Australian Study. *Journal of Neurotrauma*. Vol. 26, pp. 1623-1633

Hora, E.C.H. (2009). Adaptação Transcultural do Instrumento Family Needs Questionnaire. *Rev Lat Americana Enf* .Vol 17, N 4, pp.541-547

Hora, E.C; Sousa, RMC (2005). Os efeitos das alterações comportamentais das vítimas de trauma crânio-encefálico para o cuidador familiar. *Rev Lat Americana Enf* .Vol 13, N 1, pp.93-98

Hora, ECH; Aguiar, AFM. (2010). O paciente com hipertensão intracraniana na UTI, In: *Enfermagem em UTI: cuidando do paciente crítico*, Padilha,KG; Vattimo, MFF; Silva, SC; Kimura, M, (Ed), pp. 467-493, Manole, ISBN 978-85-204-2929-7, São Paulo

ISBN 85-334-0446-8, Brasília

Jantzen, J.P.A.H. (2007). Prevention and treatment of intracranial hypertension. *Brest Pract Res Clin Anaesthesiol*. Vol. 21 , N 4, pp. 517-38

Josephson, L (2004). Manegement of increased intracranial pressure. *Dimens crit care nurs*. Vol. 23 , N 5, pp. 194-207

Junqué, C; Bruna, O; Mataró, M (1997). Information needs of the traumatic brain injury patient's family members regarding the consequences of the injury and associated perception of physical, cognitive, emotional and quality of life changes. *Brain Inj* . Vol 11, N 4, pp. 251-8.

Kleinpell, R.M; Powers, M.J. (1992). Needs of family members of intensive care unit patients. *Applied Nursing Research*. Vol.5, N1, pp. 2-8

Kolakowsky-Hayner, SA; Miner, KD; Kreutzer, J.S. (2001). Long–term life quality and family needs after traumatic brain injury. *J Head Trauma Rehabil* . Vol. 16, N 4, pp. 374-385

Kreutzer, J.S; Rapport, L.J.; Marwitz, J.H.; Harrison-Felix, C.; Hart, T.; Glenn, M.& Hammond, F. (2009). Caregivers' Well-Being After Traumatic Brain Injury: A Multicenter Prospective Investigation. *Arch Phys Med Rehabil*. Vol. 90, pp. 938-946

Kreutzer, JS; Marwitz, J.H; Kepler K. (1992). Traumatic brain injury: family response and outcome. *Arch Phys Med Rehabil* . Vol. 73, pp.771-777

Kreutzer, JS; Serio, C.D; Bergquist, S. (1994). Family needs after brain injury: a quantitative analysis. J *Head Trauma Rehabil* . Vol. 9, N. 3: 104-115

Láinez, M.J.; Pesquera, B.L. (2011). Headache After Trauma: Physiological Considerations. *Curr Pain Headache Rep*

Livingston, M.G; Brooks, N; Bond, M.R. (1985). Three months after severe head injury: psychiatric and social impact on relatives. *J Neurol Neurosurg Psychiatry*. Vol. 48, pp. 870-875

Maas, A.; Harrison-Felix, C.L.; Menon, D.; Adelson, P.D.; Balkin,T.; Bullock, R.; Engel, D.C.; Gordon, W.; Langlois-Orman, J.; Lew, H.L.; Robertson, C.; Temkin, N.; Valadka, A.; Verfaellie, M.; Wainwright, M. & Schwab, K. (2011). Standardizing Data Collection in Traumatic Brain Injury. *Journal of Neurotrauma*. Vol. 28, pp. 177-187

Maia, C.R; Terra, M.B; Coimbra, M. (2003). Programas de auxílio aos padecentes de TCE e aos seus familiares. In: *Neuropsquiatria dos traumatismos cranioencefálicos*, Souza, C.A.C.Revinter, pp.245-262, Rio de Janeiro

Man, D (1999). Community-based empowerment programme for families with a brain injured survivor: an outcome study. *Brain Inj*. Vol. 13, N 6, pp. 443-446

Mariani , PP; Paranhos, WI. (2009). Traumatismo Cranioencefálico, In: *Atuação no trauma: uma abordagem para a enfermagem*, Sousa, RMC; Calil, AM; Paranhos, WI; Malvestio MA, (Ed.), pp. 263-88, Atheneu, ISBN 978-85-7379-309-3, São Paulo

Marsh, N.V; Kersel, D.A; Havill, J.H; Sleigh, J.W(1998b). Caregiver burden at 1 year following severe traumatic brain injury. *Brain Inj*. Vol 12, N 12, pp. 1045-59.

Marsh, N.V; Kersel, D.A; Havill, J.H; Sleigh, JW (1998a). Caregiver burden at 6 months following severe traumatic brain injury. *Brain Inj* . Vol 12, N 12, pp. 1045-59

Masel, B. & DeWitt, D.S. (2010). Traumatic Brain Injury: A Disease Process, Not an Event. *Journal of Neurotrauma*. Vol. 27, pp. 1529-1540

Mc Dowell, B. (1995).*Alternative & Complementary Therapies*,pp. 130-137.

Mello Jorge, M.H.P; Koizumi, M.S. (2004). Gastos governamentais do SUS com internações hospitalares por causas externas: análise no Estado de São Paulo, 2000. *Rev Bras Epidemiol*. Vol 7 , N 2, pp.228-238.

Mioto, R.C.T. (2004). Do conhecimento que temos à intervenção que fazemos: uma reflexão sobre a atenção as famílias no âmbito das políticas sociais. In: *Pesquisando a família: olhares contemporâneos*. Althof, C.R; Elsen, I; : Papa-Livro , Nitschke, R.G. Florianopolis,pp.107-114, ISBN 85-7291-126-X

Molloy, C.; Conroy, R.M.; Cotter, D. R. & Cannon, M. (2011). Is Traumatic Brain Injury a Risk Factor for Schizophrenia? A Meta-Analysis of Case-Controlled Population-Based Studies. *Schizophrenia Bulletin*, pp.1-7

Nampiaparampil, D. E. (2008). Prevalence of Chronic Pain After Traumatic Brain Injury: A Systematic Brain Injury. *JAMA*. Vol. 300, N 6, pp. 711-719

National Association of Emergency Medical Technicians [NAEMT].(2007) .*Atendimento Pré-hospitalar ao traumatizado-PHTLS*. Trad. de Diego Alfaro e Hermínio de Mattos Filho, Elsevier, ISBN 0-8151-4569-1, Rio de Janeiro

National Institutes Health [NIH]. (1999). Rehabilitation of Persons With Traumatic Brain Injury. *JAMA*. Vol. 282, N 10, pp. 974-983

Nieto, J.C.R; Campos, F.I.; Ospino, S.M. Sequelas Neuropsiquiátricas dos TCE. In: *Neuropsquiatria dos traumatismos cranioencefálicos*, Souza, C.A.C.Revinter, pp.89-97, Rio de Janeiro

Pelletier, P.M; Alfano, D.P.(2000). Depression, social support and family coping following traumatic brain injury. *Brain and Cognition*. Vol. 44 , N 1, pp. 45-49

Ponsford, J.; Cameron.P.; Fitzgerald, M.; Grant, M.& Mikocka-Walus, A. (2011). *Journal of Neurotrauma*. Vol. 28, pp. 937-946

Rolland, J.S. Doença crônica e o ciclo familiar. In: *As mudanças do Ciclo de Vida Familiar: Uma estrutura para a terapia familiar*, Carter, B; Goldrick, M.C. Artmed, pp. 373-391, ISBN 85-7307-833-2, Porto Alegre

Sander, A.M; Kreutzer, J.S. (1999). A holistic aprroach to family assessment after brain injury. In: *Rehabilitation of the adult and child with traumatic brain Injury*, Rosenthal, M;Griffith, E.R; Kreutzer, J.S; Pentland, B. Philadelfia: F A Davis,pp.199-215
Schreiber, S.; Barkai, G.; Gur- Hartman, T.; Peles, E. Tov, N.; Dolberg & O.T.; Pick, C.G. (2008). Long-Lasting Sleep Patterns Of Adult Patients With Minor Traumatic Brain Injury (MTBI) and non-m TBI subjects. *Sleep Medicine*. Vol. 9, PP. 481-487
Serio, C.D; Kreutzer, J.S; Witol, A.D. (1987). Family needs after traumatic brain injury: a factor analytic of the family needs questionnaire. *Brain Inj*. Vol. 11, N1, pp. 1-9.
Serna, E.C. (2005). Família do paciente de Trauma Cranioencefálico: *Adaptação Transcultural do Family Needs Questionaire e Programa de Suporte de Informação* [Tese]. Universidade de São Paulo, São Paulo
Serna, E.C.H. Sousa, R.M.C (2005). Depressão: uma possível conseqüência adversa do trauma crânio-encefálico para o cuidador familiar. *Acta Paul Enferm* Vol 18, N 2, pp.131-135
Serna, E.C.H; Sousa, R.M.C (2006). Mudanças nos papéis sociais: uma conseqüência do trauma crânio-encefálico para o cuidado familiar. *Rev Latino Am-Enfermagem*. Vol 14, N. 2, pp. 183-189
Silva, M.J; Roberts, I; Perel, P.; Edwards, P; Kenward,M.G; Fernandes,J.; Shakur, H.& Patel, V. (2009). Patient Outcome After Traumatic Brain Injury in High, Middle and Low-income countries: Analysis of Data on 8927 Patients in 46 Countries. *Internacional Journal of Epidemiology*, Vol. 38, pp. 452-458
Silva, M.R.S. (2003). *A construção da trajetória resiliente durante as primeiras etapas do desenvolvimento da criança: o papel da sensibilidade materna e do suporte social*, [Tese]. Florianópolis. Universidade Federal de Santa Catarina
Sluzki, C.E (1997). *A rede social na prática sistêmica: alternativas terapêuticas*. Caso do Psicólogo, ISBN 85-85141-77-8 São Paulo
Sousa, RMC. (2006). Traumatismo Cranioencefálico- Bases teóricas e intervenções de Enfermagem, In: *Enfermagem em neurociência: fundamentos para a prática clínica*, Koizumi, MS; Diccini MS, (Ed), pp.209-231, Atheneu, ISBN 85-7379-840-8, São Paulo
Sousa, RMC. (2009). Instrumentos de medida padronizada para diagnóstico da gravidade do trauma nas fases pré e intra-hospitalar, In: *Atuação no trauma: uma abordagem para a enfermagem*, Sousa, RMC; Calil, AM; Paranhos, WI; Malvestio MA, (Ed.), pp. 95-111, Atheneu, ISBN 978-85-7379-309-3, São Paulo
Sousa, RMC; Koizumi, MS (1998). Recuperação das Vítimas de Trauma Crânio-Encefálico entre 6 meses e 1 ano. *Arquivos Brasileiros de Neurocirurgia*. Vol 17, N 2, pp. 72-80
Souza, C.A.C. (2003). Neuropsiquiatria dos traumatismos craniencefálicos. Revinter, Rio de Janeiro
Torpy, J.M. (2003). Traumatic Brain Injury. *JAMA*. Vol. 289, N 22, pp.3038
Tyerman, A; Booth, J. (2001). Family interventions after traumatic brain injury: a service example. *Neurorehabilitation*. Vol. 16 , N 1, pp. 59-66
Walsh, F. (2005). Fortalecendo a resiliência familiar. Editora Roca, São Paulo
Watanabe, Y; Shiel, A; Asami, T; Taki, K; Tabuchi, K.(2000). An evaluation of neurobehavioural problems as perceived by family members and levels of family stress 1-3 years following brain injury in Japan. *Clin Rehabil*. Vol. 14, N 2, pp. 172-7
Wilkinson, S. (1999).Life After Brain Injury. Nursing Standart. Vol 13, N44, pp16-17.
Wright, LM; Leahey, M. (2002). Enfermeiras e famílias. *Um guia para avaliação e intervenção na família*. Trad. de Silvia M. Spada. Roca, ISBN 85-7241-346-4, São Paulo
Zasler ND, Kreutzer JS (1990). Family and sexuality after traumatic brain injury. In: *Head Injury a family matter*, Williams, J, pp.253-270.

10

Traumatic Brain Injury: Short, Long, and Very Long-Term Vocational Outcomes

Kelli W. Gary and Keith B. Wilson
Virginia Commonwealth University, The Pennsylvania State University
USA

1. Introduction

Traumatic brain injury (TBI) has proven to be a major public health problem with an annual incidence of over 1.5 million people (Langlois, Rutland-Brown, & Thomas, 2006). Medical advances have contributed to increasing the survival rate of TBI allowing many individuals with varying severities of TBI to receive treatment from the ER and be discharged immediately to their home or receive additional hospitalized treatment, but with a greater possibility to return to the community at a later time. Prevalence statistics reveal that over 3.17 million people live with TBI-related long-term disability and almost three-fourths are working-aged adults between 20 and 69 years old (Zaloshnja, Miller, Langlois, & Selassie, 2008). The statistics by Zaloshnja and colleagues indicate that a large percentage of individuals who sustain TBI will more than likely return to their community, not truly cognizant of the residual physical, cognitive, and emotional deficits that often disrupt pursuit of employment or return to productive living. This chapter provides a narrative review of research that reports short, long, and very long-term vocational outcomes for persons with brain injury and any influence of demographic and injury-related factors. Specifically, the areas to be covered are the definitions of short, long, and very-long term with regards to functional recovery from TBI, report of vocational outcomes from 3 months to 15 years post-TBI, specific demographic variables known to significantly influence vocational outcomes after TBI (e.g. age, gender, race/ethnicity, marital status, education and pre-injury employment), specific injury-related variables known to significantly influence vocational outcomes after TBI (e.g. cause of injury, injury severity, and functional status), update of disability legislation, summary of health professionals and what they contribute to the enhancement of vocational skills for individuals following TBI, and community-based interventions to improve vocational outcomes after brain injury.

2. Vocational and employment outcomes

In considering literature about vocational and employment outcomes after TBI, it is important to delineate vocation from employment to clearly understand why vocation and employment will be used synonymously throughout this chapter. The definition for vocational outcomes is typically broader than employment and employment is often included in most definitions related to vocational outcomes. From a societal perspective, vocation is considered the capacity to work and participation in work to promote full integration and participation in society (Parker, Szymanski, & Patterson, 2005). The definition by Parker et al. indicates that employment is the primary focus, but not the only one and other aspects of vocation should be taken into consideration, such as education, training and non-competitive employment. Research literature about vocational rehabilitation after traumatic brain injury note that a narrower definition of employment is necessary to produce more apparent unemployment rates than an inclusive definition. Some researchers have concluded that a true indicator of work includes only full-time and part-time employment in a competitive workforce (Kendall, Muenchberger, & Gee, 2006). However, information asserted by Kendal et al. is not the consensus of all researchers that study employment after TBI and many include competitive and non-competitive employment, and other productive activities within the definition of employment. Thus, vocational outcomes and employment outcomes are operationalized within this chapter and will be used interchangeably throughout review of the research literature.

3. Significance of employment

Prolonged consequences of TBI are typically less understood and recognized and present a substantial obstacle to recovery and community integration following an injury. The longer-term issues after TBI that are related to community integration are educational attainment, establishing a vocation, and developing and maintaining relationships. One of the most recognized long-term challenges is finding and maintaining employment and return-to-work is typically an important outcome to determine rehabilitation success post-TBI (McCrimmon, & Oddy, 2006). Productive lifestyle is a major problem area for many individuals following TBI and employment is a significant aspect of productivity and especially important to American society. Additionally, approximately 75% of survivors with TBI who suffer long-term disability are considered working-aged (e.g., between 20 and 69 years old; Zaloshjna, Miller, Langlois, & Selassie, 2008). Therefore, vocational outcomes, short and long-term, will be a major issue to address and primarily concern for a large proportion of people with TBI while re-integrating into community settings. In fact, employment is significantly related to quality of live (QOL), financial well-being, and social integration.

3.1 Employment and Quality of Life (QOL)

Employment or establishing a vocation after brain injury in intricately associated with quality of life (QOL). A study exploring the effect of employment on perceived QOL reported a strong and consistent relationship between the two variables (O'Neil et al., 1998). Similarly, life satisfaction, a concept closely related to QOL, was significantly related to the productivity domain of the World Health Organization's (WHO) International Classification of Impairments, Disabilities and Handicaps (ICIDH) in persons with TBI (Heinemann & Whiteneck, 1995). These studies suggest that employment status is highly relevant for individuals with TBI and warrants careful consideration in TBI research.

3.2 Employment and finances

Of course, one of the most essential connections is the link between employment and financial issues. Because many people with TBI experience an immediate work stoppage, financial and employment concerns are usually a major consideration. TBI necessitates a loss in the current job after returning to work, modification of the current job, etc. In addition, the loss of income for people with TBI often adds to the survivors' and caregivers' stress and threatens their economic well-being. Johnstone and colleagues (2003) concluded that during the first year after injury, TBI is associated with an estimated $642 million in lost wages. In addition, TBI has a major economic impact on society. TBI is associated with an estimated $96 million in lost income taxes and $353 million in increased public assistance (Johnstone, Mount, and Schopp, 2003). While TBI can wreck havoc on finances and employment, the residual money loss because of a TBI is further complicated by the loss in income taxes impacting more than people with TBI in the United States.

3.3 Employment and social integration

Employment has a positive effect on social integration in the community, another life dimension that contributes to the value of an individual's life. Using the Craig Handicap Assessment and Reporting Technique (CHART), researchers identified a significant positive correlation between employment and social integration for individuals with TBI that had returned to full or part-time work (O'Neill et al., 1998). Research has also measured productivity, specifically employment-related productivity, following TBI to determine its influence on societal participation, a broader concept than social integration. Whiteneck, Gerhart, and Cusick (2004) found a significant correlation between societal participation and employment/school, i.e., as productivity at work decreases, people with TBI also experience less societal participation. Clearly, the association between employment and social integration has been well established for people with TBI.

4. Short, long, and very long term category for employment

We have broadly categorized employment after TBI into short, long, and very long outcomes. This broad category is useful in organizing the large amount of research that has been published on employment post-TBI. With the inclusion of mild TBI, recovery can be rapid compared to more severe forms of this injury. Chance of good recovery for individuals who sustained mild TBI with relatively brief period of disturbed consciousness and amnesia are predicted to be as short 6 months post-injury (Stulemeijer, van der Werf, Born & Vos, 2008). However, as greater severities of TBI are taken into account, the time related to better recovery, on a relatively short-term basis, usually increases. Powell, Machamer, Temkin, and Dikmen (2001) reported that most individuals with predominately moderate TBI perceived themselves as making good recovery by 1 year post-injury. The chances of a good functional recovery after predominantly severe TBI are less likely for the first year post-injury. For example, at one year post-injury, less than one-third of 846 cases with severe TBI had good recovery, which was defined as mild or no disability and able to return to work or school (Jiang, Gao, Li, Yu, & Zhu, 2002). Given that recovery for TBI can vary widely based on a number of factors (e.g., severity, age, etc.), we categorized short vocational outcome as occurring from six months to less than 2 years post-injury. Typically by year two post-TBI, a large percentage of people with mild TBI report full recovery, suggesting that people with mild TBI resumed normal pre-morbid functional activity, although various symptoms tend to persist (e.g., headaches, dizziness, fatigue, etc.). In a meta-analysis of over 400 studies on mild TBI, noted that most studies reported good outcome short and long-term, which was by 12 months post-injury. However, there is mounting evidence that people with mild TBI have issues with memory, dizziness,

headaches, and fatigue up to five years after injury (Carroll, Cassidy, Peloso et al., 2004). The evidence by Carroll et al. provides an impetus to continue research on mild TBI for functional outcome in time periods definitely considered long-term for the mild TBI population. The years between two and ten for people who have TBI are also the time periods that many researchers use for follow-up when investigating functional outcomes after moderate to severe TBI (Dikmen, Mackamer, Powell, & Temkin, 2003; O'Connor, Colantonio, & Polatajko, 2005; Hammond, Grattan, Sasser et al., 2004). As such, we categorized long-term employment outcomes from year two to less than ten post-injury.
After ten years post-injury ten years, TBI continues to have varying effects on functional outcomes, particularly with moderate and severe injuries. Colantanio et al. (2004) defined 10 years or longer as very long term when examining functional outcomes of people with moderate to severe TBI. Her study's follow-up ranged from 10 to 24 years post-injury and found a significant amount of the study population had impairment in cognition and limitation in complex tasks related to community integration. This and other research warrant the need to investigate very long term employment outcomes after TBI.

5. Overview of employment outcomes three months to past 10 years

There is a preponderance of research exploring numerous aspects of employment in various time periods for people who have TBI. Employment outcomes after TBI have been reported starting at 3 months to 20 years post-injury. The burgeoning of research documenting employment outcomes after TBI is intuitive and statistically represents the challenges that individuals with TBI face as they attempt to enter or reenter the workforce. Summary of studies covered in the review is presented in Table 1.

5.1 Short-term employment outcomes (three months to less than two years)

Within the first year after injury, research suggests that persons with TBI have persistent difficulties returning to employment. Individuals who were not hospitalized and had mild severity of TBI generally began work one to three months after injury and a majority of those with moderate TBI typically did not begin work until six months post-injury (Boake et al., 2005). Besides the productive time (e.g. defined as time at work) that is lost immediately after injury, there are many who do not return to employment by the first year at all. Employment rates assessed at one year post-TBI with varying definitions of employment suggest that returning to employment soon after injury is challenging even with mostly mild to moderate TBI. Benedictus et al. (2010) indicated that 50% of their sample (n=434) were able to return to previous vocational activities, which consisted of work or study after final follow-up at 12 months. Similarly, Wagner et al.'s (2002) sample had a large proportion of mild to moderate injures (64%) found that 71% of sample was able to return to work within one year; however, the inflated rate is likely due to the use of a broader definition of work, which was return to pre-injury comparable work including full-time school and homemaking. Walker and colleagues (2006) reported 39% of a substantially larger multicenter sample (n=1,341) that was previously competitively employed were able to return to competitive employment at one year post-injury. Even when using a relatively unique statistical approach not consistently used in TBI and employment research, employment rates are not drastically higher or lower then previous research. Shönberger et al. (2011) found using a structural equation modeling approach that with their definition of employment (e.g., competitively employed, paid work trial, or student) 66% of a

Studies	Sample Size	Severity	Employment Definition	Findings
Short-term Employment Outcome				
Benedictus et al. (2010)	434	Mild, Moderate, Severe	Resumption of previous work or study.	50% were able to resume previous vocational activities completely after 1, 3, 6, and 12 month follow-up.
Boake et al. (2005)	210	Mild, Moderate	Return to employment.	56% began work within 6 months after injury and 61% were working at 6 months follow-up.
Johnstone et al. (2003)	35	Moderate, Severe	Competitively employed full or part-time.	31% were employed at 1 year post-injury.
Mammi et al. (2006)	80	Mild, Moderate, Severe	Work, or work with adaptations.	30% were able to return to work at 1 year follow-up.
Shönberger et al. (2011)	949	Moderate, Severe	Competitive employment, paid work trial, or student.	66% were employed post-injury at 1 year follow-up
Wagner et al. (2002)	105	Mild, Moderate, Severe	Return to pre-injury comparable work, full-time school, or homemaking.	71% were able to return to work within one year.
Walker et al. (2006)	1,341	Moderate, Severe	Competitively employment at any occupation full-time or part-time.	39% were able to return to competitive employment at 1 year post-injury.
Long-term Employment Outcomes				
Cattelani et al. (2002)	35	Severe	Employed in competitive working or studying.	54% were able to return to competitive working on studying by 20 months post-injury.
Felmingham et al. (2001)	55	Mild, Moderate, Severe	Full-time or part-time competitive employment.	34% were employed at 6 months post-injury and 46% at 2 years post-injury.

Fleming et al. (1999)	208	Severe	Returned to work (remained employed) and/or in a school/training program.	46.5% of those employed pre-injury were working at follow-up of mean 3.5 years.
Fraser et al. (2006)	140	Mild, Moderate, Severe	Working half-time or more at three to five years post-injury.	61% were working at 3-5 year follow-up.
Gollaher et al. (1998)	99	Mild, Moderate, Severe	Competitively employed or student.	36% were employed at 1 to 3 post-injury.
Parks et al. (2010)	572	Severe	Employed full-time (40) hours a week or part-time (< 40 hours a week).	52% were employed year 1, 54% years 2, and 57% year 3.
Ponsford et al. (1995)	74	Moderate, Severe	Employed full-time or part-time.	40% were employed at 2 years post-injury.
Sherer et al. (1998)	66	Mild, Moderate, Severe	[Productivity] Competitively employed; Modified jobs; In school making progress towards competitive employment.	67% were productive at follow-up an average of 30.2 months post-injury.
Shigaki et al. (2009)	49	Moderate, Severe	Competitively employed full or part-time.	38% were employed 2 year post-injury.
Whitnall et al. (2006)	549	Mild, Moderate, Severe	Employed	56% were employed 5-7 years follow-up.
Very Long-term Employment Outcome				
Avesani et al. (2005)	353	Severe	Reentered competitive employment	53% of those previously working had returned to competitive work between 2-10 years follow-up.
Franulic et al. (2004)	2002	Moderate, Severe	Employed	53.5% employed at 2 years, 55.6% at 5, and 69% at 10 years follow-up.

Hoofien et al. (2001)	76	Moderate, Severe	Regular employment in the free market, family business, in sheltered employment, volunteers, or as housekeepers for at least 4 months.	60% employed at time of follow-up at mean 14.1 years post-injury.
Johnson et al. (1998)	64	Severe	Returned to work and remained continuously employed 1 year.	43.5% employed in full-time or part-time employment at 10 years follow-up.

Table 1. Return to Work Rates for Short, Long, and Very Long Term Periods of Time Post-TBI

substantially large sample (n=949) were able to return to employment at one year post-injury. Other studies representing mild to severe injuries and with a clearer definition of employment reported rates ranging from approximately 30% to 61% (Mammi, Zaccaria, & Franceschini, 2005; Boake et al., 2005; Johnstone, Mount, & Schopp, 2003). Although employment rates vary one year after TBI, those with more accurate definitions of employment note a significant percentage of people with TBI not returning to employment 1 year after injury.

5.2 Long-term employment outcomes (two years to less than 10 years)

Since recovery for TBI, particularly for moderate to severe injuries, has shown to continue beyond one year than looking at employment outcomes during the second year presents a more realistic picture of outcome. Research, however, examining employment outcomes beyond one year and up to two years post-TBI did not look markedly different than results from year one. For example, in a study about financial and vocational outcomes regarding people with TBI, 68% (n= 49) were employed pre-injury, but only 38% reported being employed at year two follow-up (Shigaki, Johnstone, & Schoop, 2009). A longitudinal study had follow-up at 6 months and two years with interesting results. Felmingham, Baugley, and Crooks (2001) predicted employment outcome for 55 patients with mild, moderate and severe TBI and found at six months, 41% of those previously employed with TBI had regained employment and at two years the percentage had only increased to 46 percent. Ponsford et al. (1995) indicated that of the 74 participants primarily with mild and moderate injuries who were working at time of injury, 30 (40%) had returned to full-time or part-time work at two years. It appears that as the years increase, individuals with TBI continue to face challenges in a major area of productivity.

Examining employment data beyond two years and up to five years post-injury provides a unique opportunity to assess long-term employment outcomes in later stages of the recovery process. In a longitudinal study, Parks et al. (2010) had a substantially large sample (n = 572) of individuals with severe TBI and found 52% were employed at year 1, 54% at year 2, and 57% at year 3. Another study with a relatively sizeable sample (n= 290) examined employment outcomes and found 46.5% of those employed pre-injury were working 3.5 (mean/average) years post-injury follow-up. Additionally, 23 (13.5%) of people with TBI had returned to work immediately after inpatient rehabilitation but were no longer working at time of follow-up (Fleming, Tooth, Hassell, & Chan, 1999). Results in other studies with similar or slightly smaller sample sizes, which were alike in terms of analyses showed 36% to 67% employment rates for two to five years post-injury (Gollaher et al., 1998; Cattelani, Tanzi, Lombardi, & Mazzucchi, 2002; Fraser, Machamer, Temkin, Dikmen, & Doctor, 2006; Sherer et al., 1998). It is important to note, however, that samples were not always comparable, with varying degrees of severity and some including students in return to work (RTW) estimates. As the follow-up gets closer to 10 years post-injury, employment rates slightly improved. Whitnall, McMillan, Murray, and Teasdale (2006) assessed 219 young adults five to seven years after mild, moderate, and severe brain injury and indicated pre-injury 78% were in some type of working situations and that number had decreased to 56% at follow-up. However, the authors defined employment as working or seeking employment and a smaller percentage of both numbers reported that their jobs were not appropriate. The numbers presented by Whitnall and colleagues indicated that even though individuals may be further along in the post-inpatient rehabilitation process, it is not guaranteed that employment outcomes will significantly improve for people who have TBI.

5.3 Very long-term employment outcomes (ten years or greater)

There are a few studies examining employment status beyond seven years post- injury of a TBI. While some include survivors injured in earlier years, the primary objective was to assess employment in the very late stages of recovery. In fact, some researchers believe that subjects who did not return to work in the first five years were less likely to go back at all (Ip et al., 1995). When looking at employment outcomes so late post-injury, one might assume that the passage of time brings greater potential for spontaneous recovery from the injury and a possibility that the person with a TBI has had more rehabilitation and community assistance. Additionally, one might think that longer periods of ten years or more after TBI would lead to higher RTW rates when compared to follow-up periods beginning at five years or less. However, studies indicate that rates of very long-term employment are also discouraging.

Avesani et al. (2005) studied 353 patients with severe TBI that were consecutively admitted to an intensive rehabilitation unit and followed from 2-10 years post-trauma and 53% of those previously employed had returned to competitive work. Likewise, a similar study investigating employment outcomes at 2,5, and 10 years post-TBI found that over half of the sample (n = 275) returned to employment with 53.5% at 2 years, 55.6% at 5 years and 69% at 10 years), respectively (Franulic, Carbonell, Pinto, & Sepulveda, 2004). The research on TBI and employment that has had the longest follow-up to date, investigated psychosocial functioning from 10 to 20 years post-injury for 76 people with severe TBI and results revealed 46 (60.5%) were employed at time of follow-up for at least 4 months (Hoofien, Gilboa, Vakil, & Donovick, 2001). The variation in percentages may again be due to variations in sampling and sample inclusion criteria, for example, only examining the most severe cases of TBI, having relatively small samples sizes, or not distinguishing competitive from non-competitive employment. While the nature of very long-term employment for people with TBI appears uncertain, the research suggests that consequences from TBI persist and significantly affect employment even up to 20 years post-injury.

In summary, there have been many outcomes relative to people with TBI. We understand that terminology in using vocational outcomes and employment can be confusing and need clarification in the TBI literature. It is also likely that vocational outcomes relative to short and long-term time periods will be a major issue to address and a primary concern for a large proportion of people with TBI while re-integrating into community settings. Research also supports that employment is significantly related to quality of live (QOL), financial well-being, and social integration with people who may have TBI in the United States. Moreover, research supports the association between employment and social integration for people with TBI. Although employment rates vary one year after TBI injury, those with more accurate definitions of employment note a significant percentage of people with TBI not returning to employment 1 year after injury. There is much work to be done in looking at time sequence vocational and employment outcomes of people who have TBI in the United States.

6. Demographic variables that significantly influence employment outcomes

Empirical evidence suggests that various demographic variables like age, gender, race/ethnicity, marital status, education, and pre-morbid employment status significantly predict employment after TBI. When demographic variables are defined or categorized different in studies, it can significantly alter employment outcomes. Since a large majority of TBI studies covered in this review are conducted at the TBI Model Systems, the demographic variables will be definitions mostly used by their researchers (Gary et al., 2009; TBIMS National Data and Statistical Center, 2006):

Demographic Predictors of Employment Post-TBI	
Variables	**Definition**
Age	Continuous variable categorized as age in years at time of injury primarily between 16 and 65
Gender	Dichotomous variable categorized as male and female
Race/Ethnicity	Self-reported as African American (Black), White , Hispanic, Asian/Pacific Islander
Marital Status	Status of long-term union/partnership categorized as single, divorced, separated, and widowed
Education	Level of education primarily categorized as eight grade or less, grades 9 through 11, GED/high school trade school, high school diploma, some college, Associate's degree, Bachelor's degree, Master's degree, and Doctoral degree
Employment	Work status as part-time and full time competitively employed, in school progressing towards employment, and modified jobs.

Table 2. List of Demographic Predictors of Employment Post-TBI

6.1 Age

The majority of research studies investigating the relationship of age to employment after TBI have found that younger individuals post-injury have a higher probability of returning to work than those who are older. For instance, Schönberger, Ponsford, Olver, Ponsford, and Wirtz (2011) used structured equation modeling in a sample of 949 individuals with predominantly moderate to severe TBI to predict functional and employment outcome one year post-injury. They found age was a direct predictor of post-injury employment outcome;

however, age was not related to other demographic variables. Even when employment outcome have been examined 10 years post-TBI in a representative sample (n=382), younger adults are nearly 1.5 times more likely to be competitively employed than older adults (Gary et al., 2010). Some studies specified certain ages when comparing employment outcome. For example, Keyser-Marcus et al. (2002) conducted a large multiple center study where 538 subjects with moderate to severe TBI in a nationally representative sample were followed-up for return to employment at 1, 2, 3, 4, and 5 years post-injury and identified a specific age that predicted employment. Using logistic regression analyses, they found age was the most reliable predictor of RTW; whereas, individuals 40 years and older are less likely to RTW than those younger at all follow-up years. The results from other research agree younger people with TBI, are more likely to RTW compared to those who are older but studies are inconsistent and identify the cut-off age to be between 30 and 50 when predicting better employment outcome post-injury (Atchison et al., 2004; Dikman et al., 1994; Felmingham et al., 2001; Nakase-Richardson, Yablon, & Sherer, 2007). However, the larger more stringent studies identify the age of 40 as a good demarcation for predicting RTW after TBI.

6.2 Gender

The influence of gender on employment following TBI has been relatively consistent throughout the literature with males more likely to be unemployed post-TBI as opposed to females. A strong research study on RTW and occupational status one year post-TBI for a sample of over 1,300 subjects with generally moderate to severe injuries revealed that being female made significant contributions to RTW (Walker et al., 2006). In fact, the majority of studies that explored gender as a predictive factor of RTW following TBI concur that males fare worse than females post-TBI (Doctor et al., 2005; Fraser, Machamer, Temkin, Dikmen, & Doctor, 2006; Parks, Diaz-Arrastia, Gentilello, & Shafi, 2010). One large study with a significantly large sample (2,487 men vs. 957 women) with minor to severe TBI as classified by the Abbreviated Injury Score (AIS), however, has results that run counter to the majority of existing research. When considering employment as part of a multifactorial analysis, it was suggested that when other measured influences known to effect employment are held constant, women are more likely to have decreased hours of employment one year post-TBI compared to men (Corrigan et al., 2007). Although there are relatively few studies that have found gender to be predictive of RTW after TBI, most find that men are employed at lower rates than women.

6.3 Race/ethnicity

While a decade ago, there was a paucity of evidence about influence of race and ethnicity on employment outcomes after TBI, in the past ten years studies primarily about African Americans and Hispanics have surfaced. The majority of studies were conducted using the TBI Model Systems database consisting of a nationally representative and diverse sample. Rosenthal et al. (1996) examined a substantial number of minorities and whites for employment outcomes at one year post-TBI Of 109 white persons employed full time and competitively at injury, 45% were employed at 1 year post injury; for 50 minorities, 26% were similarly employed. It was noted that 20% of whites and 42% of minorities were unemployed pre-injury, and of those, 44% of whites and 69% of blacks did not return to competitive employment. Kreutzer et al. (2003) studied and found that minorities compared to non-minorities were significantly less stably employed (19% vs. 43%) and unemployed (50% vs. 31%). Although this study's primary purpose was to examine several factors that could moderate RTW and job stability (e.g., demographic and injury characteristics), it was clear that ethnicity negatively influenced employment and job stability after TBI. Arango-Lasprilla et al. (2009) extended the findings from Kreutzer and colleagues (2003) with a larger sample (n=627) and a more detailed examination of the influence of minority status on job stability. There was a clear definition of employment status with employment being dichotomized into competitively employed vs. not competitively employed. In addition, job stability was further classified as stable (competitively employed at all three follow-up visits), unemployed (not competitively employed at all three follow-up visits) and unstable (employed at any point in follow-up visit but not all). After adjusting for age, gender, marital status, education, cause of injury, pre-injury employment, length of stay, and discharge FIM scores, the odds of being unemployed in comparison to being stably employed were nearly five times greater for minorities. Additionally, minorities' odds of being unstably employed vs. stably employed and unemployed vs. unstably employed were over two times greater compared to whites.

Arango-Lasprilla et al. (2008) investigated racial (e.g., minority vs. Whites) difference in employment outcomes after TBI (n=5259) and found that controlling for a host of variables (e.g., age, marital status, gender, education, etc.), that whites are more likely to be employed compared to racial and ethnic minorities at 1 year post injury after adjusting for employment status at admissions and several controlled demographic variables. In asking questions relative to the findings, Arango-Lasprilla and his colleagues asked about the possible relationship between race, TBI, and long-term vocational retention. They also reported that "long-term employment outcomes are also not likely to be favorable for minorities" (p. 994), but that was at one year post-injury, which is not necessarily long-term as defined in this chapter. Gary et al. (2009), however, extended the findings of Arango-Lasprilla et al. (2008) with an exclusively African American sample (n=2022) taking a cross-sectional and longitudinal look at employment outcomes post-TBI. Results indicated that after adjusting for demographic and injury characteristics, the odds of not being competitively employed versus being competitively employed are 2.61, 2.10, and 3.15 times greater at years one, two, and five years, respectively for African Americans compared to whites. Although this study was the first to specifically examine employment outcomes for minorities post-TBI, the downfall is the sample was homogeneous, consisting of one minority group. Gary et al. (2010), however, examined employment outcome 10 years after TBI in a multiracial and ethnic sample (n = 382; black, Hispanic, Asian/Pacific Islander, or other) and found minorities were 2.37 times more likely to not be competitively employed versus competitively employed compared to their white counterparts. Clearly, racial and ethnic minorities are two to five times more likely to be unemployed compared to whites. The evidence is mounting, but primarily for African Americans and Whites. More research is warranted for other racial and ethnic groups and delineating the differences within ethnic groups (e.g. White Latinos vs. Black Latinos).

6.4 Marital status

Marital status has not been extensively examined after TBI. Most studies that investigated marital status and its relationship to employment post-TBI have found that being married has a positive effect on employment outcomes. For example, Walker and colleagues (2006) found, like gender, being married made a significant unique contribution to predicting RTW one year after TBI. Likewise, other studies with adequately sized nationally representative samples confirm that being married increased the likelihood of RTW and maintaining stable employment one year post-TBI (Arango-Lasprilla et al., 2008; 2009; Gary et al., 2009). While marital status has not been investigated extensively regarding people who have TBI, a consensus is beginning to emerge that being married has a positive effects on employment outcomes if you are a person with a TBI.

6.5 Education

As with many variables, education is viewed as having some effects on vocational outcomes. Gollaher and colleagues (1998) noted that education is one of the most important predictors of employment post-injury, and those with higher education were more likely to experience vocational reentry following TBI. The research confirms that employment after mild to severe injury is more likely for those who have received at least a high school education (Doctor et al., 2005; Girard et al., 1996; Sherer, Bergloff, High, & Nick, 1999; Keyser-Marcus et al., 2002; Wagner et al., 2002). Educational status also affects employment rates studied longitudinally. In a study of employment 2, 5, and 10 years after mild to severe TBI, the 10-year employed group had the highest educational attainment as well as the highest rate of job re-insertion to the same or a similar position (Franulic et al., 2004). Similarly, those with the highest levels of education were significantly more likely to sustain employment from one to three years post-TBI (Arango-Lasprilla et al., 2009; Kreutzer et al., 2003). Sherer et al. (2003) considered education to be one of the most prominent confounding factor in that it ameliorated distinct differences between racial and ethnic minorities and whites when comparing productivity outcomes that include employment.

6.6 Pre-injury employment

Among all demographic factors, pre-injury employment appears to be the most reliable predictor of RTW, and the failure to factor pre-injury employment into predictive models will likely to produce less accurate employment outcomes. A study that measured the complex interplay between various factors predicting employment after TBI at 1 year post-injury found pre-injury employment was a direct predictor of employment outcomes (Shönberger, Ponsford, Olver, Ponsford, & Wirtz, 2011). People employed prior to moderate to severe TBI were three to five times more likely to RTW than those unemployed pre-injury (Keyser-Marcus et al., 2002). Fleming et al. (1999) showed a strong influence of pre-injury unemployment and employment variables on post-injury employment. They found that only one out of 38 subjects who were unemployed prior to injury was working at follow-up; whereas, 79 out of 170 of those employed pre-injury was working post-injury. Other studies support pre-injury employment as a crucial factor for employment outcome post-TBI (Atchison et al., 2004; Arango-Lasprilla et al., 2008; Gary et al., 2010).

Some unique information is revealed when different aspects of pre-injury employment are explored in relation to post-injury, indicating the importance of considering specific characteristics of the pre-injury work experience. For example, individuals who failed to maintain stable uninterrupted employment following mild to severe TBI had pre-injury jobs that did not provide benefits. Additionally, people who were professionals or managers pre-injury were nearly three times more likely to RTW by one year post-TBI than those in manual labor positions (Machamer et al., 2005; Walker et al., 2006).

In summary, research indicates that various pre-injury demographic variables are associated with employment outcomes after TBI. Those over 40 are more likely to be unemployed post-TBI than younger individuals. Generally, males fare worse than females and those not married have less likelihood of being employed. Lower educational status is highly associated with worse employment outcomes. The strongest pre-injury predictor of employment post-TBI is pre-injury employment; those not employed pre-injury are less likely to be employed after sustaining a TBI.

7. Injury characteristics that significantly influence employment outcomes

How a TBI occurs, what severity level has the TBI been classified, and the level of disability or functional status one achieves prior to release from rehabilitation can have a significant influence on an individual with a TBI and their ability to obtain employment after injury. A large percentage of research that examines post-injury variables and of employment after TBI indicates variables for cause of injury, injury severity, and functional status as measured by valid assessments. Since a large majority of the TBI studies covered in this review are conducted at the TBI Model Systems, the injury-related variables will be definitions mostly used by their researchers (Gary et al., 2009; TBIMS National Data and Statistical Center, 2006):

Injury-related Predictors of Employment Post-TBI	
Variables	**Definition**
Cause of Injury	Categorical variable dichotomized as violent and non-violent.
Injury Severity (GCS/PTA)	(GCS) Combination of eye opening, verbal, and motor response when emerging from coma from 3 (lowest) to 15 (highest); (PTA) Duration of being disoriented in days.
Functional Status (DRS/FIM)	(DRS) Measure to assess change in function over course of recovery from coma to community ranging from 0 (no disability) to 29 (vegetative state); (FIM) Measure of independence ranging from 1 (total assist) to 7 (completely independent).

Table 3. List of Injury-related Predictors of Employment Post-TBI

7.1 Cause of injury

Regarding cause of injury, Hanlon, Demery, Martinovich, and Kelly (1999) classified type of injury into motor vehicle collision, motor vehicle-pedestrian collision, falls, assaults, injury from falling objects, and sports/recreation injuries. Results revealed that patients who experienced mild TBI from falls and those injured by falling objects had significantly worse vocational outcomes than the motor vehicle collision group. A similar study found that patients who experienced motor vehicle accidents had more positive productive outcomes than those injured from falls, other types of vehicles, motor vehicle-pedestrian accidents, and assaults (Girard et al., 1996). When classifying injuries as either intentional or unintentional, those injured intentionally were significantly more likely to be unemployed at one year post-TBI (Greenspan et al., 1996). Intentional injuries are usually violent injuries (e.g., assaults), and studies found that those who sustain TBI through violent means are less likely to be employed or productive one year post-injury compared to other etiologies of TBI (Arango-Lasprilla et al., 2008; Gary et al., 2009; Wagner et al., 2002). When violent etiology is not compared to non-violent etiology, it is not clear in TBI literature what specific cause of injury is a significant predictor of employment outcome. However, once violence is introduced in the analyses more studies concur that those who sustain TBI through violence as opposed to non-violence have worse employment outcomes.

7.2 Injury severity

Several studies have found severity of injury, as measured by GCS and PTA, predicts employment post-TBI. Scores on the GCS range from 3 to 15. Scores between three and eight indicate severe injury; 9 to 12 is moderate, and 13 to 15 is mild (Teasdale, & Jennett, 1974). PTA is considered the time elapsed from injury until recovery of full consciousness and the return of ongoing memory; it relates to severity by detailing the continued level of consciousness following the injury (Grant & Alves, 1987). GCS taken at admission and length of PTA were found to be significant predictors of employment at one year post-TBI (Cifu, et al., 1997). The GCS scores of those employed were an average of 8.9 compared to 7.6 for those unemployed, and the employed group was in PTA for an average of 25.7 days compared to 44 days for the unemployed group. Another investigation of employment one year following TBI noted that the GCS had a reliable and powerful effect; where only 25% of patients with a GCS score of eight or less returned to work by one year after injury, compared to 80% of those with scores of 13-15 (Dikmen et al., 1994). Additionally, Sherer et al. (2002) noted that when patients with shorter PTA were included in the analyses, the duration of PTA had significant and unique predictive capability of employment post-TBI. One strong comparison study of acute confusion severity with duration (measured by PTA), however, found that severity of confusion was a stronger predictor of employment outcomes 1 year post-TBI, but they still reported that PTA duration continues to be a powerful predictor (Nakase-Richardson et al., 2007).

At two years post-injury and beyond, GCS and PTA continued to contribute to employment prediction. Felmingham et al. (2001) concluded that GCS scores successfully predicted employment at two years post-injury in 72% of cases. Similarly, at three years post-injury, PTA was the strongest acute clinical predictive factor for those returning to competitive employment (Cattelani et al., 2002). Two to five years post-injury, Fleming et al. (1987) noted that shorter durations of PTA were one of the best predictors for distinguishing between those who return to work and those who do not. Vogenthaler, Smith, and Goldfader (1989) assessed RTW at four to seven years post-injury and found a strong positive correlation between the best GCS scores in the first 24 hours and employment outcomes. Severity has been shown to be a significant predictor in studies even up to 10 years post-injury (Avesani et al., 2005; Johnson, 1998; Brown, Maleck, Mandrekar et al., 2010).

7.3 Functional status

Functional status can also have a major affect on RTW outcome after TBI. Some research studies indicate that both FIM and DRS scores significantly predict employment outcomes. Walker et al. (2006) agreed that FIM discharge scores were robust RTW variables one year after moderate to severe TBI, demonstrating that those with higher discharge FIM scores were over three times more likely to RTW than those with longer lengths of stay (LOS) in rehabilitation. This study also indicated that the FIM is a better predictor of employment status than length of stay. Cifu et al. (1997) indicated that both the FIM and DRS measures at both admission and discharge influenced subsequent RTW one year after moderate to severe TBI. When exploring functional status as assessed by the FIM only, researchers found that over half of the 127 who did not return to work at one year had significant cognitive and motor limitations (Greenspan et al., 1996).

The DRS is often chosen in TBI literature to accompany or replace the FIM when measuring functional status. Gollaher and colleagues (1998) suggested that both admission and discharge DRS scores significantly predict employment one to three years after mild to severe TBI, with discharge scores being better predictors than admission scores. DRS and FIM scores from admission, discharge, and one year post-injury were investigated to determine job stability from one to four years post-TBI. DRS scores at one year after primarily moderate to severe TBI proved to be the most impressive predictor; 78% of those with no impairment and none with severe impairment were stably employed (Kreutzer et al., 2003). Other studies concur that DRS and FIM are strong injury-related variables that predict employment post-TBI, but the discharge scores should be used instead of admission scores (Sherer, Sander, Nick et al., 2002; Kosch, Browne, King et al., 2010).

In summary, primarily, injury-related variables, including etiology, severity of injury, and functional status are significantly related to RTW post-TBI. Additionally, the most prominent cause of injury related to employment after TBI is violent etiology. Severity of injury has been shown to be a powerful predictor of employment up to 10 years post-injury; typically those with a GCS of eight or less and PTA of 26 days or more have worse outcomes. Furthermore, functional status can significantly predict employment several years post-TBI with discharge FIM and DRS scores proven to be better predictors than admission scores.

8. Disability legislation

Since TBI often results in cognitive and emotional deficits that are not always apparent to the physical eye, there can be misconceptions about the capability of those who sustain the injury. These misconceptions can come from those in the general public and even professionals that do not have the expertise to deal with TBI. For example, in a qualitative exploratory study about misconception after brain injury, participants reported that because their cognitive disabilities were not easily recognizable they were not really expected to have long-term consequences or received more active pressure from friends, family, and work to perform to standards that they could not realistically achieve (Swift, & Wilson, 2001). Given that many individuals with TBI that recover well from acute problems and could likely enter or reenter the workforce, this population can be prone to various forms of employment discrimination. McMahon et al. (2005) found in an US Equal Employment Opportunities Commission (EEOC) study with a sample of 2,037 individuals with TBI that employment discrimination for this group is more likely to occur after employment has been obtained as opposed to during the hiring process. This evidence is why disability legislation is imperative for people with TBI who have aspirations to be employed with the same rights and benefits as the non-injured general population. The American Disabilities Act (ADA) of 1990 (Public Law 101-336), is such legislation, that is the result of federal legislators' efforts to ensure employment rights, advocacy, and support for people with brain injury and other disabling conditions (109 United States. Office of Disability Employment Policy, 1992). Title 1 of the ADA protects people with brain injury who were employed prior and wish to return to their previous position or be reassigned in another area. In addition, the ADA provides protection for those with brain injuries who were never employed prior to injury, but wish to pursue a job after the injury has occurred. The ADA covers individuals with brain injury that meet essential job functions, which is being qualified for the job and has a declared disability from brain injury as established by law (109 United States. Office of Disability Employment Policy 1992). Once the person with a brain injury is covered and the employer falls into the category in which they must adhere to ADA guidelines (e.g., employers with 15 or more employees), they are protected in the following areas:

- Unfair treatment because of your disability.
- Harassment by managers, co-workers, and others in the workplace because of your disability.
- Denial of reasonable workplace accommodation that you need.
- Retaliation because you complained about job discrimination.

The ADA was also amended in 2008 (effective January 1, 2009) and the changes have major implications for people with disabilities resulting from brain injury. The amended ADA law still retains the former definition of disability, which is "a physical or mental impairment that substantially limits one or more life activities; a record of such impairment; or being regarded as having such impairment", but it expands the definition meaning so it can be applicable to those with impairment that were not covered in the earlier interpretation of disability (Thomas, & Gostin, 2009).

Since research suggests that persons with TBI are more likely to be discriminated against after the employment occurs compared to other aspects of employment discrimination (e.g., hiring, harassment, etc.; McMahon et al., 2005), a major issue for the employees with TBI is the retention of employment. It has been documented that challenges for individuals with TBI are not just subject to returning to or obtaining employment, but having a significant degree of job stability (Kreutzer et al., 2003; Pössl et al., 2001; Mackamer et al., 2005). As such, one of the most important strategies covered under the ADA, that could assist with the retention of individuals with TBI in employment settings is the right to reasonable accommodations. It is important to note that the ADA *only* requires an employer to provide reasonable accommodations that would not cause undue hardship (e.g., lack of financial resources by employer to provide accommodations). Such accommodations that would benefit individuals with TBI at work are the following (Program on Employment and Disability, 2000).

- Memory aids
- Timers
- Wheelchair accessibility
- Visual aids
- Work task modification
- Environmental changes

These accommodations can enhance productivity for people with brain injury on the job. It can make work tasks easier and more amenable for individuals with disabilities.

9. Health professions in preparing people with brain injury for employment

There are a myriad of health professionals that work across the continuum of service delivery systems who are directly and indirectly involved in treatment of individuals with TBI that ultimately will lead to enhanced vocational outcome. Service providers vary coming from the acute stages of the rehabilitation process to community-based settings.

However, each profession has a unique set of skills that addresses the physical, cognitive, and emotional sequalae that primarily results from TBI and potentially interfere with productivity. Table 4 list health professionals who are prominent in acute care to community-based settings.

Physiatrists and rehabilitation nurses who specializes in physical medicine and rehabilitation typically provide services in acute care and rehabilitation settings right after initial trauma of individuals with TBI has occurred. The effect of early rehabilitation by specialized medical staff can be paramount in recovery and functional outcomes of people with TBI. This presents a case for better chances to achieve greater long-term function, such as employment and other areas of productivity. Studies have indicated that there is a positive effect on the functional outcome and discharge disposition of those with TBI who receive early specialized physical medicine and rehabilitation care as opposed to less formal specialized medical care (Mackley, 1994; Wagner, Fabio, Zafonte et al., 2003; Zhu, Poon, Chan, & Chan, 2007).

Health Professionals Involved in Return to Work after TBI	
Profession	**Related Roles**
Physiatrists	Specialize in medical services and can perform independent medical evaluations in area of physical medicine and rehabilitation with emphasis on restoration of function.
Rehabilitation Nurses	Gives specialized nursing care to individuals with physical disabilities and/or chronic conditions and help promote restoration and optimal health.
Social Workers	Provides resources specialized for brain injury, be a liaison between healthcare system and family, and facilitate discharge planning by linking to community based services.
Occupational Therapists	Use specialized skills to focus on reengaging in meaningful activities and address barriers to participation in work environment through home and workplace modification and strategies for independent living.
Physical Therapists	Use specialized skills to overcome debilitating physical deficits resulting from brain injury and promote functional mobility and use of physical modalities and assistive technology.
Speech Therapists	Use specialized skills to address communication and cognitive deficits that would enhance productive and functional living.
Vocational Rehabilitation Counselors	Uses specialized skills to be directly involved in the education, employment training, and consistent progress of vocational placement after brain injury.

Table 4. List of Health Professional Involved in Return to Work after TBI

Since social work has numerous roles related to education, resource allocation, and being a liaison between health setting and caregivers and their specialized services is vital to the care, support and transition of individuals with TBI. Although social work services may not seem directly linked to enhancing skills related to employment, they can, in fact, provide important information and referrals that would assist with transition of individuals with TBI back into employment settings (Wagner, Fabio, Zafonte et al., 2003).

The majority of therapeutic teams that service individuals with TBI in physical medicine and rehabilitation settings consist of occupational and physical therapists, and speech and language pathologists. These professions are essential to the rehabilitation process and to progressing individuals with TBI towards employment. For example, research notes the effectiveness of the specialized assessments and interventions delivered by therapy professions that would assist clients with brain injury transition and obtain meaningful occupation (Duff & Proctor, 2002; McCullah, 2007; Phipps, 2007).

One most the important professionals directly related to enhancing the vocational outcomes of people with brain injury are vocational rehabilitation counselors. The specific roles of vocational counselors are to educate, train, educate, and monitor those with disabilities in vocational situations. This profession is very useful for many individuals with TBI who may desire to enter the workforce after an unexpected injury and alteration of functional skills. It has been found that vocational rehabilitation services were positive predictors of job placement and employment status for individuals with TBI (Gamble & Moore, 2003).

In summary, numerous health professionals work to improve the life and well being of persons with TBI. Although some work more in multidisciplinary settings in acute and inpatient care and some work more in the community based settings, collectively their efforts assist in progressing individuals with TBI towards vocational goals, which helps improve overall quality of life.

10. Intervention to increase employment for people with brain injury

The majority of this chapter has focused on employment rates and factors that predict employment, but emphasis should not only be placed on the research that report statistics related to employment post-TBI, but also research that is attempting to rectify the problems related to obtaining and maintain employment post-injury. Interventions are particularly needed due to the residual problems related to brain injury that typically interferes with successful return to work and the maintenance of employment. Ideally, interventions both post-rehabilitation and community-based can be designed to address and ameliorate problems with return to work and educate the employee with brain injury and employer so that the work environment can be amenable to this population and more efficient for all those involved. In addition, there must be research to evaluate and report the efficacy of utilizing these interventions. There are quite a few studies that employ vocational services to intervene and assist people with brain injury return to employment, but few actual interventions have been specifically developed and evaluated in research to address problems of employment in this population. One such intervention was developed in an outpatient rehabilitation setting. Guérin et al. (2006) developed an intervention for individuals with mild TBI to enhance vocational outcomes in Québec, Canada. Primarily, their intervention starts by indentifying the over-arching problem that seems to affect daily life after injury. Next, short-term objectives are developed by the treatment team and client, followed by development of a framework for return to work involving the client and employer. Constant encouragement and advice is given to assist person in maintaining contact with employer and creating an employment milieu until the client is able to return to work. Likewise, another intervention was developed that indirectly addressed employment through goal attainment, which included sustaining employment. Muenchberger et al. (2011) developed a structured community-based intervention called Skills to Enable People with brain injury in their communities (STEPS). This was a 6 week program that was delivered in a group setting involving person with brain injury and family. A workbook was used that covered 6 sessions related to education about brain injury, setting goals, maintaining relationships, identifying and working through problems, and exploring activities. The problem with the STEPS program and the intervention for mild TBI is that both were developed and implemented in countries outside the US (Australia and Québec, respectively).These setting are different than the US and may be less applicable to people who live in the US due to resources and service provisions. However, Niemeier et al. (2010) were very successful at implementing a community based intervention specifically designed for improving productivity and employability following brain injury. Using a 20 session manualized approach; the Virginia Clubhouse Vocational Transitions (VCVTP) program was implemented in six clubhouses in the state of Virginia to transition severely injured people with brain injury living in the community to working as a volunteer, in competitive employment full or part-time, or an education or training program. The program had modest significant treatment effect for employment status and productivity. Overall, there is a dearth of interventions for employment after brain injury that is being adequately evaluated and published in the research literature. There is distinct need to continue development and research in this area.

11. Future research

This chapter has reviewed the majority of employment research conducted on individuals with TBI in the last 15 years. Clearly from this review, there is continued need for longitudinal research with multiple follow-up periods to elucidate expected employment trends and changes to employment over time with the same co-hort of participants. Additionally, more prospective research that examines employment 10 to 20 years post-injury with a large enough sample that attrition will not significantly bias results. Research with mixed methodology will help to identify challenges to employment and additional variables, after brain injury by understanding the breadth of the issues in more explicit detail. With additional knowledge about employment after brain injury, more interventions can be developed that will address identified issues and make transition back to employment settings after TBI more successful.

12. Conclusion

In summary, TBI can have a devastating effect on employment and vocational skills that potentially will extend for many years post-injury. Although employment rates vary due to numerous pre-injury and post-injury factors (e.g., severity, cause of injury, pre-injury employment status), the majority of research using different definitions of employment identify rates to be around 40-60%. The enactment of solid federal legislation that aims to protect individuals with disabilities resulting from brain injury and a variety of health professionals especially skilled to adequately treat this population makes the climate right for unique employment interventions and continued research to profoundly affect the quality of life for those living with brain injury.

13. References

Arango-Lasprilla, J., Ketchum, J. M., Gary, K. W., Kreutzer, J. S., O'Neil-Pirozzi, T.,M., Wehman, P., Jha, A. (2009). The influence of minority status on job stability after traumatic brain injury. *PM & R: The Journal of Injury, Function, and Rehabilitation, 1*(1), 41-49.

Arango-Lasprilla, J.C., Ketchum, J.M., Williams, K., Kreutzer, J.S., Marquez, C., O'Neil-Pirozzi, T.M., Wehman, P. (2008). Racial differences in employment outcomes after traumatic brain injury. *Archives of Physical Medicine Rehabilitation, 89*(5), 988-995.

Atchison, T. B., Sander, A. M., Struchen, M. A., High, W. M., Jr., Roebuck, T. M., Contant, C. F., et al. (2004). Relationship between neuropsychological test performance and productivity at 1-year following traumatic brain injury. *Clinical Neuropsychologist, 18*(2), 249-265.

Avesani, R., Salvi, L., Rigoli, G., & Gambini, M. G. (2005). Reintegration after severe brain injury: A retrospective study. *Brain Injury, 19*(11), 933-939.

Benedictus, M. R., Spikman, J. M., & van der Naalt, J. (2010). Cognitive and behavioral impairment in traumatic brain injury related to outcome and return to work. *Archives of Physical Medicine and Rehabilitation, 91*(9), 1436-1441. doi:10.1016/j.apmr.2010.06.019

Boake, C., McCauley, S. R., Pedroza, C., Levin, H. S., Brown, S. A., & Brundage, S. I. (2005). Lost productive work time after mild to moderate traumatic brain injury with and without hospitalization. *Neurosurgery, 56*(5), 994-1003; discussion 1994-1003.

Cattelani, R., Tanzi, F., Lombardi, F., & Mazzucchi, A. (2002). Competitive re-employment after severe traumatic brain injury: Clinical, cognitive and behavioural predictive variables. *Brain Injury, 16*(1), 51-64.

Cifu, D. X., Keyser-Marcus, L., Lopez, E., Wehman, P., Kreutzer, J. S., Englander, J., et al. (1997). Acute predictors of successful return to work 1 year after traumatic brain injury: A multicenter analysis. *Archives of Physical Medicine and Rehabilitation, 78*(2), 125-131.

Catalano, D., Pereira, A. P., Ming-Yi Wu, Ho, H., & Chan, F. (2006). Service patterns related to successful employment outcomes of persons with traumatic brain injury in vocational rehabilitation. *NeuroRehabilitation, 21*(4), 279-293.

Corrigan, J. D., Lineberry, L. A., Komaroff, E., Langlois, J. A., Selassie, A. W., & Wood, K. D. (2007). Employment after traumatic brain injury: Differences between men and women. *Archives of Physical Medicine and Rehabilitation, 88*(11), 1400-1409.

Dikmen, S. S., Temkin, N. R., Machamer, J. E., Holubkov, A. L., Fraser, R. T., & Winn, H. R. (1994). Employment following traumatic head injuries. *Archives of Neurology, 51*(2), 177-186.

Doctor, J. N., Castro, J., Temkin, N. R., Fraser, R. T., Machamer, J. E., & Dikmen, S. S. (2005). Workers' risk of unemployment after traumatic brain injury: A normed comparison. *Journal of the International Neuropsychological Society, 11*(6), 747-752.

Duff, M. C., Proctor, A., & Haley, K. (2002). Mild traumatic brain injury (MTBI): Assessment and treatment procedures used by speech-language pathologists (SLPs). *Brain Injury : [BI], 16*(9), 773-787. doi:10.1080/02699050210128870

Felmingham, K. L., Baguley, I. J., & Crooks, J. (2001). A comparison of acute and postdischarge predictors of employment 2 years after traumatic brain injury. *Archives of Physical Medicine and Rehabilitation, 82*(4), 435-439.

Fleming, J., Tooth, L., Hassell, M., & Chan, W. (1999). Prediction of community integration and vocational outcome 2-5 years after traumatic brain injury rehabilitation in Australia. *Brain Injury, 13*(6), 417-431.

Franulic, A., Carbonell, C. G., Pinto, P., & Sepulveda, I. (2004). Psychosocial adjustment and employment outcome 2, 5 and 10 years after TBI. *Brain Injury, 18*(2), 119-129.

Fraser, R., Machamer, J., Temkin, N., Dikmen, S., & Doctor, J. (2006). Return to work in traumatic brain injury (TBI): A perspective on capacity for job complexity. *Journal of Vocational Rehabilitation, 25*(3), 141-148.Gary, K. W., Arango-Lasprilla, J., Ketchum, J. M., Kreutzer, J. S., Copolillo, A., Novack, T. A., & Jha, A. (2009). Racial differences in employment outcome after traumatic brain injury at 1, 2, and 5 years postinjury. *Archives of Physical Medicine & Rehabilitation, 90*(10), 1699-1707.

Gamble, D., & Moore, C. L. (2003). The relation between VR services and employment outcomes of individuals with traumatic brain injury. *Journal of Rehabilitation, 69*(3), 31.

Gary, K. W., Arango-Lasprilla, J., Ketchum, J. M., Kreutzer, J. S., Copolillo, A., Novack, T. A., & Jha, A. (2009). Racial differences in employment outcome after traumatic brain injury at 1, 2, and 5 years postinjury. *Archives of Physical Medicine & Rehabilitation, 90*(10), 1699-1707. doi:10.1016/j.apmr.2009.04.014

Gary, K. W., Ketchum, J. M., Arango-Lasprillac, J., Kreutzer, J. S., Novack, T., Copolillo, A., & Deng, X. (2010). Differences in employment outcomes 10 years after traumatic brain injury among racial and ethnic minority groups. *Journal of Vocational Rehabilitation, 33*(1), 65-75. doi:10.3233/JVR-2010-0516

Girard, D., Brown, J., Burnett-Stolnack, M., Hashimoto, N., Hier-Wellmer, S., Perlman, O. Z., et al. (1996). The relationship of neuropsychological status and productive outcomes following traumatic brain injury. *Brain Injury, 10*(9), 663-676.

Gollaher, K., High, W., Sherer, M., Bergloff, P., Boake, C., Young, M. E., et al. (1998). Prediction of employment outcome one to three years following traumatic brain injury (TBI). *Brain Injury, 12*(4), 255-263.

Grant, I., & Alves, W. (1987). *Psychiatric and psychosocial disturbances in head injury.* New York: Oxford University Press.

Greenspan, A. I., Wrigley, J. M., Kresnow, M., Branche-Dorsey, C. M., & Fine, P. R. (1996). Factors influencing failure to return to work due to traumatic brain injury. *Brain Injury, 10*(3), 207-218.

Hammond, F. M., Grattan, K. D., Sasser, H., Corrigan, J. D., Rosenthal, M., Bushnik, T., & Shull, W. (2004). Five years after traumatic brain injury: A study of individual outcomes and predictors of change in function. *NeuroRehabilitation, 19*(1), 25-35.

Hanlon, R. E., Demery, J. A., Martinovich, Z., & Kelly, J. P. (1999). Effects of acute injury characteristics on neuropsychological status and vocational outcome following mild traumatic brain injury. *Brain Injury, 13*(11), 873-887.

Heinemann, A. W., & Whiteneck, G. G. (1995). Relationships among impairment, disability, handicap, and life satisfaction in persons with traumatic brain injury. *Journal of Head Trauma Rehabilitation, 10*(4), 54-63.

Hoofien, D., Gilboa, A., Vakil, E., & Donovick, P. J. (2001). Traumatic brain injury (TBI) 10-20 years later: A comprehensive outcome study of psychiatric symptomatology, cognitive abilities and psychosocial functioning. *Brain Injury, 15*(3), 189-209.

Ip, R. Y., Doran, J., & Schentag, C. (1995). Traumatic brain injury: Factors predicting return to work to school. *Brain Injury, 9*(5), 517-532.

Jiang, Ji-Yao, Gao, Guo-YI, Li, Wei-Ping, Yu, Ming-Kun, Zhu, Cheng, Early predictors of prognosis in 846 cases of severe traumatic brain injury. *Journal of Neurotrauma,* 19(7): 869-874, 2002

Johnson, R. (1998). How do people get back to work after severe head injury? A 10 year follow-up study. *Neuropsychological Rehabilitation, 8*, 61-79.

Johnstone, B., Mount, D., & Schopp, L. H. (2003). Financial and vocational outcomes 1 year after traumatic brain injury. *Archives of Physical Medicine and Rehabilitation, 84*(2), 238-241.

Kendall, E., Muenchberger, H., & Gee, T. (2006). Vocational rehabilitation following traumatic brain injury: A quantitative synthesis of outcome studies. *Journal of Vocational Rehabilitation, 25*(3), 149-160.

Keyser-Marcus, L. A., Bricout, J. C., Wehman, P., Campbell, L. R., Cifu, D. X., Englander, J., et al. (2002). Acute predictors of return to employment after traumatic brain injury: A longitudinal follow-up. *Archives of Physical Medicine and Rehabilitation, 83*(5), 635-641.

Kreutzer, J. S., Marwitz, J. H., Walker, W., Sander, A., Sherer, M., Bogner, J., et al. (2003). Moderating factors in return to work and job stability after traumatic brain injury. *Journal of Head Trauma Rehabilitation, 18*(2), 128-138.

Kosch, Y., Browne, S., King, C., Fitzgerald, J., & Cameron, I. (2010). Post-traumatic amnesia and its relationship to the functional outcome of people with severe traumatic brain injury. *Brain Injury, 24*(3), 479-485.

Langois, J., Rutland-Brown, W., & Thomas, K. (2006). Traumatic brain injury in the United States: Emergency department visits, hospitalizations, and deaths. In C. US Dept Health & Human Services, National Center for Injury Prevention and Control (Ed.). Atlanta, (GA).

Machamer, J., Temkin, N., Fraser, R., Doctor, J. N., & Dikmen, S. (2005). Stability of employment after traumatic brain injury. *Journal of the International Neuropsychological Society, 11*(7), 807-816.

Mackay, L. E. (1994). Benefits of a formalized traumatic brain injury program within a trauma center. *The Journal of Heald Trauma Rehabilitation,* 9(1), 11-17.

Mammi, P., Zaccaria, B., & Franceschini, M. (2006). Early rehabilitative treatment in patients with traumatic brain injuries: Outcome at one-year follow-up. *Europa Medicophysica, 42*(1), 17-22.

McCrimmon, S., & Oddy, M. (2006). Return to work following moderate-to-severe traumatic brain injury. *Brain Injury : [BI], 20*(10), 1037-1046.

McCulloch, K. (2007). Attention and dual-task conditions: Physical therapy implications for individuals with acquired brain injury. *Journal of Neurologic Physical Therapy : JNPT, 31*(3), 104-118. doi:10.1097/NPT.0b013e31814a6493

McMahon, B. T., West, S. L., Shaw, L. R., Waid-Ebbs, K., & Belongia, L. (2005). Workplace discrimination and traumatic brain injury: The national EEOC ADA research project. *Work (Reading, Mass.), 25*(1), 67-75.

Muenchberger, H., Kendall, E., Kennedy, A., & Charker, J. (2011). Living with brain injury in the community: Outcomes from a community-based self-management support (CB-SMS) programme in australia. *Brain Injury: [BI], 25*(1), 23-34.

Nakase-Richardson, R., Yablon, S. A., & Sherer, M. (2007). Prospective comparison of acute confusion severity with duration of post-traumatic amnesia in predicting employment outcome after traumatic brain injury. *Journal of Neurology, Neurosurgery, and Psychiatry, 78*(8), 872-876. doi:10.1136/jnnp.2006.104190

Niemeier, J. P., DeGrace, S. M., Farrar, L. F., Ketchum, J. S., Berman, A. J., & Young, J. A. (2010). Effectiveness of a comprehensive, manualized intervention for improving productivity and employability following brain injury. *Journal of Vocational Rehabilitation, 33*(3), 167-179.

Nakase-Richardson, R., Yablon, S. A., & Sherer, M. (2007). Prospective comparison of acute confusion severity with duration of post-traumatic amnesia in predicting employment outcome alter traumatic brain injury. *Journal of Neurology, Neurosurgery & Psychiatry, 78*(8), 872-876.

O'Connor, C., Colantonio, A., & Polatajko, H. (2005). Long term symptoms and limitations of activity of people with traumatic brain injury: A ten-year follow-up. *Psychological Reports, 97*(1), 169-179.

O'Neill, J., Hibbard, M. R., Brown, M., Jaffe, M., Sliwinski, M., Vandergoot, D., et al. (1998). The effect of employment on quality of life and community integration after traumatic brain injury. *Journal of Head Trauma Rehabilitation, 13*(4), 68-79.

Parker, R. M., Szymanski, E. M., Patterson, J. B. (2005) editors. *Rehabilitation counseling: basics and beyond*. 4th ed. Austin: Pro-Ed. Inc. ISBN number 0-89079-987-3.

Parks, J. K., Diaz-Arrastia, R., Gentilello, L. M., & Shafi, S. (2010). Postinjury employment as a surrogate for functional outcomes: A quality indicator for trauma systems. *Baylor University Medical Center Proceedings, 23*(4), 355-358.

Phipps, S., & Richardson, P. (2007). Occupational therapy outcomes for clients with traumatic brain injury and stroke using the canadian occupational performance measure. *The American Journal of Occupational Therapy.: Official Publication of the American Occupational Therapy Association, 61*(3), 328-334.

Ponsford, J. L., Olver, J. H., Curran, C., & Ng, K. (1995). Prediction of employment status 2 years after traumatic brain injury. *Brain Injury, 9*(1), 11-20.

Pössl, J., Jürgensmeyer, S., Karlbauer, F., Wenz, C., & Goldenberg, G. (2001). Stability of employment after brain injury: A 7-year follow-up study. *Brain Injury, 15*(1), 15.

Powell, J. M., Machamer, J. E., Temkin, N. R., & Dikmen, S. S. (2001). Self-report of extent of recovery and barriers to recovery after traumatic brain injury: A longitudinal study. *Archives of Physical Medicine and Rehabilitation, 82*(8), 1025-1030. doi:10.1053/apmr.2001.25082

Program on Employment and Disability. (June 2000). Working effectively with employees who have sustained a brain injury. [Brochure]. Retrieved from http://www.eric.ed.gov/ERICWebPortal/search/detailmini.jsp?_nfpb=true&_&ERICExtSearch_SearchValue_0=ED415595&ERICExtSearch_SearchType_0=no&accno=ED415595

Rosenthal, M., Dijkers, M., Harrison-Felix, C., Nabors, N., Witol, A. D., Young, M. E., et al. (1996). Impact of minority status on functional outcome and community integration after traumatic brain injury. *Journal of Head Trauma Rehabilitation, 11*(4), 69-79.

Sherer, M., Nick, T. G., Sander, A. M., Hart, T., Hanks, R., Rosenthal, M., et al. (2003). Race and productivity outcome after traumatic brain injury: Influence of confounding factors. *Journal of Head Trauma Rehabilitation, 18*(5), 408-424.

Sherer, M., Sander, A. M., Nick, T. G., High, W. M., Jr., Malec, J. F., & Rosenthal, M. (2002). Early cognitive status and productivity outcome after traumatic brain injury: Findings from the TBI model systems. *Archives of Physical Medicine and Rehabilitation, 83*(2), 183-192.

Sherer, M., Bergloff, P., High, W., Jr., & Nick, T. G. (1999). Contribution of functional rating to prediction of long term employment outcome after traumatic brain injury. *Brain Injury, 13*(12), 973.

Schönberger, M., Ponsford, J., Olver, J., Ponsford, M., & Wirtz, M. (2011). Prediction of functional and employment outcome 1 year after traumatic brain injury: A structural equation modelling approach. *Journal of Neurology, Neurosurgery, and Psychiatry, 82*(8), 936-941.

Shigaki, C. L., Johnstone, B., & Schopp, L. H. (2009). Financial and vocational outcomes 2 years after traumatic brain injury. *Disability & Rehabilitation, 31*(6), 484-489.

Stulemeijer, M., van der Werf, S., Borm, G. F., & Vos, P. E. (2008). Early prediction of favourable recovery 6 months after mild traumatic brain injury. *Journal of Neurology, Neurosurgery, and Psychiatry, 79*(8), 936-942. doi:10.1136/jnnp.2007.131250

Swift, T. L., & Wilson, S. L. (2001). Misconceptions about brain injury among the general public and non-expert health professionals: An exploratory study. *Brain Injury : [BI], 15*(2), 149-165. doi:10.1080/026990501458380

TBIMS National Database and Statistical Center. (2006). *Traumatic Brain Injury Model Systems National Database Syllabus*. Englewood, CO: Craig Hospital.

Teasdale, G., & Jennett, B. (1974). Assessment of coma and impaired consciousness: A practical scale. *Lancet, 2*(7872), 81-84.

United States. Office of Disability Employment Policy. (1992). *The american with disabilities act public law 101-336*. Washington, D.C.: U.S. Department of Labor, Office of Disability Employment Policy.

Vogenthaler, D. R., Smith, K. R., Jr., & Goldfader, P. (1989). Head injury, a multivariate study: Predicting long-term productivity and independent living outcome. *Brain Injury, 3*(4), 369-385.

Wagner, A. K., Hammond, F. M., Sasser, H. C., & Wiercisiewski, D. (2002). Return to productive activity after traumatic brain injury: Relationship with measures of disability, handicap, and community integration. *Archives of Physical Medicine and Rehabilitation, 83*(1), 107-114.

Walker, W. C., Marwitz, J. H., Kreutzer, J. S., Hart, T., & Novack, T. A. (2006). Occupational categories and return to work after traumatic brain injury: A multicenter study. *Archives of Physical Medicine and Rehabilitation, 87*, 1576-1582.

Whiteneck, G. G., Gerhart, K. A., & Cusick, C. P. (2004). Identifying environmental factors that influence the outcomes of people with traumatic brain injury. *The Journal of Head Trauma Rehabilitation, 19*(3), 191-204. Guérin, F., Kennepohl, S., Léveillé, G., Dominique, A., & McKerral, M. (2006). Vocational outcome indicators in atypically recovering mild TBI: A post-intervention study. *NeuroRehabilitation, 21*(4), 295-303.

11

Driving After Traumatic Brain Injury: Closing the Gap Between Assessing, Rehabilitating and Safe Driving

Sylvain Gagnon[1], Andrea Jane Hickey[1] and Shawn Marshall[2]
[1]*School of Psychology, University of Ottawa, Ontario*
[2]*The Rehabilitation Centre of the Ottawa General Hospital, Ottawa, Ontario*
Canada

1. Introduction

The privilege of driving a vehicle is often a fundamental part of individuals' daily lives. For many individuals who have suffered a traumatic brain injury (TBI), the ability to return to driving post TBI is an integral step to recovering independence and enhancing community reintegration (Rapport et al., 2008). Approximately 50% of TBI survivors with moderate to severe injuries resume driving, often irrespective of medical-legal evaluations (Fisk, Schneider, & Novack, 1998; Lew et al., 2005; Tamietto et al., 2006).

Evidently, helping TBI survivors return to safe driving plays a pivotal role in their path to recovery and reintegration to the community. A proper assessment of a TBI survivor's strengths and weaknesses can help prevent harm to the driver and other members of society and further enable their return to productive roles, work, and other favored activities. For instance, Kreutzer and colleagues (2003) revealed that the ability to drive post TBI is an independent moderator for employment stability. Determining whether a TBI survivor is safe or unsafe to drive remains a challenging issue since driving is a functional task with varying levels of complexity that can be potentially compensated for if impairments exist. Unfortunately, two negative outcomes may occur as a result of inaccurate driving assessment. The first negative outcome may be removing the privilege to drive from a TBI survivor who is either safe to drive, or could become safe to drive after retraining or further recovery (false positive result). The second outcome is a false negative result where the brain injury survivor is a potentially unsafe driver who is allowed to resume driving. Previous research suggests that TBI drivers tend to receive greater traffic violations (Haselkorn et al., 1998), tend to drive slower (in a simulated environment; Stinchcombe et al., 2008), and perhaps most importantly, have an increased crash risk compared to uninjured controls (e.g., Formisano et al., 2005; Lundqvist et al., 2008; but see Haselkorn et al., 1998; Schultheis et al., 2002). For example, Schanke and colleagues (2008) assessed driving behaviour of TBI survivors both pre and post injury. Results indicated that the accident rate of the TBI survivors was twice as high as that of the general population. Cyr and colleagues (2009) observed that in a simulated driving environment, TBI survivors who had returned to driving, compared to uninjured controls, were significantly more likely to crash in reaction to a surprising and challenging event.

Similar findings were obtained by Lew and colleagues (2005) in a small sample of TBI survivors.

Driving a car is certainly one of the most cognitively complex daily activities. It requires the integration of continuously changing visual-perceptual stimuli, swift information processing, and correct motor responses. The elements of a roadway environment can vary in complexity from one moment to another or from one geographical location to another. Because of the continuously changing nature of the driving environment (e.g., other drivers and road users' reactions, road conditions, etc.), driving reactions cannot be fully predicted. Indeed, even if a large portion of driving responses can be planned in advance based on the anticipation of events, many reactions must be activated spontaneously and rapidly in response to unanticipated events (Michon, 1985). Consequently, driving requires good judgment and decision making. All of the above ultimately lead to safe reactions behind the wheel.

According to Michon's (1985) hierarchical model of driving which includes strategic, tactical and operational levels, safe driving requires the ability to correctly perform each level of driving as well as optimal interactions between the various levels (see Figure 1). Unfortunately, TBI survivors may have difficulty in executing a variety of the necessary driving abilities for safe driving, including adequate and rapid processing of simultaneous inputs and anticipation of danger (Van Zomeran, Brouwer, & Minderhoud, 1987). Additionally, due to the sensori-motor and cognitive sequelae (including impairments of vision, attention, speed, and executive functions) frequently observed in TBI survivors, inappropriate driving reactions can be observed, even in TBI survivors who have been deemed fit to drive (Innes et al., 2007; Cyr et al., 2009). Evidently, the difficulty in assessing the driving ability of TBI survivors' consists of pinpointing which abilities are impaired and whether these impairments will translate into unsafe reactions behind the wheel.

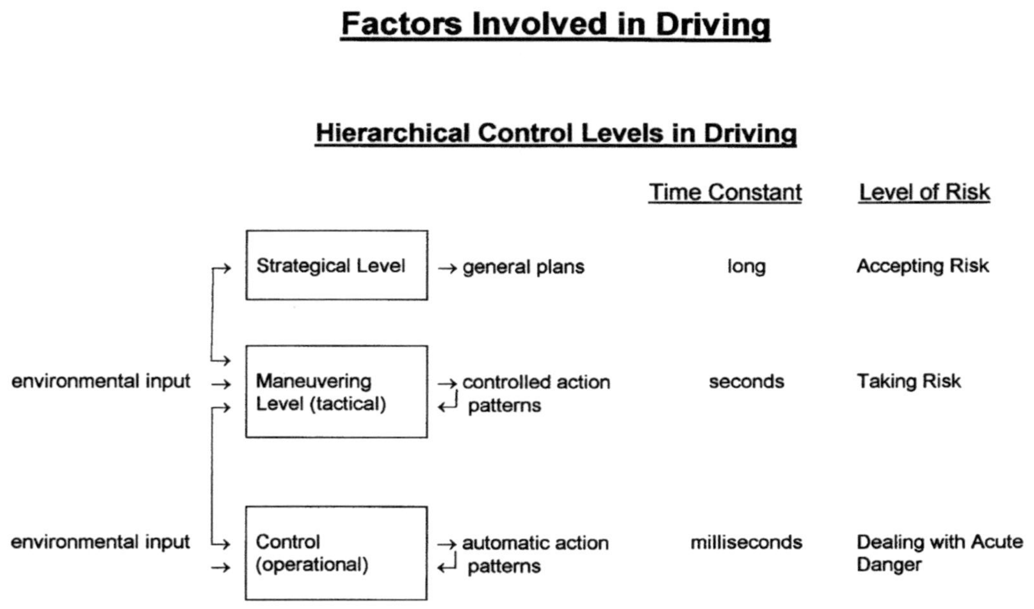

Fig. 1. Factors involved in driving according to Michon (1985).

2. The constellation of cognitive deficits observed in TBI survivors that may affect driving

The challenging problem that clinicians routinely face concerns the heterogeneous nature as well as the severity of cognitive deficits induced by a TBI (Schretlen & Shapiro, 2003). Individual differences are the hallmark of TBI. Further, cognitive recovery post TBI is not uniform across individuals and cognitive domains. Generally, TBI survivors exhibit deficits in attention, executive functions, processing speed, and memory (Hart et al., 2005; Lengenfelder et al., 2002; Madigan et al., 2000; Schretlen & Shapiro, 2003). Millis and colleagues (2001) found that reasoning and problem solving skills significantly differ between TBI survivors 5 years post injury. These cognitive and physical deficits are typically chronic and as expected, even 10 years post injury, TBI survivors may continue to demonstrate deficits in processing speed, memory, and executive function (Draper & Ponsford, 2008).

3. Assessment of TBI survivors using a generic approach

As indicated above, determining the capacity to drive post TBI poses a significant burden for rehabilitation professionals. To date, no commonly agreed upon best-practice guidelines are available to direct the assessment of driving ability post TBI and significant controversy exists regarding the most appropriate way to assess fitness to drive (Yale et al., 2003). The cognitive functions of TBI drivers are often assessed using 'generic' off-road tests that were not originally designed to assess driving competency and the specific cognitive requirements necessary for safe driving (e.g., Ball et al., 1988). The reliability, validity, and clinical effectiveness of these procedures have yet to be fully established. A recent systematic literature review indicated that studies have yet to provide evidence-based data that support the use of generic cognitive assessment tools to predict the driving abilities of TBI survivors (Classen et al., 2009). The lack of evidence-based data can be explained by at least four factors: 1) Generic cognitive/neuropsychological tests do not fully consider the heterogeneity of the cognitive deficits observed in TBI survivors and by the same token neglect to acknowledge the individual differences; 2) the lack of a sufficient generalizability between the cognitive functions assessed by these tests and those that are necessitated while driving; 3) Generic tests do not consider the continuous interaction between the cognitive processes involved in driving reflecting the need for the ability to shift and divide attention; and 4) the rather exclusive use of the on-road assessment to ultimately predict safe driving.

Current assessment procedures typically include a combination of off-road testing, including neuropsychological/cognitive tests and on-road testing. Simulator assessment is occasionally used (Cox et al., 2010; Lew et al., 2005) but its relevance will be detailed later in this chapter.

Off-road assessments are commonly used to assess cognitive, physical, and motor ability. These tests are often used as a primary screening assessment. They can also help identify the principal limitations of survivors and can help anticipate the difficulties they might have once behind the wheel. Typically, the first step in assessing TBI survivors' fitness to drive is through a neuropsychological exam (Côté, Syam, Vogel, & Cowper, 2007). Examples of neuropsychological tests include: the Trail Making test parts A and B, the Rey Complex Figure test, and the Clock Drawing test. Although these tests can discriminate between TBI survivors with different ability levels required for safe driving and are moderately correlated with driving ability (Marottoli et al., 1994), these tests alone cannot sufficiently determine fitness to drive (Schanke & Sundet, 2000; Classen et al., 2009) in all survivors, but can assist in estimating degree of recovery in order to prompt timing of further driving assessment. Another common test used to evaluate driving fitness is the Useful Field of View (UFOV; Owsley et al., 1991; Fisk et al., 2002). The UFOV assesses many important skills associated with safe driving, including visual processing speed and visual attention. It has been developed to assess fitness to drive in older drivers but has also been used to assess TBI survivors. The test has been found to be moderately associated with on-road driving performance (Myers et al., 2000; Novack et al., 2006). In fact Novack et al. (2006) found that the second subtest of the UFOV (divided attention subtest) did predict on-road driving performance of moderate to severe TBI individuals.

In sum, the results of cognitive tests can be used to determine whether someone is truly unable to drive when results demonstrate a significantly impaired ability. However, survivors for whom it is impossible to reach a decision about their driving based on the results of cognitive testing alone, need further clinical assessment, often in the form of an on-road driving assessment (Schanke & Sundet, 2000). The on-road driving assessment test may also be used to determine whether a potential driver can deploy compensatory strategies in order to overcome some of their limitations (Lew et al., 2009).

The on-road test which is typically administered by a driving rehabilitation specialist is the gold standard for driving assessment post TBI (Korner-Bitensky et al., 1994; Odenheimer et al., 1994). Although the on-road test demonstrates excellent face validity, some limitations have been raised (Lew et al., 2005). For instance, appropriate standardization between individuals and across assessment centres cannot always be achieved. Most importantly, the on-road test does not allow for the assessment of reactions in response to challenging or critical situations, impeding upon its predictive validity. This limitation is of most importance as TBI survivors most often demonstrate great difficulty in response to novel or challenging events (Couillet et al., 2000; Draper & Ponsford, 2008). Due to the nature of the on-road test, and the inability to assess driving behavior in response to more challenging events, there is a risk that TBI survivors could be granted license renewal, when in fact they may not be safe to drive. Few studies have assessed the predictive validity of the on-road test to real-world driving performance in people with TBI, which is necessary as drivers do not always drive as they do on the on-road test (Fox, Bowden, Smith, 1998; Lew et al., 2005).

4. A specificity-based approach: Unifying cognitive testing, driving assessment and retraining

The generic approach, as described above, operates in a highly structured sequential manner: tests of cognitive functions are administered first and are followed by the on-road test if necessary. On-road testing is often expensive, time consuming, and the safety of the driver and other road users is not always guaranteed. The on-road test is the final confirmation of driving ability. However, as mentioned previously, the generic approach may not provide sufficient information in regards to the specific limitations of the brain injury survivor. The content of the on-road driving assessment is not specifically adapted to the documented cognitive deficits of each individual, thus the observed relationship between test results and driving performance could be limited.

The importance of employing an approach that is customized to a TBI survivor's symptom profile has been raised by Lew and colleagues (2005). Such an approach favours a flexible perspective to the assessment of driving safety that combines the cognitive assessment, the driving assessment, and perhaps the rehabilitation potential and needs of the individual. Ideally, the driving challenges of the brain injury survivor should be known even before cognitive testing occurs. Once the driving difficulties are circumscribed, the cognitive underpinnings of these errors should be identified, ideally leading to a specific 'cognitive' profile. A better characterization of the limitations of a TBI survivor could translate into an adapted retraining effort that could combine a cognitive retraining protocol within a driving context.

For the purpose of supporting the specificity-based approach, we will use the concept of attention to highlight the challenges associated with its assessment and how the proposed approach could lead to a more sophisticated understanding of the attention deficits of TBI survivors and how they might influence driving.

5. The specificity-based approach applied to deficits of attention in TBI

Attention can be broadly defined as the ability to receive and process information from the environment while filtering out irrelevant input (Trick et al., 2004). More recent models incorporate a strategic control dimension to attention (Whyte et al., in press). In such perspectives, sustaining attention to a task, inhibiting irrelevant input that induces distractions, shifting attention as a function of the changing goals and priorities of an individual, and manipulating currently processed information are also active attention processes (Whyte et al., in press). Within this context, the contribution of attention processes to safe driving is considerable. Most importantly, this conception of attention better incorporates the complexity of driving and the cognitive flexibility that it requires. It also allows one to explore more specifically why TBI survivors with attention deficits tend to have difficulty driving. Arguably, a TBI could disrupt several subcomponents of attention, given its diffuse nature, thereby altering a survivor's driving ability.

Attention is critical for safe driving. It is needed not only to respond to a continuously changing environment but also to allow one to rapidly and flexibly shift focus from one activity to another. A driver's lack of attention has been frequently cited as a major cause of motor vehicle accidents (Langham et al., 2002). More specifically, divided attention, which refers to the ability to simultaneously carry out two competing tasks (Van Zomeren & Brouwer, 1994), has been commonly considered to be central to safe driving (Trick et al., 2004). In TBI, impaired performance on tasks requiring divided attention has been documented (Lengenfelder et al., 2002). For example, Dockree et al. (2006) found that more mistakes were made by TBI survivors in a sustained attention task that also included a dual task, compared to the same sustained attention task that did not include a dual task.

An important element of the specificity-based approach consists of documenting the specific driving difficulties even before executing cognitive testing. Arguably, the on-road test cannot be used for that purpose; it is designed to assess driving safety not to document the specific difficulties of a TBI survivor. Moreover, due to safety reasons, the standard on-road driving assessment does not incorporate situations that would allow one to assess strategic control (e.g. ignoring distractor stimuli); and behavioral flexibility (reacting to surprising events). Simulator testing is a flexible, ecological tool that may be a valid replacement for the on-road test.

6. Using the simulator to uncover the driving limitations of TBI survivors

Simulator testing utilizes virtual reality technology to assess the driving behaviour of individuals. Driving simulation provides a convenient and safe method for assessing driving behaviors. Unlike the on-road test, the simulator allows for the assessment of a driver's behaviour in response to challenging or critical situations (Cyr et al., 2009), and further allows for standardized and objective testing across individuals (e.g., same conditions regardless of location, weather, traffic density and examiner).

Evidence indicating that simulator testing is a valid *substitute* for real-world driving is still lacking. However the results of recent studies do indicate that driving behaviour within a simulated context is similar to driving behaviour on-road (Lew et al., 2005; Bella, 2008) and can predict on-road driving behaviour (de Winter et al., 2009; Bedard et al., 2010) even five years post brain injury (Hoffman & McDowd, 2010). Indeed, the ability to test an individual's response to challenging situations may make simulated driving a more sensitive assessment technique in comparison to traditional on-road assessments (Lew et al., 2009). It is also likely that the variables examined within a simulator assessment differ substantially from those examined in a standard on-road assessment. For instance, variables such as speed maintenance, lane deviation, steering and pedal control can be quantified. This could eventually explain why the correlation between the results of simulator and on-road assessment are low or at best moderate (Lew et al., 2009). Arguably more research is needed to discern the validity between simulator and on-the-road studies versus meaningful outcomes such as violation and collision rates for TBI survivors after return to driving.

Another interesting feature of simulator testing is its flexibility. Indeed, simulator testing allows for the development of scenarios that can target specific aspects of attention. This can be achieved in at least two different ways. The first approach consists of developing scenarios that will incorporate situations that will require the execution of a set of responses that rely on a specific cognitive process. In a study by Bélanger, Gagnon, & Yamin (2009), older individuals were required to react to specific challenging situations. The situations varied in terms of speed of response, planning ability, and strategic control. Results indicated that older individuals were great planners and could react quickly to a challenging situation that required sudden braking (e.g., pedestrian crossing). Their capacity to anticipate a risky situation is a dominant feature of their driving style. Interestingly, when tested in a situation that required strategic control of attention (steering and braking), older adults tended to crash more often than younger drivers. The second approach consists of merging cognitive assessment and driving. This has been frequently done in the field by testing the capacity to divide attention while driving. A classic paradigm consists of assessing the ability to detect visual stimuli or to react to sound while driving (e.g., Cantin et al., 2009; Lengenfelder et al., 2002). In one such study, Cyr et al. (2009), assessed whether divided attention performance of TBI survivors while driving the simulator was correlated with the risk of crashing in response to challenging events. The results indicated that TBI survivors were more likely to crash, and further, crash rate was best predicted by the divided attention scores as assessed in the simulator. The divided attention scores were not moderated by reaction time test results nor by processing and attention scores from the UFOV test.

Attention control in TBI survivors can also be deduced from their visual exploration via an eye-tracking device coupled with a highly controlled simulator environment. Milleville-Pennel et al. (2010) recently assessed the visual exploration of TBI survivors while driving within a simulated context, and related these findings to neuropsychological test results.

Interestingly, TBI survivors exhibited a reduction in the number of visual zones explored as well as a reduction of the explored distance. Further, these TBI survivors also exhibited deficits in divided attention as assessed via the Test for Attentional Performance (Zimmermann et al., 2007).

The above research illustrates that the inclusion of a simulator protocol can provide a unique ecological opportunity for an in-depth cognitive assessment of safe driving in TBI survivors. The research to date is minimal but suggests that a driving simulator can help clinicians better determine survivors driving difficulties. Due to the heterogeneity of deficits in TBI survivors, assessment needs to be made on a case by case basis and the simulator assessment should be tailored to reflect a survivor's specific cognitive profile. Moreover, because errors in attention tend to be made primarily in relatively novel or complex situations and/or when demands on cognition are increased (e.g., dual task) (Lengenfelder et al., 2002), readiness to drive can only be fully determined in novel as well as complex driving environments. Evidently, driving simulators can be used in that regard. Their potential as an assessment tool is enormous (Lew et al., 2009) if used within the logic of the specificity-based approach. However, if simulator testing merely copied the on-road assessment it is unlikely that the results would lead to a better understanding of the unique challenges of a given individual; results would more closely resemble those yielded by the generic approach. Although time and money could be saved, the idea of replicating the on-road test in a simulator does not reflect what a simulator based assessment can ultimately deliver.

7. Closing the gap between assessment, rehabilitation and safety

Ponsford (2008) summarized that "despite the large number of attention rehabilitation studies conducted to date, there is still limited evidence of their success". Thus the issue appears to be one of specificity, not quantity. Indeed, recent research suggests that by creating more specific approaches to rehabilitation, such as the utilization of a training program focused on one specific impairment (i.e., one impaired attentional process), significant improvements can be made by TBI survivors. Strum and colleagues (2003) found that by implementing a *specific* re-training program designed to improve *specific* attention deficits (e.g., divided attention), TBI survivors improved significantly more when tested on that specific aspect of attention, compared to when TBI survivors received a general re-training program (Test for Attentional Performance). More recently, Coulliet et al. (2010) found that TBI survivors with divided attention deficits (as assessed by the Divided Attention subtest of the Test for Attentional Performance) improved significantly on tests of divided attention after receiving a specific rehabilitation program for divided attention. TBI survivors were trained on two tasks separately; once competency was reached on both tasks individually, TBI survivors were instructed to complete the two tasks simultaneously. The tasks consisted of both paper and pencil tests as well as computerized testing (e.g., go no-go task, verbal fluency, word sorting). The program consisted of six weeks of 1-hour individual training sessions, 4 times a week.

8. How can this idea of testing specific deficits translate into driving assessments and retraining?

The current assessment tools used to determine fitness to drive, although able to discern between differing driving abilities, do not necessarily assess specific deficits associated with driving. Based on the idea that specificity-based interventions are more effective rehabilitation tools compared to more general interventions, future research should assess whether a specificity-based approach can be more effective in determining fitness to drive post TBI. To that regard, Bouillon et al. (2006) have suggested that the content of a driving competency assessment should vary according to the specific diagnosis of the individual. Driving simulators also have the potential to be excellent training devices to help improve on-road driving performance by providing practice within a range of driving scenarios. Indeed, simulator training has been found to improve on-road driving abilities (Cox et al., 2010). In a randomized controlled trial, Akinwuntan and colleagues (2005) used the driving simulator as a training device to demonstrate that it can improve the rate of those who return to driving after stroke. More specifically, TBI survivors who received 5 weeks, (15-hour/week) of training in the simulator, were significantly more likely to pass a follow-up official pre-driving assessment and were legally allowed to resume driving, compared to TBI survivors who received driving-related cognitive tasks. Furthermore, simulator training may also improve complex neurocognitive skills. Rosen (2005) has likened the driving simulator to a mental "treadmill" as it challenges brain functioning across many levels and systems. Just as running on a treadmill utilizes several bodily systems (e.g., the respiratory and muscular systems), the driving simulator pushes several cognitive components (e,g., attention, vision) to work together.

The use of driving simulators may prove to be the most ideal method to asses and rehabilitate specific deficits associated with driving. For example, Kewman et al. (1985) developed a simulator based retraining procedure for TBI survivors to improve specific skills of functional significance involved in driving. The training consisted of exercises to improve attentional and visuomotor skills necessary for driving, focusing on visuomotor tracking and divided attention. Driving was broken down into simple components, and shaping procedures were then used to help participants gain the skill as they practiced. Such training resulted in better on-road driving performance, compared to the control group that receive no specific skill training, but rather just practiced driving.

A better understanding of the limitations of a TBI survivor can also lead to the selection of a more effective rehabilitation approach. Therefore, one could determine whether it is better to favor a compensatory retraining approach or one that emphasizes the retraining of the impaired cognitive functions (Boelen, et al., 2011; Lew et al., 2009).

In conclusion, the standard generic approach to driving assessment in TBI survivors could sometimes lead to inaccurate decisions regarding their driving safety. The specificity-based approach consists of developing an assessment and retraining procedure within a driving context that is ecological and customized to the individual's limitations. We believe that this approach should revolve around the simulator as an assessment/retraining tool. We used some research examples on attentional deficits and driving in TBI to demonstrate that this approach could potentially lead to more reliable decisions regarding driving safety. However, the specificity-based approach as well as the use of the simulator is definitely not limited to the assessment and rehabilitation of attention deficits. Other processes such as visual detection, speed of processing and even awareness deficits could be assessed within the simulator and examined within a specificity-based approach. The research in this area also has to generate evidence-based data to support its relevance. For instance, assessment results yielded by the generic and the specificity-based approaches should ultimately be validated against real world driving outcomes.

9. Acknowledgement

The Ontario Neurotrauma Foundation supported this work through a summer scholarship awareded to AJH.

10. References

Akinwuntan, A. E., De Weerdt, W., Feys, H., et al. (2005). Effect of simulator training on the driving ability of stroke patients: a randomized controlled trial (RCT). *Neurology, 65,* 843–850.

Ball, K. K., Beard, B. L., Roenker, D. L., Miller, R. L., & Griggs, D. S. (1988). Age and visual search: Expanding the useful field of view. *Journal of the Optical Society of America, 5,* 2210–2219.

Bédard, M. B., Parkkari, M., Weaver, B., Riendeau, J., & Dahlquist, M. (2010). Assessment of driving performance using a simulator protocol: validity and reproducibility. *Am J Occup Ther, 64*(2), 336-340.

Bélanger, A., Gagnon, S., & Yamin, S. (2010). Capturing the serial nature of older drivers' responses towards challenging events: a simulator study. *Accid Anal Prev, 42*(3), 809-817.

Bella, F. (2008). Driving simulator for speed research on two-lane rural roads. *Accident Analysis and Prevention, 40,* 1078–1087.

Boelen, D.H., Spikman, J.M., & Fasotti, L. (2011). Rehabilitation of executive disorders after brain injury: Are interventions effective? *Journal of Neuropsychology, 5,* 73- 113.

Bouillon L, Mazer B, Gelinas I. (2006). Validity of the cognitive behavioral driver's inventory in predicting driving outcome. *American Journal of Occupational Therapy, 60,* 420–427.

Cantin, V., Lavallière, M., Simoneau, M., & Teasdale, N. (2009). Mental Workload when driving in a simulator: Effects of age and driving complexity. *Accident Analysis and Prevention, 41*(4), 763-771.

Classen, S., Levy, C., McCarthy, D. *et al.* (2009). Traumatic Brain Injury and Driving Assessment: An Evidence-Based Literature Review. *American Journal of Occupational Therapy, 64,* 580-591.

Côté, M. J., Syam, S. S., Vogel, W. B., & Cowper, D. C. (2007). A mixed integer programming model to locate traumatic brain injury treatment units in the Department of Veterans Affairs: A case study. *Health Care Management Science, 10*(3), 253–267.

Couillet, J., Soury, S., Lebornec, G., Asloun, S., Joseph, P. A., Mazaux, J. M., & Azouvi, P. (2010). Rehabilitation of divided attention after severe traumatic brain injury: A randomised trial. *Neuropsychological Rehabilitation, 20,* 321-339.

Couillet, J., Leclercq, M., Martin, Y., Rousseaux, M., & Azouvi, P. (2000). Divided attention after severe diffuse traumatic brain injury. *European Brain Injury Association Meeting.* Paris.

Cox, D. J., Davis, M., Singh, H., Barbour, B., Nidiffer F .D., Trudel, T., Mourant, R., & Moncrief, R. (2010). Driving rehabilitation for military personnel recovering from traumatic brain injury using virtual reality driving simulation: A feasibility study. *Mil Med, 175*(6), 411-416.

Cyr, A. A., Stinchcombe, A., Gagnon, S., Marshall, S., Hing, M. M., & Finestone, H. (2009). Driving difficulties of brain-injured drivers in reaction to high-crash-risk simulated road events: A question of impaired divided attention? *Journal of Clinical & Experimental Neuropsychology, 31*, 472-482.

De Winter, J. C. F., de Groot, S., Mulder, M., Wieringa, P. A., Dankelman, J., & Mulder, J. A. (2009). Relationships between driving simulator performance and driving test results. *Ergonomics, 52*(2), 137-153.

Dockree, P.M., Bellgrove, M. A., O'Keeffe, F. M., Moloney, P., Aimola, L., Carton, S., & Robertson, I. H. (2006). Sustained attention in traumatic brain injury (TBI) and healthy controls: enhanced sensitivity with dual-task load. *Exp Brain Res, 168*, 218-229.

Draper, K., & Ponsford, J. (2008). Cognitive Functioning Ten Years Following Traumatic Brain Injury and Rehabilitation. *Neuropsychology, 22*, 618-625.

Fisk, G. D., Novack, T., Mennemeier, M., & Roenker, D. (2002). Useful field of view after traumatic brain injury. *Journal of Head Trauma Rehabilitation, 17*(1), 16–25.

Fisk, J., Schneider, & Novack, T. (1998). Driving following traumatic brain injury; prevalence, exposure, advice and evaluation. *Brain Injury, 12*, 683–695.

Formisano, R., Bivona, U., Brunelli, S., Giustini, M., Longo, E., & Taggi, F. (2005). A preliminary investigation of road traffic accident rate after severe brain injury. *Brain Injury, 19*, 159–163.

Fox, G. K., Bowden, S. C., & Smith, D. S. (1998). On-road assessment of driving competence after brain impairment: review of current practice and recommendations for a standardized examination. *Arch Phys Med Rehabil, 79*(10), 1288-1296.

Hart, T., Whyte, J., Kim, J., & Vaccaro, M. (2005). Executive Function and Self-awareness of "Real-world" Behavior and Attention Deficits Following Traumatic Brain Injury. *Journal of Head Trauma Rehabilitation, 20*(4), 333-347.

Haselkorn, J. K., Mueller, B. A., Rivara, F. A. (1998). Characteristics of drivers and driving record after traumatic and nontraumatic brain injury. *Archives of Physical Medicine & Rehabilitation, 79*, 738–742.

Himanen, L., Portin, R., Isoniemi, H. et al. (2006). Longitudinal cognitive changes in traumatic brain injury: A 30-year follow-up study. *Neurology, 66*, 187-192.

Hoffman, L. & McDowd, J. M. (2010). Simulator driving performance predicts accident reports five years later. *Psychology and Aging, 25*(3), 741-745.

Innes, C. R., Jones, R. D., Dalrymple-Alford, J. C., Hayes, S., Hollobon, S., Severinsen, J., et al. (2007). Sensory-motor and cognitive tests predict driving ability of persons with brain disorders. *Journal of the Neurological Sciences, 260*, 188–198.

Kewman, D. G., Seigerman, C., Kinter, H., Chu, S., Henson, D., & Reeder, C. (1985). Simulation training of psychomotor skills: Teaching the brain-injured to drive. *Rehabilitation Psychology, 30*, 11-27.

Kreutzer, J. S., Marwitz, J. H., Walker, W, Sander, A., Sherer, M., Bogner, J., Fraser, R., & Bushnik, T. (2003). Moderating factors in return to work and job stability after traumatic brain injury. *J Head Trauma Rehabil, 18*(2), 128–38.

Korner-Bitensky, N., Sofer, S., Kaizer, F., Gelinas, I., & Talbot, L. (1994). Assessing ability to drive following an acute neurological event: Are we on the right road? *Canadian Journal of Occupational Therapy, 61*(3), 141–148.

Langham, M., Hole, G., Edwards, J., & O'Neil, C. (2002). An analysis of 'looked but failed to see' accidents involving parked police cars. *Ergonomics, 45*, 167–185.

Lengenfelder, J., Schultheis, M. T., Al Shihabi, T., Mourant, R., & DeLuca, J. (2002). Divided attention and driving: A pilot study using virtual reality technology. *Journal of Head Trauma Rehabilitation, 17*, 26–37.

Lew, H. L., Poole, J. H., Lee, E. H., Jaffe, D. L., Huang, H., & Brodd, E. (2005). Predictive validity of driving-simulator assessments following traumatic brain injury: A preliminary study. *Brain Injury, 19*, 177–188.

Lew, H. L., Rosen, P. N., Thomander, D., & Poole, J. H. (2009). The potential utility of driving simulators in the cognitive rehabilitation of combat-returnees with traumatic brain injury. *J Head Trauma Rehabil, 24*(1), 51-56.

Liddle, J., & McKenna, K. (2003). Older drivers and driving cessation. *British Journal of Occupational Therapy, 66*(3), 125–132.

Lundqvist, A., Alinder, J., & Ronnberg, J. (2008). Factors influencing driving 10 years after brain injury. *Brain Injury, 22*, 295-304.

Madigan, N. K., DeLuca, J., Diamond, B. J., Tramontano, G., & Averill, A. (2000). Speed of information processing in traumatic brain injury: Modality-specific factors. *Journal of Head Trauma Rehabilitation, 15*, 943–956.

Marottoli, R. A., Cooney, L. M., Wagner, R., et al. (1994). Predictors of automobile crashes and moving violations among elderly drivers. *Ann Intern Med, 121*(11) 842-846.

Mathias, J. L. & Wheaton, P. (2007). Changes in attention and information-processing speed following severe traumatic brain injury: A meta-analytic review. *Neuropsychology, 21*, 212-223.

Michon, J. (1985). In L. Evans & R. Schwing, (Eds.), *Human behaviour and traffic Safety* (pp. 485-520). New York: Plenum Press.

Milleville-Pennel, I., Pothier, J., Hoc J. M., & Mathe, J. F. (2010). Consequences of cognitive impairments following traumatic brain injury: Pilot study on visual exploration while driving. *Brain Injury, 24*, 678–691.

Millis, S. R., Rosenthal, M., Novack, T. A., Sherer, M., Nick, T. G., Kreutzer, J. S., et al. (2001). Long-term neuropsychological outcome after traumatic brain injury. *J Head Trauma Rehabil, 16*(4), 343-355.

Myers, R. S., Ball, K. K., Kalina, T. D., Roth, D. L., Goode, K. T. (2000). Relation of useful field of view and other screening tests to on-road driving performance. *Perceptual and Motor Skills, 91*(1), 279-290.

Novack, T. A., Banos, J. H., Alderson, A. L., Schneider, J. J., Weed, W., Blankenship, J., et al. (2006). UFOV performance and driving ability following traumatic brain injury. *Brain Injury, 20*(5), 455–461.

Odenheimer, G. L., Beaudet, M., Jette, A. M., Albert, M. S., Grande, L., & Minaker, K. L. (1994). Performance-based driving evaluation of the elderly driver: Safety, reliability, and validity. *Journal of Gerontology, 49*A(4), 153–159.

Owsley, C., Ball, K., Sloane, M. E., Roenker, D. L., & Bruni, J. R. (1991). Visual/cognitive correlates of vehicle accidents in older drivers. *Psychol Aging, 6*(3), 403-15.

Ponsford, J. (2008). Rehabilitation of attention following traumatic brain injury (2nd). Cognitive Neurorehabilitation, (pp. 507-521) New York: Cambridge University Press

Rapport, L. J., Bryer, R. C., & Hanks, R. A. (2008). Driving and community integration after traumatic brain injury. *Arch Phys Med Rehabil, 89*(5), 922-930.

Rosen PN. Simulators can be thought of as a "treadmill" for the brain. Presented at: Driving Simulation Users Group's Third Bi-annual Driver Assessment Meeting; 2005; Rockport, Me.

Schanke, A. K. Rike, P. O., Molmen, A., Osten, P. E. (2008). Driving behaviour after brain injury: a follow-up of accident rate and driving patterns 6-9 years post injury. *Journal of Rehabilitation Medicine, 40*(9), 733-736.

Schanke, A. K., & Sundet, K. (2000). Comprehensive driving assessment: Neuropsychological testing and on-road evaluation of brain injured patients. *Scandinavian Journal of Psychology, 41*(2), 113–121.

Schneider, J. J., & Gouvier, W. D. (2005). Utility of the UFOV test with mild traumatic brain injury. *Applied Neuropsychology, 12*, 138–142.

Schretlen, D.J., & Shapiro, A.M. (2003). A quantitative review of the effects of traumatic brain injury on cognitive functioning. *International Journal of Psychiatry, 15*, 341-349.

Schultheis, M. T., Matheis, R. J., Nead, R., & DeLuca, J. (2002). Driving behaviors following brain injury: Self-report and motor vehicle record. *J Head Trauma Rehabil, 17*(1), 38–47.

Stinchcombe, A., Yamin, S., Cyr, A-A., Gagnon, S., Marshall, S., Man-Soon Hing, M., & Finestone, H. (2008). Examination of Traumatic Brain Injured Drivers' Behavioural Reactions to Simulated Complex Roadway Events. *Advances in Transportation Studies an international Journal, Special Issue*, 5-17.

Sturm, W., Fimm, B., Cantagallo, A., Cremel, N., North, P., Passadori, A., et al. (2003). Specific Computerized Attention Training in Stroke and Traumatic Brain-Injured Patients. *Journal of Neuropsychology, 14*, 283-292.

Tamietto, M., Torrini, G., Adenzato, M., Pietrapiana, P., Rago, R., & Perino, C. (2006). To drive or not to drive (after TBI)? A review of the literature and its implications for rehabilitation and future research. *NeuroRehabilitation, 21*, 81-92.

Trick, L. M., Enns, J. T., Mills, J., & Vavrik, J. (2004). Paying attention behind the wheel: A framework for studying the role of attention in driving. *Theoretical Issues in Ergonomics Science, 5*, 385–424.

Van Zomeren, A. H., & Brouwer, W. H. (1994). Clinical neuropsychology of attention. New York: Oxford University Press.

Van Zomeren, A.H., Brouwer, W.H., & Minderhoud, J.M. (1987). Acquired brain damage and driving: A review. *Archives of Physical Medicine and Rehabilitation, 68*, 697-705.

Whyte, J., Ponsford, J., Watanabe, T., & Hart, T. (in press). Traumatic brain injury. In W. R. Frontera, J. D. Delisa, B. M. Gans, N. A. Walsh, & L. Robinson (Eds.), Physical medicine and rehabilitation: Principles and practice (5th ed.): Lippincott, Williams and Wilkins.

Yale, S. H., Hansotia, P., Knapp, D., & Ehrfurth, J. (2003). Neurologic conditions: Assessing medical fitness to drive. *Clinical Medicine and Research, 1*(3), 177–188.

Zimmermann P, Fimm B. Test for Attentional Performance (TAP)–Version 2.01. Vera Fimm, psychologische Testsysteme, Freiberg; 2007.

Part 3

Prevention

12

Helmet Use for the Prevention of Brain Injuries in Motorcycle Accidents

Concepció Fuentes-Pumarola, Carme Bertran, M. Eugènia Gras, Sílvia Font-Mayolas, David Ballester, Mark J. M. Sullman and Dolors Juvinyà
University of Girona
Spain

1. Introduction

The results of numerous studies show the effectiveness of helmets in avoiding or reducing the severity of injuries in a motorcycle accident (Hundley et al., 2004; Keng, 2005; La Torre, 2003; León & Hernández, 2004; Liu et al., 2004). Despite the proven effectiveness of helmets in avoiding or reducing the severity of brain injuries and legislation requiring their use by both motorcycles drivers and passengers in Spain since 1992, research has found that 29% of those killed in motorcycle accidents in 2007 were not wearing a helmet at the time of the accident (Spanish Interior Ministry, 2008). Similar legislation exists in most European countries.

One model that can be used to predict risk and prevention behaviour among drivers is Bandura and Walters (1963) socio-behavioural approach. According to this model, a large proportion of social learning takes place through observing the real actions of others and the consequences these have (Bandura, 1986) Social approval for a specific conduct may change a risk behaviour, principally among young people and adolescents. According to the socio-behavioural model, adolescents' use of a helmet when riding a motorbike is related to their beliefs regarding friends and relatives' use of the same protective headgear.

Other theoretical approaches, such as Bayés (1992) illness prevention model, postulate that the immediate consequences of past conducts are the most relevant variables in predicting future behaviour. Adolescents will therefore tend to produce behaviours which have immediate positive consequences or avoid immediate negative consequences.

Various different studies have identified a number of variables related to adopting preventive behaviours when driving, including: social influence (Bianco et al., 2005, State of Hawaii Department of Transportation, 2004; Canada Safety Council, 2006; Fuentes, 2007; Fuentes et al., 2010), belief in the effectiveness of the behaviour (Gras et al., 2007; Fuentes, 2007; Fuentes et al., 2010) and the immediate consequences of its use (Block, 2001; Chiliaoutakis et al., 2000; Cunill et al., 2004; Cunill et al., 2005).

If we focus on gender, according to a recent study (Fuentes et al.,2010) young men ride motorcycles more frequently than young women (23.4% vs. 6.9%) ($p < 0.05$) and eight out of every ten male and female adolescents say they always wear a helmet when riding a motorbike, with no differences by gender.

The main reason adolescents who ride motorbikes wear a helmet is the safety it provides (87.2%), whereas there are three reasons for not wearing one: the characteristics of the journey (it being short, for example) (34.8%), not having one (30.5%) and its use bothering drivers (21.7%) (Fuentes et al. , 2009).

2. Consequences of motorcycle accidents

The most common injuries caused by motorcycle accidents are lower limb contusions, abrasions and fractures due to direct impact with another vehicle or a secondary fall and sliding on the floor or flying through the air. In the case of frontal collision with a fixed obstacle, diaphyseal fractures of both femurs can be caused by the driver being projected over the handlebars. Also frequent are fractures of vertebral bodies, whether affecting the medulla or not, from falling in front of the motorbike and colliding with an obstacle (Figure 1), and skin abrasions and injuries due to severe friction and tearing of the skin with deep wounds from impact with fixed barriers on the road (Hernando, 2001). The poorly named "protective barriers" are the cause of 50% of serious injuries suffered by motorists and 20% of deaths in motorcycle accidents. This is why motorists are demanding a double safety barrier on roads to prevent these acting as knife blades.

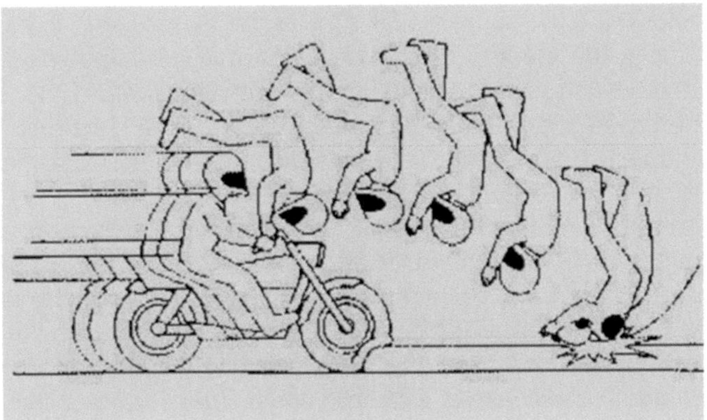

Fig. 1. Mechanism producing fractures in motorcycle accidents.

Other types of injury are traumatic brain injuries (TBI) and traumatic facial injuries (Figure 2). The term TBI includes all cases in which, following a traumatism, victims present one or some of the following symptoms: loss of consciousness, post-traumatic amnesia, convulsive seizure, laceration of the frontal scalp, brain injury or cranial and/or facial fracture (Net & Marruecos-Sant, 2001). In an epidemiological study conducted in San Diego (USA), TBI was defined as any physical injury or functional deterioration of the cranial content, secondary to a brusque interchange of mechanical energy. This definition takes into account external causes that may provoke concussion, contusion, haemorrhaging or laceration of the brain, cerebellum and encephalic trunk as far as the first cervical vertebra (Kraus et al., 1984).

The estimated incidence of TBI in Spain is 200 cases/100,000 inhabitants, of which 90% receive hospital medical attention. Incidence is higher among men than women, by a ratio of 3:1, particularly in the 15 to 25 age range. Approximately 10% of TBI is considered serious, 10% moderate and 80% mild. The most frequent causes are traffic accidents (73%), followed by falls (20%) and sports injuries (5%). Motorbike accidents are mainly found among the

under 25s and car accidents in adults (Ezpeleta, 2002). Differences are observed according to gender, with drivers who crash or lose control of the vehicle predominantly being men, and women predominant among injured companions (Muñoz & Murillo, 1993).
According to other data, 6% of TBI are suffered by motorcyclists (Gennarelli et al., 1994). TBI are the primary cause of death and disability in people aged under 45 (Goikoetxea & Aretxe, 1997).

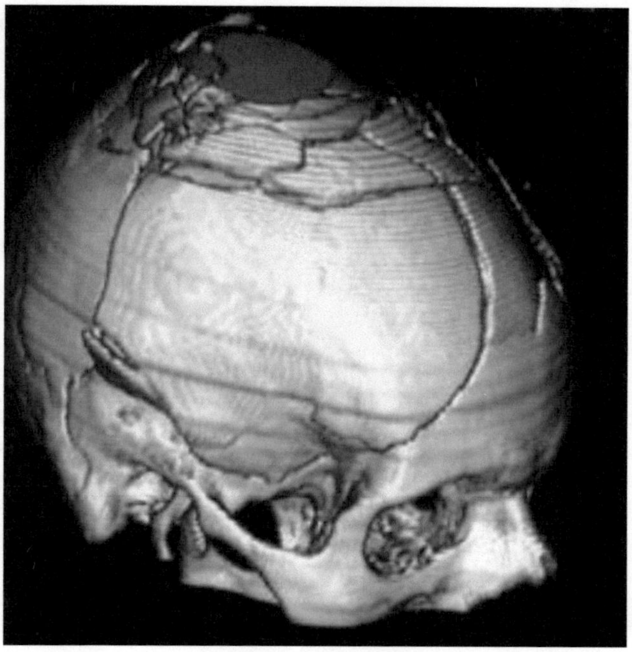

Fig. 2. Cranial fractures due to a frontal fall from a motorcycle without a helmet

The severity of TBI is measured neurologically using the Glasgow Coma Scale (ECG) (Moore et al., 2003). Another scale for measuring trauma severity is the Injury Severety Score (ISS) (Jaramillo et al., 2001). This instrument considers injuries in different regions of the body and the result is obtained by applying the Abbreviated Injury Scale (AIS).
We must not forget possible sequelae caused by injuries resulting from traffic accidents. In a study conducted by the Legal Medicine Institute in Castelló (Spain) for the period 1995 to 2000 evaluating bodily damage caused by traffic accidents, for all types of accidents (work-related and non work-related) an average of one sequela per accident was observed. Over 50% of car and motorbike accidents did not have sequelae. However, the type of accident with most sequelae, 21 to be precise, was caused by the motorcycle accident (De Luís, 2003).
The approximate distribution of results and sequelae in patients with severe TBI is: death, 30-36%; persistent vegetative state, 5%; severe disability, 15%; moderate disability, 15-20% and satisfactory recovery, 25%. In patients with moderate TBI, the distribution of results and sequelae is as follows: death or persistent vegetative state, 7%; severe disability, 7%; moderate disability, 25%, and satisfactory recovery, 60% (Moore et al., 2004).
Other types of sequelae to take into account in TBI are psychological and behavioural disorders persisting over time (Brooks et al., 1996).

Another aspect that has been studied in victims with injuries and sequelae due to traffic accidents is what is known as "social pain", which includes hospitalisation, sick leave, professional incapacity and the need for third party involvement and adapted housing and vehicles. In a study conducted in Spain, 2,180 accident victims were monitored over 4 years, 500 with severe sequelae. Of the overall sample, 15% required hospitalisation, this figure rising to 37% among the 500 most severe cases. The type of vehicle or means of transport in which most social pain was observed was motorcycle accidents or walking. The study differentiates between injuries and sequelae. It is observed that injuries provoking extreme social pain among accident victims are located in the central nervous system (SNC)/spinal medulla, peripheral nervous system (SNP) and ocular system. On the other hand, the sequelae that provoke extreme social pain are related to the SNC/spinal medulla, visual apparatus, significant aesthetic damage and head /cranium /face (Consultrans & UVAME, 2005, as cited in Rodríguez, 2005) .

All of the above costs money, not only in health expenditure but also due to social and work-related consequences. In the aforementioned Consultrans and UVAME study (2005, as cited in Rodríguez, 2005), a cost of over 100,000 euros per accident was estimated. Other authors, as well as demonstrating that victims of motorcycle accidents not wearing a helmet suffer more severe injuries than those who are wearing one, regardless of alcohol or drug consumption, also observe that the cost to society of motorcycle drivers having accidents without a helmet represents 70 million dollars annually (some 53 million euros) and, of this amount, some 30 million (over 22 and a half million euros) was not covered by private insurance. This represents a small burden for society, 25 cents (19 euro cents) annually per citizen, which is why the authors state that whether to wear a helmet or not can be seen as an issue for individuals, with few social connotations (Heller & Jacoby, 2005; Hundley et al., 2004).

3. Active and passive safety measures in motorcycle riding

Two concepts exist in traffic road safety: active and passive safety.

Active safety is the set of design elements, systems or concepts incorporated into the vehicle which ensure its correct functioning when in use (European Automobile Commissariat [CEA], 2005). These include the brakes, tyres, lights and mirrors, which help the driver to avoid accidents when the motorcycle is in use. Motorcycles are manufactured in accordance with safety regulations and contain a whole series of elements which, if subject to any type of modification or adaptation, lose their effectiveness and endanger the life of the driver and any other public highway users. These elements are: size and weight, number of seats, engine capacity, maximum speed and level of environmental pollution. It should be observed that the motorcycle must also pass periodical checks and maintenance in order for the safety elements to work properly. Those elements that require periodical checks are basically the mirrors, lights, brakes, suspension, tyres, engine and bodywork.

Passive safety elements are those which are designed to protect the integrity of the user in the event of an accident. In the case of motorcycle drivers, the main passive safety element is without doubt the helmet. Results from numerous studies demonstrate the effectiveness of helmets in avoiding or reducing the severity of injuries in the event of traffic accidents for two-wheeled vehicles (Hundley, et al. 2004; Keng, 2005; La Torre, 2003; León & Hernández, 2004; Liu et al., 2004; Nakahara et al., 2005; Norvell & Cummings, 2002; Peek-Asa et al., 1999; WHO, 2003).

4. Bandura and Walters' socio-behavioural model

Bandura and Walters (1974) base their work on the operant learning model, and award significant importance to social variables in acquiring new behaviours.

Bandura (1987) proposes that behaviours are learnt by observing others (modelling).

Operant conditioning models behaviour in the same way a sculptor models a mass of clay (Skinner, 1953, as cited in Bandura, 1974). A powerful modelled influence can simultaneously modify the observer's behaviour, thought patterns, emotional responses and judgements (Rosenthal & Bandura, 1978, as cited in Bandura, 1987). Much of social learning takes place on the basis of observing the real behaviours of others and the consequences they lead to.

Many theorists have considered modelling to be imitation, and that this plays a very important role in acquiring deviant and adapted behaviour (McBrearty et al., 1961, as cited in Bandura, 1974). When we refer to learning by imitation, the cultural importance of learning by observation is most clearly demonstrated in anthropological explanations of the socialisation process in other societies. For example, in many languages the word "teach" is the same word for "show", and in many cultures children do not do what adults tell them to do, but rather what they see them do (Reichar, 1938, as cited in Bandura, 1974). Bandura insists that in acquiring a skill, more than a response to imitation, modelling constitutes a rule of learning (Bandura, 1987). With advances in technology, more trust is increasingly being placed in the use of symbolic models, such as plastic models (audiovisual media). Motivating factors and anticipation of positive or negative reinforcement increase or reduce the likelihood of responses to observation, which are the essential aspect of learning by imitation.

Three effects derive from observing models of learning behaviour:

1. The observer acquires new responses that did not previously exist in their repertoire, giving rise to the modelling effect, where the model has to exhibit very new responses and the observer reproduce them identically.
2. Observing models may strengthen or weaken inhibitory responses; here the provoked responses already existed in the subject's repertoire and do not have to be identical to those of the model.
3. Observing a model may at times provoke previously learned imitation responses in the observer because the perception of certain behaviours acts as a trigger for responses of the same kind.

The characteristics of the observer influence modelling. These are the result of their reinforcement histories and will determine to what extent they will have a tendency to imitate.

According to Bandura and Walters' model, the best way to promote helmet use among adolescents and young motorcycle drivers is to provide them with models of this type of behaviour.

5. Bayés' illness prevention model

The Illness Prevention Model (Bayés, 1992; 1995) is structured into three time phases: past, present and future (Figure 3).

According to Bayés (1992), the past includes all prior knowledge and specific baggage (information, emotional reactivity, interactive style, functional skills) subjects have in their personal history.

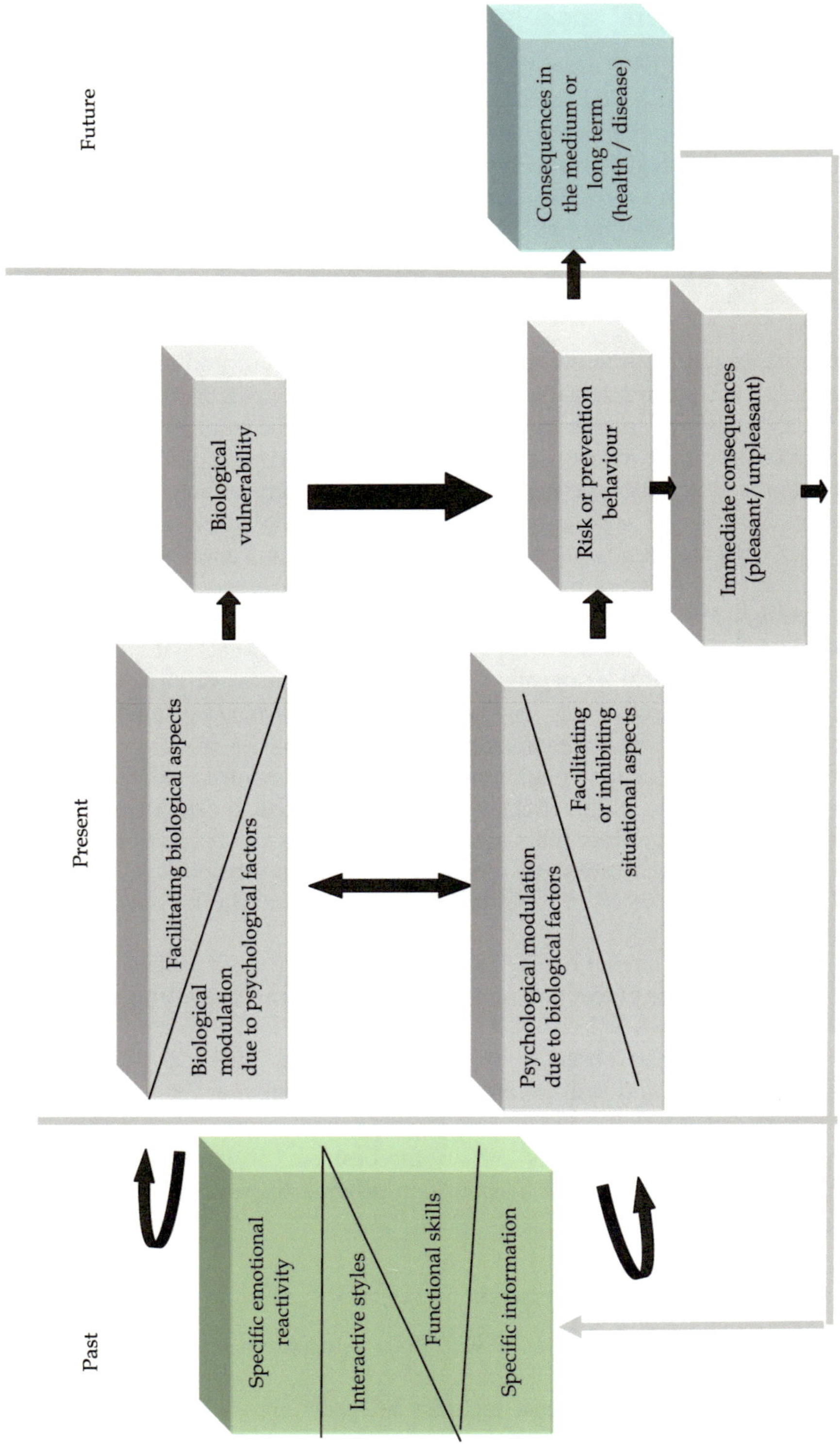

Fig. 3. Illness Prevention Model (Bayés, 1992 cited as Rodríguez Marín, 1994)

Information refers to questions such as to the extent to which the subject knows what effective preventive behaviours are and how to effect them, what signs indicate the existence of risk, or the immediate and delayed consequences of the behaviour.

For example, with regard to helmet use, young people must know that wearing one is an effective behaviour in absorbing the effect of blows in the event of an accident or avoiding being fined by the police. They must also know how to detect when the risk of an accident or fine is greater (for example, when riding at faster or slower speeds, in urban or rural areas, etc.) and the short and long-term consequences of using a helmet (annoyance, more severe injury in the event of an accident, etc.). According to Bayés (1992), information is a necessary but not sufficient condition for predicting preventive behaviour: it is a reality that practically all adolescents "know" that the helmet is an effective preventive measure in reducing injuries in the event of a motorcycle accident and what consequences not wearing one may have in this case; but having this information does not guarantee its use.

6. Helmet use among adolescents

A study conducted on a sample of 874 students (46.8% male; average age 15.08; SD = 0.82) in public secondary schools in the city of Girona (Spain) (Fuentes, 2007; Fuentes et al., 2010) evaluated such variables as frequency of motorcycle use (every day, more than once a week, once a week, less than once a week, or never), wearing a helmet when riding a motorcycle or as a passenger (always, sometimes or never), belief in the effectiveness of helmet use (0 = not effective at all / 10 = extremely effective) and belief in its use among friends and family members (always, sometimes or never).

The results indicate that young men use motorcycles more often than young women (23.4% vs. 6.9%) ($p < 0.05$) and 8 out of every 10 adolescents say they always wear a helmet when riding a motorcycle, with no differences by gender. Self-informed helmet use increases with age, rising from 66.6% at 14 to 85.7% at 16 or over ($p < 0.05$ (Table 1). Adolescents who always wear a helmet consider it to be more effective than those who use it only sometimes or never (Table 2).

	Age	Drivers	Passengers
Motorcycle use	14	29.2% (n=63)	58.4% (n=128)
	15	37.8% (n=152)	66.7% (n= 268)
	16 or over	44.6% (n=112)	71.8% (n=181)
	Total	37.4% (*n*=327)	66.0% (*n*=577)
Helmet use	14	66.6% (n=44)	72.6% (n=93)
	15	76.3% (n=116)	79.8% (n=214)
	16 or over	85.7% (n=96)	86.7% (n=157)
	Total	78.28%(*n*=256)	80.4% (*n*=464)

Table 1. Motorcycle and helmet use, by age (Fuentes et al., 2010).

Additionally, social influence is the variable that best predicts helmet use on all occasions: 56.5% of adolescents who always wear one believe that their friends do too, whilst this is true for only 13.5% of those who do not always wear one ($p < 0.05$); for family members, the percentages are 94.8% and 69.8%, respectively ($p < 0.05$) (Figure 4).

In this study, 66% of the participants reported riding a motorcycle as passengers quite frequently, with no gender differences. These findings are remarkably similar to a study of

Italian adolescents, which found that 66% of their participants reported using motorcycles as drivers or passengers (Bianco et al., 2005). However, the present findings are considerably higher than those found in a study of the general public conducted by the Directorate General of Traffic (2003), where the percentage was less than 20%. This leads us to conclude that adolescents travel by motorcycle far more often than older people, who may have access to other types of vehicles. Thus, prevention campaigns aimed specifically at this sector of the population would be an appropriate way to improve motorcycle safety overall.
Among the adolescents in this sample, motorcycle use increased with age, both as drivers and passengers. Furthermore, helmet use, particularly among passengers, also increased with age. These results differ from those found by Plieggi et al. (2006), but are in agreement with those found by other researchers. For example, in a study carried out in India, the prevalence of various health-risk behaviours among the adolescent student population (such as not using a helmet) was found to be significantly associated with lower ages and the male gender (Sharma et al., 2007). In addition, a recent Taiwanese study of accidents involving motorcyclists has also found that young male drivers were more likely to disobey traffic regulations (Hsin-Li & Tsu-Hurng, 2007).

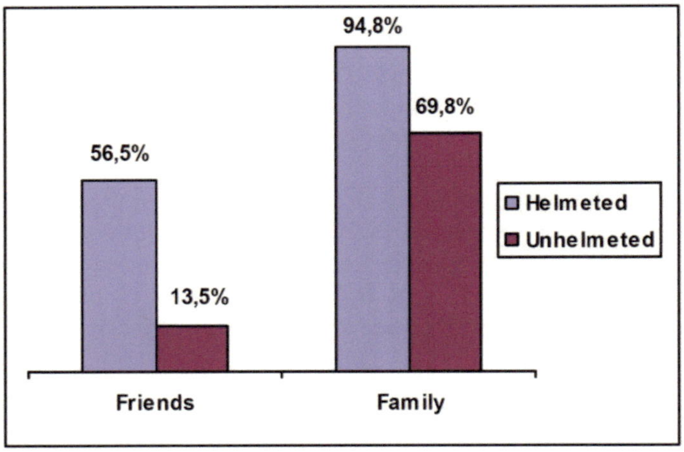

Fig. 4. Belief in the use of a helmet by friends and family members according to helmet use by adolescents (Fuentes et al., 2010).

The safety of the helmet is the main reason why adolescent motorcycle drivers use this preventive measure (87.2%). Other reasons are shown in Table 3, classifying users according to whether they are drivers or passengers. By contrast, three reasons are given for not wearing one: the characteristics of the journey (for example, short) (34.8%), not having one (30.5%) and the fact that it is annoying to use (21.7%) (Fuentes et al., 2009). Table 4 shows the distribution of motorcycle users (drivers and passengers, according to helmet use) (Fuentes et al; 2009).
These results agree with those obtained in previous studies. According to research conducted by the Directorate General of Traffic (2003), journeys undertaken by adolescents using a helmet correctly are longer on average (16.5 km) than those undertaken by adolescents who do not wear one or do so incorrectly (8.4 km). Paradoxically, according to reports from the Catalan Traffic Service (Larriba et al., 2006), in Catalonia 93.3% of motorcycle accidents take place in urban areas.

GENDER	HELMET USE	DRIVERS		PASSENGERS	
		Mean (SD)	N	Mean (SD)	N
Male	ALWAYS	8.7 (1.3)	164	8.6 (1.3)	212
	OMETIMES OR NEVER	7.7 (2.7)	41	7.9 (2.4)	54
	Total	*8.5 (1.7)*	*205*	*8.5 (1.6)*	*266*
Female	ALWAYS	8.5 (1.9)	84	8.5 (1.5)	244
	SOMETIMES OR NEVER	7.7 (2.2)	19	7.3 (2.3)	47
	Total	*8.3 (1.9)*	*103*	*8.3 (1.7)*	*291*
TOTAL	ALWAYS	8.7 (1.5)	248	8.5 (1.4)	456
	SOMETIMES OR NEVER	7.7 (2.5)	60	7.6 (2.4)	101
	Total	*8.5 (1.8)*	*308*	*8.4 (1.7)*	*557*

Table 2. Means and standard deviations for beliefs about the helmet's effectiveness, by helmet use and gender, for motorcycle drivers and passengers (Fuentes et al., 2010).

Adolescents generally reported that helmets are effective in preventing serious injuries or even death in the case of an accident, and both drivers and passengers who report using them tend to give helmets higher effectiveness scores than those who do not use a helmet regularly. In the case of passengers, males believed more strongly in the effectiveness of helmet-use, although this difference did not result in greater use of these safety devices by males. Previous research on other safety devices, such as car seat belts, has also found that belief in the effectiveness of the device is a significant predictor of its use among car drivers (Gras et al., 2007).

The results of research by Fuentes et al. (2010) support Bandura's social cognitive theory (1990), as belief in the effectiveness of a helmet was strongly related to engaging in the preventive behaviour of wearing a helmet. Consequently, disseminating information that highlights and proves the effectiveness of helmet-use can strongly encourage greater use of this device by adolescents.

Adolescents believe their relatives use helmets more frequently than their friends do. The perception that relatives, who are generally adults, take more precautions than young people has been confirmed by other researchers (Bianco et al., 2005; Canada Safety Council, 2006; State of Hawaii Department of Transportation, 2004; Lajunen & Räsänen, 2001) and accident data. This again highlights the excessive risks taken by young people, especially males (Goldenbeld et al., 2008; Hsin-Li & Tsu-Hurng, 2007; Sharma et al., 2007).

Adolescent motorcycle drivers who reported that most of their friends use helmets when riding motorcycles adopt this safety measure more frequently than those who do not believe their friends use them. In fact, belief in helmet use by friends was the best predictor of helmet use by adolescents on all occasions. This relationship was also found between adolescents' self-reported helmet use and whether or not they believe their relatives use a helmet. This variable also predicted helmet use among adolescent motorcycle drivers. In accordance with Bandura and Walters (1979) and Bayés (1995) these results back the hypothesis of social influence as a relevant variable for predicting preventative behaviour, and are in agreement with the findings of other researchers in relation to: helmet use (e.g. Bianco, 2005; Canada Safety Council, 2006; State of Hawaii Department of Transportation, 2004: Plieggi, et al. 2006); seat belt use (Chliaoutakis et al., 2000; Cunill et al., 2004; Gras et al., 2007; Harrison et al., 2000); and in relation to driving style and how this effects the number of motoring offences committed by children and their parents (Beck et al., 2001a,b; Bianchi & Summala, 2004; Shopeet al., 2001).

REASONS FOR WEARING A HELMET	DRIVERS	PASSENGERS
Safety reasons	217 [87.2%]	360 [84.7%]
Legal reasons, fines or obligation	23 [9.2%]	42 [9.9%]
The death of a friend in an accident	3[1.2%]	6[1.4%]
Driver-related	-	4[0.9%]
Other reasons	6[2.4%]	13[3.1%]
Total	249[100%]	425[100%]

Table 3. Distribution of motorcycle users according to reasons for wearing a helmet

REASONS FOR NOT WEARING A HELMET	DRIVERS	PASSENGERS
Characteristics of the journey (short or rural)	16 [34.8%]	13 [18.8%]
Not having one	14 [30.5%]	45[65.2%]
Annoying	10 [21.7%]	4 [5.8%]
Other reasons	6 [13%]	7 [10%]
Total	46 [100%]	69 [100%]

Table 4. Distribution of motorcycle users according to reasons for not wearing a helmet

Another study on 500 adolescents attending secondary schools in the county district of La Selva (Girona, Spain) (49.5% male, average age = 14.19; SD = 0.76) analysed variables such as: helmet use the last time they rode a motorcycle, intention to use one next time they travel with this vehicle, expectations regarding the results of using this safety measure, expectations regarding self-efficacy in using one, some immediate negative consequences (annoying, messes up your hair) and the belief that friends and family also use one (Cunill, 2009).

Eight of every ten adolescents say they used a helmet the last time they rode a motorcycle. These data are similar to those found in the study conducted by Fuentes, et al. (2010), where this variable was recorded using a scale with three values: always, sometimes and never, considering only those participants who say they "always" use a helmet.

Those adolescents who used a helmet on their last journey by motorcycle believed more in its effectiveness for avoiding serious injuries or death in the event of an accident and perceive themselves as having more self-efficacy in using one in the future compared to those who did not use one.

In addition, adolescents who did not use a helmet on their last journey consider that using them is more annoying, unnecessary if riding in the city and that wearing one unbuckled is effective in avoiding injuries in the event of an accident, more than those who did use one.

7. Conclusions

Programmes and campaigns promoting helmet use should take into account the modelling effect peer role models and other models have on adolescent helmet use. In addition, faced with the problem that motorcycle accidents among adolescents represents, it is advisable to remind parents, legal guardians and other relatives of the strong influence they have on adolescents' driving behaviour, and to start educational programmes before adolescents begin driving vehicles.

Results of different studies into helmet use suggest the following different preventive actions for increasing use and avoiding possible brain injury in the event of an accident:

- Improve helmet design to make them more comfortable.
- Use positive social influence to increase helmet use, employing models who are important points of reference for young people's behaviour (singers, sportsmen and women, etc.).
- Remind parents of adolescents that in their vehicle driving behaviour they are also modelling behaviour for their children.
- Continue to create programmes aimed at health professionals that enable them to act as agents involved in educating young people with regard to risk prevention behaviour when riding a motorbike. Said educational intervention should take place in primary, secondary and tertiary healthcare.
- Promote further research into potentially avoidable injury and mortality from traffic accidents in order to design new prevention strategies.

These actions may help to prevent important sequelae of brain injury and reduce mortality among adolescents on the roads.

It is therefore essential to ensure the involvement in this endeavour of teaching professionals, educators, health professionals and associations and bodies involved in the prevention of risk behaviour in adolescents and vehicle use.

8. References

Hundley, J.C., Kilgo, P.D., Miller, P.R., Chang, M.C., Hensberry, R.A., Meredith, J.W., & Hoth, J.J. (2004). Non-helmeted motorcyclists: a burden to society? A study using the National Trauma Data Bank. *The Journal of Trauma*, 57(5),944-949.

Jaramillo, F.J., González, G., Vélez, P., Bran, M.E., Restrepo, D. &Duque, A. (2001). Factores de riesgo asociados con letalidad y complicaciones tempranas en pacientes con trauma craneoencefálico cerrado. *Colombia Médica*, 32(1), 49-56.

Keng, S.H. (2005). Helmet use and motorcycle fatalities in Taiwan. *Accident Analysis and Prevention*, 37(2) 349-55.

Kraus, J.F., Black, M.A., Hessol, N., Ley, P., Rokaw, W., Sullivan, C., Bowers, S., Knowlton, S. & Marshall, L. (1984). The incidence of acute brain injury and serious impairment in a defined population. *American Journal of Epidemiology*, 119(2), 186-201.

La Torre, G. (2003). Epidemiologia degli incidenti con ciclomotore in Italia: efficacia del casco nel ridurre numero e gravità dei traumi cranici. *Recenií Progressi in Medicina*, 94(1),1-4.

Lajunen, T., & Räsänen, M. (2001). Why teenagers owning a bicycle helmet do not use their helmets. *Journal of Safety Research*, 32(3), 323-332.

Larriba, J., Canales, G. & Duran, A. (2006). *Homo transitus*. Servei Català de Trànsit. Barcelona. Spain.

León, M.E., & Hernández, J.A. (2004). Uso de un casco adecuado y su relación con fracturas craneofaciales en motociclistas de Cali. *Colombia médica*, 35(3,1), 10-15.

Liu, B., Ivers, R., Norton, R., Blows, S., & Lo, S.K. (2004). Helmets for preventing injury in motorcycle riders. *Cochrane Database Syst Rev. 2004*; (2):CD004333.

Moore, E.E., Mattox, K.L. i Feliciano, D.V. (2004). *Manual del Trauma* (4a ed). Mc.Graw Hill. Méjico.

Muñoz Sánchez, M.A. i Murillo Cabezas, F. (1993). Traffic accidents. Comparitive analysis of hospital records vs police records. *Medicina Intensiva*, 17,(supl)103.

Nakahara, S., Chadbunchachai, W., Ichikawa, M., Tipsuntornsak, N., & Wakai, S. (2005). Temporal distribution of motorcyclist injuries and risk of fatalities in relation to age, helmet use, and riding while intoxicated in Khon Kaen, Thailand. *Accident Analysis & Prevention*, 37(5), 833-842.

Norvell, D.C., & Cummings, P. (2002). Association of helmet use with death in motorcycle crashes: a matched-pair cohort study. American Journal of Epidemiology, 156(5).

Net, A. & Marruecos-Sant, L. (2001). *El paciente traumatizado*. Springer-Verlag Ibérica. Barcelona. Spain.

Peek-Asa, C., McArthur, D.L., & Kraus, J.F. (1999). The prevalence of non-standard helmet use and head injuries among motorcycle riders. *Accident Analysis & Prevention*, 31(3), 229-233.

Plieggi, C., Bianco, A., Nobile, C.G.A., & Angelillo, I.F. (2006). Risky behaviours among motorcycling adolescents in Italy. *The Journal of Pediatrics*, 148, 527-532.

Rodríguez, J.M. (2005). El reto de sobrevivir, In: *Tráfico, 12-18*. 12.12.2006. Available from: http://www.dgt.es/revista/num183/interior.html?s=../archivo/pages/index.html

Sharma, R., Grover, V.L., &, Chaturvedi, S. (2007). Health-risk behaviors related to road safety among adolescent students. *Indian Journal of Medical Sciences*, 61 (12), 656-662.

Shope, J.T., Waller, P.F., Raghunathan, T.E., & Patil, S.M. (2001). Adolescent antecedents of high-risk driving behavior into young adulthood: substance use and parental influences. *Accident Analysis and Prevention*, 33, 649-658.

Spanish Interior Ministry (2008). Nota de Prensa, *Balance de seguridad vial: 316 fallecidos menos en 2006*. Author. Madrid. Spain.

State of Hawaii Department of Transportation (2004). *Motorcycle Helmet Integration report.* Hawaii: SMS Research and Marketing Services.

WHO (2003). Informe sobre la salud en el mundo. Epidemias mundiales desatendidas: tres amenazas crecientes. In *WHO,* 10.01.05, Available from: http://www.who.int/whr/2003/chapter.6/es/print.html.

Bandura, A., & Walters, R.H. (1963). *Social learning and personality development.* New York: Holt, Rinehart and Winston.

Bandura, A., & Walters, R.H. (1974). *Aprendizaje social y desarrollo de la personalidad.* Alianza Universidad. Madrid. Spain.

Bandura, A. (1986). *Social fundations of thought and action: a social cognitive theory.*Englewood Cliffs, Prentice-Hall.NJ.

Bandura, A. (1987). *Pensamiento y acción. Fundamentos sociales.* Ed. Martínez Roca. Libros universitarios y profesionales. Barcelona. Spain.

Bayés, R. (1992). Aportaciones del análisis funcional de la conducta al problema del sida. *Revista Latinoamericana de Psicología.* 24(1-2):35-56.

Bayés, R. (1995). *Sida y psicología.* Martínez Roca. Barcelona. Spain.

Beck, K. H., Shattuck, T., & Raleigh, R. (2001b). Parental predictors of teen driving risk. *American Journal of Health Behavior,* 25 (19),10-20.

Beck, K. H., Shattuck, T., & Raleigh, R. (2001b). A comparison of teen perceptions and parental reports of influence on driving risk. *American Journal of Health Behavior,* 29 (1), 73-84.

Bianchi, A., & Summala, H. (2004). The "genetics" of driving behavior: parents' driving style predicts their children's driving style. *Accident Analysis and Prevention,* 36, 655-659.

Bianco, A., Trani, F., Santoro, G., & Angelillo, I.F. (2005). Adolescents' attitudes and behaviour towards motorcycle helmet use in Italy. *European Journal of Pediatrics,* 164(4), 207-211.

Block, A.W. (2001). 1998 *Motor Vehicle Occupant, Safety Survery*: Volume 2 Sealt Belt Report. National Highway Traffic Safety Administration, U.S. Department of Transportation.

Brooks, N., Campsie, L., Symington, C., Beattie, A. i McKinlay, W. (1986). The Five year outcome of severe blunt head injury: a relative's view. *Journal of Neurology, Neurosurgery & Psychiatry,* 49(7), 764-770.

Canada Safety Council (July 2002). *Helmets: attitudes and actions. Survey finds most kids wear helmets, most adult don't.* Vol. XLVI (3), 2002.

Comisariado Europea del Automóvil (CEA) (2005). 23.07.2005, Available from: http://www.seguridad-vial.net/seguridad_activa.html

Chliaoutakis, J.E., Gnardellis, C., Drakou, I., Darviri, C., & Sboukis, V. (2000). Modeling the factors related to the seatbelt use by the young drivers of Athens. *Accident Analysis and Prevention,* 32, 815-825.

Cunill, M. (2009). Comportamientos de riesgo en la adolescencia. Paralelismos entre el uso del casco y el uso del preservativo. Tesis doctoral. Universitat de Girona. In: *Tesis en red.* 27.06.2011, Available from: http://www.tesisenred.net/

Cunill, M., Gras, M.E., Sullman, M.J.M., i Planes, M. (2005). *Seat belt use by Spanish adolescents.* En: L. Dorn (ed.) Driver behavior training (pp.223-232) Vol.II. Cornwall: Ashgate.

Cunill, M., Gras, M.E., Planes, M., Oliveras,C., i Sullman , M.J.M. (2004). An investigation of factors reducing seat belt use amongst Spanish drivers and passengers on urban roads. *Accident Analysis and Prevention,* 36(3) 439-445.

De Luis, M.J. (2003). La valoración del daño corporal por accidente de tráfico en el instituto de medicina legal de Castellón, tras la ley 30 de 1995. Tesi doctoral. Universitat de Valencia. In: *TDX*, 27.06.2011, Available from: http://www.tdr.cesca.es/

Directorate General of Traffic (2003). *Uso del casco en motocicletas y ciclomotores: resultado de una campaña especial.* S.G. de Investigación y Formación Vial.

Ezpeleta, D. (2002). Apuntes de Neurología. Traumatismo craneoencefálico. In: *Apuntes de Neurología, capítulo 13*, 26.02.2006, Available from: http://www.infodoctor.org/neuro/cap13.htm

Fuentes, C. (2007). Factors relacionats amb l'ús del casc en adolescents i aspectes canviants desprès d'un accident amb ciclomotor. Tesi doctoral. Universitat de Girona. In: *TDX*, 27.06.2011, Available from: http://www.tdr.cesca.es/

Fuentes, C., Gras, M.E., Font-Mayolas, S., Bertrán, C., Ballester, D. & Juvinyà, D. (2009). Uso del casco en adolescentes usuarios de ciclomotores en la ciudad de Gerona, 2006. *Revista Española de Salud Pública*, 83, 877-889.

Fuentes, C., Gras, M.E., Font-Mayolas, S., Bertrán, C., Sullman M.J.M. & Ballester, D. (2010). Expectations of efficacy, social influence and age as predictors of helmet use in a sample of Spanish adolescents. *Transportation Research Part F*, 13(5), 289-296.

Gennarelli, T.A., Champion, H.R., Copes, W.S. i Sacco, W.J. (1994). Comparison of mortality, morbidity, and severity of 59,713 head injured patients with 114.447 patients with extracranial injuries. *The Journal of Trauma*, 37(6), 962-968.

Goikoetxea, X. i Aretxe, J. (1997). Traumatismo craneoencefálico, In: *Atención inicial al politraumatizado*, Ed. Polikalte, pp.(207-224), Estella.

Goldenbeld, C., Twisk, D., & Houwing, S. (2008). Effects of persuasive communication and group discussions on acceptability of anti-speeding policies for male and female drivers. *Transportation Research, Part F*, 11, 207-220.

Gras, M.E., Cunill, M., Sullman, J.M., Planes, M. &Font-Mayolas, S. (2007). Predictors of seat belt use amongst Spanish drivers. *Transportation Research Part F.*, 10, 263-269.

Harrison, W.A., Senserrik, T.M., & Tingvall, C. (2000). *Development and Trial of a Method to investigate the acceptability of Seat Belt Reminder Systems.* Report 170. Monash University Accident Research Centre, July.

Heller, M. & Jacoby, J. (2005). Helmet versus unhelmeted motorcyclist: a dime's worth of difference. *The Journal of Trauma*, 58(5), 1091-1902

Hernando, A. E. (2001). *Biomecánica del trauma*, In: Net, A. y Marruecos-Sant, L. El paciente politraumatizado. Barcelona: Springer.

Hsin-Li C., & Tsu-Hurng Y. (2007) Motorcyclist accident involvement by age, gender and risky behaviors in Taipei, Taiwan. *Transportation Research Part F*, 10 (2): 109-122.